SOCIAL PERSPECTIVES ON DEATH AND DYING
FOURTH EDITION

SOCIAL PERSPECTIVES ON DEATH AND DYING

FOURTH EDITION

Jeanette A. Auger and Kerstin Roger

with contributions by
Zohreh BayatRizi, Rita Giancola,
Audrey Medwayosh and Catherine White

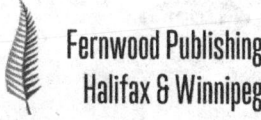
Fernwood Publishing
Halifax & Winnipeg

Copyright © 2026 Jeanette A. Auger and Kerstin Roger

All rights reserved. No part of this book may be reproduced or transmitted in any form by any means without permission in writing from the publisher, except by a reviewer, who may quote brief passages in a review. The publisher expressly prohibits the use of this work in connection with the development of any software program, including, without limitation, training a machine learning or generative artificial intelligence (AI) system.

Development editor: Errol Sharpe
Copyediting: Brenda Conroy
Cover photo: Megan Lutz
Cover design: John van der Woude
Text Design: Lauren Jeanneau
Printed and bound in Canada

Published by Fernwood Publishing
2970 Oxford Street, Halifax, Nova Scotia, B3L 2W4
Halifax and Winnipeg
www.fernwoodpublishing.ca

Fernwood Publishing Company Limited gratefully acknowledges the financial support of the Government of Canada through the Canada Book Fund and the Canada Council for the Arts. We acknowledge the Province of Manitoba for support through the Manitoba Publishers Marketing Assistance Program and the Book Publishing Tax Credit. We acknowledge the Nova Scotia Department of Communities, Culture and Heritage for support through the Publishers Assistance Fund.

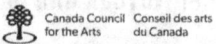 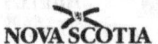 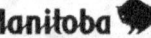

Library and Archives Canada Cataloguing in Publication
Title: Social perspectives on death and dying / Jeanette A. Auger and Kerstin Roger ; with contributions by Zohreh BayatRizi, Rita Giancola, Audrey Medwayosh and Catherine White.
Names: Auger, Jeanette A., 1945- author | Roger, Kerstin, 1966- author.
Description: Fourth edition. | Includes bibliographical references and index.
Identifiers: Canadiana 20250311399 | ISBN 9781773638072 (softcover)
Subjects: LCSH: Death—Social aspects. | LCSH: Death—Social aspects—Canada.
Classification: LCC HQ1073 .A93 2026 | DDC 306.9—dc23

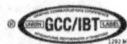

CONTENTS

Acknowledgements xi

ONE: Beginnings 1
The Text Within: My First Experiences with Death (Jeanette) 5
The Text Within: My First Experiences with Death (Kerstin) 7
Why Study Death and Dying? 8
    Personal Reasons *8*
    Academic Reasons *9*
    Institutional Reasons *9*
Who Studies Death and Dying? 9
Where Is Death and Dying Studied? 9
How Is Death and Dying Studied? 10
Disciplinary Approaches to Death and Dying 10
    Psychological Studies *10*
    Sociological Studies *11*
    Literary and Aesthetic Studies *14*
    Philosophical Studies *14*
    Theological Studies *15*
Conclusion 16
Self-Reflection and Thoughtful Conversations 16
In-Class Assignments 16

TWO: Your Experiences and Perceptions of Death and Dying 17
Personal Experiences with Death Exercise 17
Reflecting on Our Dying Exercise 18
Fears of Dying Exercise 19
Loss Awareness Exercise 19
    Loss Inventory *19*
    Responding to World Events that Impact Our Lives *19*
Conclusion 20

THREE: Key Concepts in the Maze of Death and Dying 21
Definitions and the Diagnosis of Death 23
The Non-Beating Heart Donor Controversy 24
Organ Donation, Body Brokers and the Transplant Tourist Industry 27
Types of Death 30
Social Rules of Death 30
Nearly Dead 31
Process of Dying 31
After Death 31
Conclusion 32
Self-Reflection and Thoughtful Conversations 32
In-Class Assignments 32

FOUR: Historical Attitudes Toward Death and Dying 33
Historical Perceptions of Death and Dying 36
Care of the Dead 39
Historical Definitions of Death 42
Contemporary Western Views of Death 44
Critical Moments in Canada — HIV/AIDS and COVID-19 46
Conclusion 48
Self-Reflection and Thoughtful Conversations 48
In-Class Assignments 48

FIVE: Types of Death and Dying 49
Clinical/Brain Death 49
Emotional/Psychological Death 50
Spiritual Death 50
Social Death 51
Stages of Death and Dying 51
Personal/Structural Elements 52
Good Deaths versus Bad Deaths 52
Death Education 55
Conclusion 56
Self-Reflection and Thoughtful Conversations 56
In-Class Assignments 56

SIX: Hospice Palliative Care 57
Hospice Palliative Care: An Overview 59
Hospice Chronology: Europe 60
The Impact of the COVID-19 Pandemic on Hospice Palliative Care 65
The Impact of Medical Assistance in Dying on Volunteers in Hospice Palliative Care ... 67
The Work of a Palliative Care Volunteer 69
Conclusion 70
Self-Reflection and Thoughtful Conversations 70
In-Class Assignments 70

SEVEN: Medical Assistance in Dying and Euthanasia 71
Canadian Hospice and Palliative Care Association 74
Current Controversies 75
Types of Euthanasia 76
A Canadian Leader: Dr. Jocelyn Downie 77
Conclusion 80
Self-Reflection and Thoughtful Conversations 80
In-Class Assignments 81

EIGHT: Death Education and the Arts (Rita Giancola) 82
Visual Arts 83
    Painting *83*
    Photography *84*
    Sculpture *84*

Music 85
    Classical Music 85
    Contemporary Music 86
    Cultural 87
Media 87
    Film 88
    Television 89
    Animation 90
    Theatre 90
    Musicals 93
    Dance 96
    Literature 97
Conclusion 98
Self-Reflection and Thoughtful Conversations 99
In-Class Assignments 99

NINE: Drug and Opioid Deaths in Canada 100

Conclusion 105
Self-Reflection and Thoughtful Conversations 106
In-Class Assignments 106

TEN: Cross-Cultural Variations in Death and Dying (Zohreh BayatRizi) 107

Religion 109
Language and Art 109
Food 111
Clothing 111
Grief across Cultures 111
    Cultural Scripts and Ritual Frameworks 112
    Cultural Policing of Grief 114
    Grief Pathology and Cultural Considerations for Bereavement Support 116
Multicultural Death and Grief Practices in Canada 117
    Religious and Cultural Diversity in Canada 117
    End-of-Life Care and Cultural Diversity in Canada 120
Conclusion 122
Self-Reflection and Thoughtful Conversations 123
In-Class Assignments 123

ELEVEN: Indigenous Perspectives on Death and Grief (Audrey Medwayosh) 124

Colonial History 124
Social Determinants of Health 125
Indigenous Mortality Rates and the Social Determinants of Health 126
    Rates of Homicide, Suicide and Other Violent Deaths 127
    Infant Mortality Rates 128
Medical Racism 128
Contemporary Indigenous Approaches to Death Care 129
    Indigenous Funeral Homes 129
    Death Doulas and End-of-Life Care 130
Indigenous Mortality Pre- and Post-Contact 131

Grieving Practices Prior to Colonization 132
   Traditional Anishinaabe Funerals *133*
Contemporary Indigenous End-of-Life Rituals 134
   Contemporary Anishinaabe Funerals *135*
Intangible, Symbolic and Ambiguous Losses 136
   Disenfranchised Grief *137*
   Why Should We Care? *137*
Culture as Healing 138
   Culture for Addiction Treatment *138*
The Text Within: Love and Humour Through the Darkness (Audrey) 139
Conclusion 140
In-Class Assignments 140
Self-Reflection and Thoughtful Conversations 141
Chapter 11 References 141

TWELVE: The Changing Face of Cremation, Funeral and Burial Practices 144

The Impact of COVID-19 on the Funeral Industry 146
Final Disposition Services 149
Behind the Scenes in the Funeral Parlour 154
Living Funerals and Wakes 157
Cemeteries 158
   Graveyard Symbols *158*
   Grave Blankets *160*
Cards of Condolence 160
Conclusion 161
Self-Reflection and Thoughtful Conversations 161
Visit Your Local Cemetery 161

THIRTEEN: Legal and Ethical Issues in Death and Dying 162

Living Wills and Advance Health-Care Directives 162
Preparing a Legal Will 163
The Text Within: Completing a Health-Care Directive (Jeanette) 164
Ethical Wills 164
Organ Donations 165
Financial Planning 166
Charitable Donations 167
Preparing Your Own Death Plan 168
Conclusion 169
Self-Reflection and Thoughtful Conversations 170
In-Class Assignments 170

FOURTEEN: Causes and Prevention of Suicide in Canada *(Catherine White)* 171

The Text Within: Encounters with Suicide (Catherine) 171
Theoretical Perspectives 174
   Risk Factors and Protective Factors *175*
   High-Risk Groups *178*
Suicide Among Indigenous Peoples 178
Suicide Among the 2SLGBTQ+ Community 180
Suicide Among the Armed Forces and Veterans 181

Suicide Among Prison Inmates 183
Suicide Prevention Spectrum 184
Conclusion 189
Self-Reflection and Thoughtful Conversations 190
In-Class Assignments 190

FIFTEEN: Dealing with Grief and Bereavement 191
Social Responses 192
Physical Responses 193
Emotional Responses 193
Spiritual Responses 193
Reconnecting 194
Types of Grief and Bereavement 195
Grief Walking Groups 196
Cyber-Grieving 197
Grief Doulas 197
Music Thanatology Doulas 198
Death Dinners and Grief Cafés 198
Living with Loss 200
Assisting the Dying Person 201
Children and Grief 202
The Loss of a Child 203
Losing a Pet 203
Grief in Old Age 204
Grief as an Opportunity for Growth 205
Conclusion 205
Self-Reflection and Thoughtful Conversations 205
In-Class Assignments 206

SIXTEEN: Reviving Interest in Death and Dying and Immortality 207
Demographics 209
Politics 210
Religion 210
Law 211
Medicine 211
The Quest for Immortality: Life Everlasting, Could We Really Live Forever? 212
    Cryonic Suspension 212
    Bionic Limbs 214
    Deathbots 216
Cultural Differences in the Quest for Immortality 216
The Text Within: Nothing Stays the Same (Jeanette) 218
Conclusion 218
Self-Reflection and Thoughtful Conversations 218
In-Class Assignments 219

Select Bibliography 220

Index 249

*We dedicate this book to the memory of our mothers,
Bronislava Ruth Auger, 1916–1947,
and Gisela Stieber Roger, 1932–2021.
Jeanette also dedicates this book to her brother
John Sleznikas, who died at two months old in 1942.*

ACKNOWLEDGEMENTS

First, we thank our co-contributors, Dr. Zohreh BayatRizi, Rita Giancola, Audrey Medwayosh and Dr. Catherine White, for their valuable contributions and support of this edition. We also thank the students in our Death and Dying classes for their creative insights and feedback on the previous editions. Jeanette thanks Kerstin for her support in agreeing to co-edit this edition with her and adding her teaching, research and personal experiences to the book. We are grateful to Dr. Lindsay Allen for meticulous proofreading. We thank our format specialist, Terry Aulenbach, for his efficiency and helpful suggestions regarding the layout of the manuscript and for producing the index. The anonymous reviewers of the book provided thoughtful and positive suggestions to improve the book, and we thank them for their helpful contributions. Our publisher, Errol Sharpe of Fernwood, has always been a huge supporter of this book and of Jeanette's other publications, and we are grateful to him, Beverley Rach, Brenda Conroy, Deb Mathers and the entire Fernwood team.

Chapter One

BEGINNINGS

> Dying is a universal life passage that can be seen as natural: the final state of living. However, dying is also a major existential crisis for most people and usually represents a crisis point for both the dying person and for his or her family. (Latimer 1995: 362)
>
> To be concerned with death and its celebration is not "morbid." It is proper to reflect on a certainty of life. All healthy and vigorous civilizations of the past have apprehended the significance of death. (Curl 1993: 366)

SINCE THE FIRST EDITION OF THIS BOOK was published in 2000, the field of thanatology has expanded greatly, with courses on a variety of death- and dying-related topics taught in universities and colleges across Canada and elsewhere. For example, Tyndale University in Toronto and King's University College in London, Ontario, offer certificate programs in thanatology. The University of Ottawa, the University of Calgary, and Dalhousie University provide programs in end-of-life studies. The Network for End-of-Life Studies, based at Dalhousie, has been doing research on end of life since the mid-1990s. The Ontario Institute for Studies in Education (OISE) has a grief studies certificate program. These examples are just a few of the many academic courses in Canada related to the study of death and dying, palliative care and hospice, end-of-life care, grief and bereavement and related topics. In the previous three editions of this book, Jeanette A. Auger covered as many of the issues in the field as possible. In this revised edition, we continue in this vein, recognizing the broad and complex events that have occurred since the first edition was published. Jeanette is pleased to be co-editing this edition with Dr. Kerstin Roger, a professor in the College of Community and Global Health at the University of Manitoba.

In 2000, when the first edition was published, there were no death cafés, living wakes, death ambassadors, death dinner groups, grief walks, grief gatherings, grief wells, deathbots, death journeyers, death midwives or death doulas. Things have changed considerably since then! Collective grief was manifest after the COVID-19 outbreak, not just in Canada but across the world, where, according to the World Health Organization (WHO) in 2023, over seven million people died. In Canada, the number was more than fifty-five thousand. At the very beginning of the pandemic, older adults were particularly vulnerable to being abandoned in long-term care and left to die. The pandemic is still amongst us, and the COVID-19 dashboard (World Health Organization 2023) provides weekly updates on the latest number of cases.

Since the first, second and third editions of this book were published in 2000, 2007 and 2019, we have witnessed on a global scale more hurricanes, tsunamis, floods and other disasters, as well as increased acts of terrorism, wars, civil unrest, and, and often, because of these conflicts, increasing numbers of refugees and migrants coming to our country for safety. Another issue which concerns Canadians is the opioid crisis, especially in major cities. Every day we hear news about death, such as in the genocide in Gaza, the wars in Ukraine and Sudan, gun-related deaths in the United States, political violence in Haiti and elsewhere, the murders of Indigenous women and girls in Canada, and the mass graves of children who attended residential schools (which resulted in the Every Child Matters social movement and in turn helped create the annual Day of Truth and Reconciliation in Canada on September 30). These and other world disasters that cause death and suffering have created a pandemic of anxiety and grief not seen to the same extent for many years. Individuals are more aware of the suffering of others and, in some cases, join with like-minded individuals in their communities and beyond to grieve and try to improve situations as best they can.

These tragic and often preventable deaths are a daily reminder of the prevalence of the shadow of death in the midst of life. These events also challenge those working in the health and social services sector to provide more culturally aware and sensitive care to immigrants from war-torn countries and to those suffering from mental health issues and the impacts of racism, transphobia and poverty. Many of these death events come to us through the lens of television, radio and the internet, and we thus become passive consumers of tragedy, sometimes with difficulty separating reality from entertainment. For some of us, grief fatigue overrides our desire to be informed about world events.

As a result of the growth in academia in the study of death- and dying-related topics and to recognize the contributions of others in the field across Canada, this edition includes material written by others: Dr. Zohreh BayatRizi, an associate professor at the University of Alberta, Dr. Catherine White, a mental health practitioner in New Brunswick, Audrey Medwayosh, an Anishinaabe and member of the Wasauksing First Nation in Perry Sound, Ontario, and Rita Giancola, a former high school teacher, musical and theatre composer, and an April 2024 master's degree graduate from York University.

Canadians have long been involved in both public and academic debates about matters related to death and dying. As part of the background research for the first edition of this book, Jeanette reviewed over a thousand articles from the previous thirty years dealing with these topics. These articles were found in publications in all the health and social science fields as well as in journals related to sociology, philosophy, psychology, theology, ethics, geography, law, literature and multiculturalism. Jeanette also used numerous internet sites, books, reports, monographs, radio and television news items, newspaper and magazine articles, and a small selection of video and audio tapes.

One of the major areas of social change regarding issues related to death and dying is the emerging pan-death movement, which aims to assist individuals through what they see as the three levels of death: *before* death, at the diagnoses of a life-threatening, terminal illness; *during* the death process, through active dying and then death; and *after* the death, when funeral rites, burial or cremation services are held. Preferring the term "deathing," the Canadian Integrative Network for Death Education and Alternatives (n.d.) provides the following rationale:

> We often use this term, instead of "death and dying" (which is out of order chronologically!), to indicate that we understand the journey to include all of the process (i.e., a verb, rather than a noun) between preparing choices in advance, terminal diagnosis, active dying, the moment of death, post-deathcare, and funerals/memorials for the Death Journeyer — as well as those who care about them.

In this book we explore and critically discuss key topics in terms of what they tell us about the social changes that may occur in the Canadian environment as we know it. Will we continue to be a death-denying and death-defying culture, or will we embrace death as but another part of life, as part of the cycle of nature, as believed by Indigenous Peoples and other cultures and individuals? This book examines the world of death and dying through a lens that sees these concepts as socially constructed, engaged with by us as individuals moving about our everyday lives and also as impacted by social determinants of health and their own long histories around the globe. From a sociological perspective, death and dying are not clearly defined and articulated abstract concepts but rather an array of social behaviours, expectations, rules and obligations that occur in different cultures as the result of the end of an individual's life.

According to Statistics Canada (2025), the number of deaths per year has been on an upward trend for several years, the result of a growing and aging population. Between July 1, 2022, and June 30, 2023, 330,380 people died in Canada. In 2023, the ten major causes of death in this country were as follows: 1) malignant neoplasms (cancer), 2) diseases of the heart, 3) accidents (unintentional injuries), 4) cerebrovascular diseases, 5) chronic lower respiratory diseases, 6) COVID-19, 7) diabetes mellitus, 8) influenza and pneumonia, 9) Alzheimer's, 10) chronic liver disease cirrhosis (Statistics Canada 2023). Between January 2016 and March 2025, the number of deaths due to opioids rose yearly, with a total of 53,821 such deaths in that period. The majority, 73 percent, were males, and eighteen people a day die from opioid poisoning in this country (Health Canada 2025). While opioid deaths are not included in the top ten causes of death, they are still of great concern to citizens and governments at all levels, as we discuss in Chapter 8.

Inherent in this book is a subtext about our personal experiences with the subject matter at hand, a way of making visible our connections with the topic and of owning what we know — our "epistemology," as it is called in the social sciences. Epistemology refers to how we know what we know. From where, whom and under what social, cultural, historic and geographic circumstances do we gain our experiences and understanding of how the world works? What are the characteristics, limits and methods of knowing something? When we identify these factors, it helps us understand who we are. It also helps us make choices about which parts of our knowledge base we want to hold on to and which we can let go of. When we read most academic texts, the author's experience is hidden and, although they have a voice, we are unable to separate their experiences from their facts. We didn't want to write that kind of book because part of our writing goals includes telling you who we are. Writing and reading are interactive processes; they represent a relationship.

You, as the reader, and we, as writers, engage in a relationship of interaction. As students in the classroom, you also engage with your peers and the instructor in a similar relationship. Therefore, throughout the text, we include in-class assignments aimed at encouraging you to reflect upon and share your experiences with each other. We want to share ours with you too. So, where appropriate, we have included a section in each chapter called "The Text Within." This helps you to understand who we are and where we are coming from, and because of these experiences, why we write as we do.

> **The Text Within: My First Experiences with Death (Jeanette)**
>
> I was born on March 19, 1945, in England (a significant date for many reasons). I was baptized in the Roman Catholic faith, and those familiar with this religion may know that in England, St. Joseph's Day is March 19 and that St. Joseph is the patron saint of a happy death. Although I no longer practise any organized religious activities, I still like to think that my interest and work in death and dying was fated to be by higher forces!
>
> My birth came shortly after the end of the Second World War, in a place called Braintree, Essex, a rural part of the country. My family lived in London's East End, but due to the bombing, pregnant women were sent off to have their babies outside of London. My mother had tuberculosis when I was born, a disease she probably contracted, like so many others in England, from sleeping in air raid shelters in the Underground. She died two years later in a hospice, a few days before my second birthday.
>
> I grew up in Shoreditch, in the East End of London, where death was a constant shadow looming over us. All the children I went to school with had lost family members in the war. We played on bomb sites that had once been people's homes, factories and shops. Because our area had housed several factories, it had been bombed many times. When I was a child, a favourite showing-off spot to friends and acquaintances (and as a very young child to the man who came to collect the football pools money!) was the repaired hole in the downstairs hallway where a bomb had gone through the floor on its way to the cellar. Apparently, the bomb was dropped in 1944 and had gone right through the window above the door and landed on the hallway floor. The brown scorch marks on the wooden floor were a testament to what my parents always referred to as good old British luck. In the basement that was no longer used by any but the mice and the family cat that chased them, overhead windows were still painted black as part of the blackout procedures required during the war years.

I grew up then in a time of mourning, as many of my Jewish friends did, whose families still relived the Holocaust daily. My family was Lithuanian on my mother's side and French Canadian on my father's. All my family members longed for a past that they could not return to in their lifetime. So, death was a part of my life at a very young age and has been with me ever since.

My public school was St. Monica's in Hoxton, a fifteen-minute walk from my home. There were no buses or trains going there from my house because there were no such things as school buses in England. The school was across the street from a small park that had once been the burial pit for victims of the Black Death (bubonic plague), which swept across Europe killing hundreds of thousands in the fourteenth century.

When I was fifteen and still active in the church, I became a volunteer at St. Joseph's Hospice in London, working predominantly with dying children whose mothers had been prescribed the drug thalidomide during pregnancy. It was during this time that my interest in working with the dying was sparked, and even then, I was convinced that we needed to provide more sensitive care to the dying and their important ones and that we couldn't do this work very well in hospital settings.

Within the traditions of my families of origin, it was normal and appropriate for people to die in their own homes rather than in hospitals or nursing homes. Friends and relatives came to the family home to pay their last respects to the old ones. Daily life was going on around them as Lithuanian cabbage soup cooked on the stove, my brother listened to his records, my parents were glued to the latest episode of *The Archers* (a popular nightly radio show in Britain, then and now), and I was downstairs reading. Grandparents, aunts and uncles were waked in our living room, and these elderly relatives had died in their own beds.

Death was very much part of life and in our homes, always visible and present, not hidden as it is today. Children were always present at funerals and invited to kiss the dead relatives before the coffin lid was closed. We attended the wakes afterwards and learned that although death was a sad event within the family, it was also a time to celebrate life and to remember the good times we had shared.

Growing up in the particular time and place that I did, in a country steeped in thousands of years of history and mourning for its many dead, caused me to wonder about the role of death in our lives, the kind of work that death makes necessary for the living, and the social changes that death brings about, not just for immediate family and friends but for entire communities, cultures and regions.

The Text Within: My First Experiences with Death (Kerstin)

I remember the first time when I was a child that a dear pet died. It was a guinea pig which used to run around free in our yard, and we loved it. It was always quite resilient, scaring off cats who tried to poach it, hiding in the foot-high, palm tree–like weeds and popping out with a fierce determination as needed to scare off predators. This tiny, soft and vulnerable creature put on a good defence! When Toto died, I was beside myself with grief, and it took me years to understand that when our pets die, we can experience a lot of grief, and we learn about ourselves and letting go, possibly feeling the sadness we have carried over from other meaningful human relationships. I believe that all our relationships, big and small, human and natural, inanimate and filled with life, create opportunities for personal growth and living our own lives in a better way — and death is no different.

I always knew and heard a lot about death growing up since my family stems from Europe and lived there through many tragedies in and around the Second World War. As a Canadian student in public school, I learned very little initially about the way in which Indigenous Peoples in Canada had been harmed. It simply wasn't in the school curriculum! Developing a deeper knowledge as an adult about colonization and its traumatic impact on Indigenous Peoples was truly alarming and is a continual reminder about the role governments can play in both the destruction and also the promotion of a human being's value and the meaning of their very lives.

My interest in death became more focused when, at twenty-one, I went alone to Calcutta and worked with Mother Teresa in the House of the Destitute and the Dying for three months. I became a psychotherapist in downtown Toronto at one point in my life after being a musician, a consultant, and later an educator and a researcher. I lost both of my parents (my father in later years to a heart attack), and I was an at-home care provider during COVID for my mom, who unexpectedly got cancer. I have gone through other losses of people very near and dear to me and supported others in the same way.

Throughout, I never let go of the importance of understanding the big impact that end-of-life decision making has on others, and what personal, social and institutional factors shape those decisions. I have done research on caregiving, on families and chronic illness, on end-of-life decision making, on palliative care and more recently on the impact of legalizing MAID (medical assistance in dying) in Canada. We all need to be healers and receivers of care at different times in our lives; we all need to be conscientious clinicians and health-care providers or educators and clergy; and we all need to know that life and death are deeply intertwined in this shared time on Earth. Death teaches us many things — about the short time we have to live, love and share joy in our communities!

WHY STUDY DEATH AND DYING?

When someone we love dies, we engage in a process through which we try to make sense of that death. Whether we knew the person or not, as in the case of celebrities, the death causes us to reflect on and remember our past. Death reconnects us to a string of memories and relationships; it takes us into our pasts and helps us come to terms with the passing of the years. In this sense, death provides psychological work for us to do to come to terms with the loss.

The end of life is a complex and difficult subject. While media stories on the end of life are common, final decisions around death and dying are personal and shaped by the cultures in which we live. There are many reasons to study these topics. Some include the following, and you could add your own to the list too.

Personal Reasons

Many of us study death and dying because of our personal experiences or infatuation with or interest in the topic. What are your reasons? Here are some reasons why academics and students want to study and reflect on these topics:

- to heal a loss that has not been resolved, resulting in unfinished business;
- to come to terms with the fear of death;
- to be able to help others deal with death;
- to learn about the history of social practices.

Academic Reasons

Many academic disciplines have long traditions of studying death and dying. All branches of the humanities, social sciences and basic sciences are involved with the study of death and dying in some way, from laboratory-based experiments in biology and medicine to pharmacological studies of drugs to alleviate pain and symptoms; from in-depth interviews with the dying and their important ones in psychology, sociology and anthropology; to the need for an understanding of the religious, cultural and spiritual needs of the dying on the part of pastoral care counsellors and others in the field of theology. Supernatural issues are often of interest to students, but so also are grief and how funerals operate. While science is involved in a variety of examinations of issues related to death and dying, many are concerned with the prolongation of life. However, medical advances that prolong life also create ethical, legal and practical dilemmas about who may end the life of another, as well as how and when. The topics scientists in all disciplines are interested in include:

- causes of death, types of death, chronic and acute pain and symptom management, treatment and cures;
- prevention of death due to accidents, drug and alcohol abuse, suicide and illness;
- training techniques to prepare caregivers and others in the "helping professions" to assist the dying;
- changes in life expectancy and mortality rates.

Institutional Reasons

Many institutions are involved in care for the dying and deceased, ranging from those involved in medicine, ethics, law, spirituality and religion, counsellors, social workers and those working in the funeral industry. The types of issues these professionals pursue include everything from the emotional, physical, cultural, economic and spiritual costs of prolonging life to end-of-life issues such as medically assisted death, legal issues and the final disposition of the dead.

WHO STUDIES DEATH AND DYING?

Many people choose to study death and dying, either for personal reasons such as their own mortality or that of those they love, or because their profession, vocation or field of academic inquiry requires it. Although all citizens may be interested in death and dying for personal reasons, scientists normally engage in more rigorous and systematic examinations of the topics. Others are just fascinated by knowing more about what happens when we die. Scientists and others who choose to study the dying process and death include sociologists, gerontologists, medical professionals, social planners and journalists, funeral directors and psychologists, spiritual advisors, criminologists and workers in emergency measures, the military and the police.

WHERE IS DEATH AND DYING STUDIED?

Death and dying are studied in a variety of laboratory, medical, legal, university and colleges, scientific and everyday settings, some of which include the following:

- in classrooms and people's homes;
- in the "field," e.g., in archaeology and anthropology;
- in literature, art, film, theatre and other popular culture sources;
- in pharmaceutical companies and laboratories and a variety of medical settings;
- in coroners' and medical examiners' offices and crime laboratories.

HOW IS DEATH AND DYING STUDIED?

When death and dying are studied, regardless of whether the methods used are qualitative (such as observations, case studies, interviews, ethnographies and so on) or quantitative (using surveys, questionnaires, theoretical models and such), in all cases our understanding and awareness of these processes are enhanced. Because of these studies, different treatment options may be available, we may become more aware of the options facing those with life-limiting illnesses in terms of where they choose to die, and we may assess and evaluate care of the dying in our own homes and our own communities.

DISCIPLINARY APPROACHES TO DEATH AND DYING

Within the realm of academia, several disciplines are concerned with the topics of death and dying. Whether these courses and programs are provided within specific schools, such as thanatology, palliative care, nursing, medicine or social work, or in more general programs, such as arts and the humanities and social, environmental or biological sciences, each discipline approaches the topic from a unique perspective. Sometimes there is an overlap between disciplines, and this assists in being able to examine issues from different perspectives, thus providing a more detailed and thorough account of the phenomenon. Below are just some of the disciplinary approaches to the study of death and dying.

Psychological Studies

Psychology is both an academic discipline and an applied field of research and treatment involving the study of the mind, brain and behaviour in both humans and non-humans. Psychology is also interested in a variety of human activities, including the ways in which people deal with the challenges of everyday life and the diagnosis and treatment of mental illness. Psychologists are primarily interested in the mental processes and behaviours of individuals, whether alone or in groups. Death possesses many faces and meanings, and perceptions of it vary across cultures and historical time periods. It is obviously too intricate to be the province of any one discipline. Nevertheless, psychology's contributions to the topic have succeeded in increasing understanding of the mind and body mechanisms which enable people to deal with death and bereavement.

Most of us experience anxiety over our own death and those of the people we love at some time in our lives. How we manifest this in our daily lives is of interest to psychologists and those who provide care to the terminally ill and their loved ones. "Thanatophobia" is the term used by some psychologists and counsellors who work with and for persons dealing with the loss of self and loved ones to explain the excessive and incapacitating fear of death of others or the self. Psychologists Rachel Menzies and Ross Menzies (2020) reviewed studies from several countries examining death anxiety and its treatments during the COVID-19 pandemic and concluded:

> The recent COVID-19 pandemic has caused an understandable surge in anxiety across the globe. Much of the behavioural response to COVID-19 can be understood through the lens of terror management theory, which argues that death anxiety drives much of human behaviour. From this perspective, reminders of death (of which there are many in the current pandemic), produce increases in attempts to avoid a physical death (such as by wearing protective gear or self-isolating) or ensure a symbolic immortality (such as by bolstering one's cultural worldviews, and aggressing against those that threaten them). Death anxiety, which has recently been proposed to be a transdiagnostic construct, appears to be more relevant now than ever before. In addition to predicting anxiety related to COVID-19, fear of death has also been shown to play a causal role across a number of mental health conditions.

All the death anxiety studies confirm that individuals share similar elements of fear regarding not only their own deaths but also those of others.

Sociological Studies

Sociologists are interested in the ways in which human beings socially construct the worlds in which we live. Dying, death and bereavement do not occur in a vacuum. How individuals and groups experience these phenomena is influenced by the social context in which they occur as well as their cultural, religious and social values. Sociologists are also concerned with the rules and regulations (both visible and implied) that govern our everyday activities. Because sociology is primarily the science of everyday life and social change, it brings an especially useful set of ideas, concepts and descriptions about the study of death and dying.

Sherwin Nuland highlights the significant change in dying in recent times:

> We have created the method of modern dying. Modern dying takes place in the modern hospital, where it can be hidden, cleansed of its organic light ... and finally packaged for modern burial. We can now deny the power not only of death but of nature itself. We hide our faces from its face, but still we spread our fingers just a bit, because there is something in us that cannot resist a peek. (Nuland 1995: 113)

From a sociological perspective, we recognize that death and dying will occur for each of us, and when this happens, an entire infrastructure of social and personal institutions will come to act on our behalf. If we deconstruct the notions of death and dying as two separate yet connected events, we crisscross the institutions of the family, whether we define this term biologically, socially or chosen; health care, whether provided in hospital, hospice, palliative care unit, nursing home or an in-home care program; law, in terms of wills and estate planning; the professions, especially medical personnel and funeral directors; religion, whether denominational or alternative; social attitudes about so-called "good" and "bad" deaths and so on. In fact, the gamut of sociological investigations can be applied to the concepts of death and dying.

Robert Kastenbaum discusses what he calls a "societal death system," which shows the interconnectedness of life events and death. Included in this death system are the following:

- *Warning and predicting death*: This refers to the varied organizations within a society that warn individuals or collectives about impending dangers, such as weather forecasting agencies, emergency personnel and social media. It also includes laboratories and physicians that interpret test results to patients.
- *Caring for the dying*: This category offers a good example of cultural change. The hospital was considered ineffective by many in caring for the dying, so new cultural forms such as hospice, at-home and palliative care emerged to fulfil this function.

- *Disposing of the dead*: This area includes practices that surround the removal of a body, rituals and methods of disposal. Since every culture, religious, ethnic and age group has its own meaningful ways to dispose of the dead, this can lead to strains when opinions differ.
- *Social consolidation after death*: When a person dies, other members of the society, such as the family or the work unit, adjust and come together. Part of the death system which enables people to deal with death includes self-help groups, counsellors, religious organizations and so on.
- *Making sense of death*: Every society develops ways to understand and make sense of loss. One of the values of funeral and celebration-of-life rituals is that they allow for a death to be interpreted within a given faith, culture or philosophical viewpoint.
- *Killing*: Every death system has norms that indicate when, how and for what reasons individuals or other living creatures can be killed. International treaties define what weapons and what killings are justifiable in war. Different cultures determine the crimes an individual can be executed for, as well as the appropriate methods of execution. Cultures, too, determine the reason and ways that animals may be killed (adapted from Kastenbaum 2001).

Further to his ideas about a death system, Kastenbaum also suggests that there are at least three ways to think about death — as an event, a condition or a state of non-existence (Corr 2014).

When we deal with death and dying from a sociological perspective, we see death not as a given but rather as a socially constructed and maintained phenomenon. Death then doesn't just happen: there are processes involved that include behaviours, expectations, beliefs, rituals and a vast array of everyday social practices that constitute a death. When we die, decisions must be made about disposal: whether to have a traditional or alternate funeral; whether to bury or cremate; whether to embalm and have an open casket or have memorial services and so on. There are many decisions to make, both before and after death occurs.

We all die! When we examine the sociology of death and dying, we recognize that there are both personal, experiential features of learning as well as structural, scientific ones. Physical death is an essentially social experience that takes place in two realms of reality: the structural/public and the personal/private. In the personal/private realm, the reality of death is often hidden from public view and from those unknown to the deceased and their family. This is less so when the death occurs because of a crime, suicide, murder, military manoeuvre or tragic accident. In those cases, media coverage may move the private grief of family, friends and coworkers into the public arena. In the structural/public realm, death becomes a matter for public discourse while the infrastructure of goods and services provided by the death industry goes to work on our behalf.

To learn how others in our society deal with death, we need to examine our own thoughts, feelings and fears. As well, by looking at the death practices of other cultures, we can learn, in a comparative way, about our own. Death is part of our history. Much of the study of archaeology, palaeontology and geology is about creatures and people who have died. We discover information about our predecessors and other cultures by digging into their pasts both metaphorically and physically. Through examining ancient tombs and burial sites, we have learned much about earlier civilizations. Cadavers help us deal with the future in terms of finding "cures" for diseases, and we can learn much from these contexts.

Literary and Aesthetic Studies

Those involved in the field of literary and aesthetic studies are interested in the social production of works of art, the meaning and symbols that authors and artists use to display emotion, behaviour and feelings about the human journey and the ways in which art and literature contribute to a society's understanding of life and death. Some of the ways in which these topics are studied include the role of and presentation, past and present, of death in literature, in the visual arts and in in film.

Philosophical Studies

Philosophers are interested in the moral, ethical and values-based ideas upon which societies are created and maintained. They may also be concerned with matters such as the role of the state and religion in matters concerning the end of life. The International Association for the Philosophy of Death and Dying is a global organization of some two hundred scholars who are interested in the investigation of philosophical questions surrounding death and dying. Among the topics they explore are the metaphysics of death, including personal identity criteria for declaring death. They consider issues such as the possibility and/or desirability of immortality, and the meanings of death and life. They also explore reactions to death and dying (e.g., grief, Ars moriendi and the "good death"), ethical controversies related to death (e.g., suicide, organ donation, abortion, capital punishment, etc.) and clinical and biomedical issues related to death and dying.

Theological Studies

Theologians are interested in the study of the role of religions, the sacred and spirituality in the everyday lives of members of societies. They are also concerned with the values and beliefs of individuals and the ways these impact the choices they make. Some of the topics of interest to theologians include the following:

- the origins of belief in heaven and hell and cross-cultural equivalents;
- near-death experiences;
- religious rituals concerning death and beyond;
- the portrayal of death in religious texts, symbols, artifacts and teachings.

Jane Littlewood points out that "the general attitude of western societies towards death is characterized by fear and shame" (1993: 69). Even though we are a death-denying society, in the United States the average child TV viewer will have seen ten thousand deaths by the time they are thirteen. These deaths are often devoid of feelings, suffering and grief. This attitudinal pattern of death as denied or forbidden, and yet also a source of great fascination and mystery, is what Geoffrey Gorer (1965) defines as the "pornography of death." Because most deaths in Western societies take place outside of our homes and communities, in hospitals, nursing homes and other care settings, the living are separated from the dead. Death work, such as preparing the body for disposal, is now normally conducted by strangers. In many ways, death is an absent intruder in our lives — present but ignored.

For most of us, when death touches our lives in personal ways, we engage in a conspiracy of silence, not wanting others to feel too sorry for us. We want recognition for our loss, but we do not want to draw attention to ourselves and our loved ones. In Jeanette's experience with bereaved individuals, she often hears them say they don't want others to "make a fuss." We wear a mask of coping because in our culture, dependence on others and appearing weak are negative signs. Yet everyone dies! The only absolute fact we may learn from this book is that each one of us will die.

CONCLUSION

Sociology is not about reinforcing the status quo but about unpacking and critically analyzing how, where and why we practise the rituals of death and dying that we do. In this chapter we introduce you to some of the key issues in the various disciplines which examine and discuss a variety of topics related to death and dying. In the following ones, we are social detectives discovering clues about the social processes and behaviours involved in death and dying.

SELF-REFLECTION AND THOUGHTFUL CONVERSATIONS

1. What social issues have changed our thinking about death and dying over the past twenty years?
2. Why and in what ways is Canada a death-denying society?
3. How are your views about death different than the views of your grandparents?
4. Why is there a renewed interest in the topics of death and dying?

IN-CLASS ASSIGNMENTS

1. Bring items to class that discuss death and dying in Canada, such as newspaper or magazine articles. What do they tell you about common notions of these concepts?
2. Write down a list of positive and negative thoughts associated with death. What are the similarities and differences between the items on your list?
3. If you were dying, what three things, events or behaviours would you most want to be remembered for?

Chapter Two

YOUR EXPERIENCES AND PERCEPTIONS OF DEATH AND DYING

TO UNDERSTAND THE EXPERIENCES OF OTHERS, to be able to relate to them and be empathetic, it is important to know how *you* feel about death and dying. Our experiences shape how we see those of others. If you are like most Canadians, you fear death. Perhaps what is more frightening than death itself is the process of dying, whether it be at home, in a hospital, nursing home or assisted-living facility, in a hospice or palliative care unit or because of an accident, murder or other catastrophe. Even though we may be pain- and symptom-free and comfortable in our surroundings, we may still experience death anxiety, and why shouldn't we? Everything and everyone we love will be gone from us when we experience what some see as the final loss — death itself.

The learning objectives of the following exercises are aimed at helping you to reflect on your experiences and learn from them in terms of helping yourself and perhaps others to become more comfortable and familiar with death. You may complete the following exercises by writing, or if you prefer, by drawing a picture of your experiences or making a sound or body posture that most accurately portrays how you feel or have felt.

PERSONAL EXPERIENCES WITH DEATH EXERCISE

This first exercise is designed to have you recall past experiences. Try to reflect on what your feelings were at the time when the deaths occurred.

1. My first experience with death was when I was _____ years old.
2. Describe what happened, where and when.
3. Describe how you felt at the time.
4. I dealt with this death by feeling or doing what?
5. Friends and family who have died include:

6. My own life was in danger when _____.
7. What activities did you engage in to help you deal with these deaths?
8. Was there anyone specific whom you turned to when these deaths occurred?
9. How did and does your family of origin deal with death, dying and the experience of grief?
10. Do you think that your first experience with death might influence the way you interact with dying or grieving people now? If so, how?
11. How have your thoughts and feelings about death changed since your first encounter with it?
12. Are there specific religious, ethnic and cultural rituals around death and dying in your family of origin?

REFLECTING ON OUR DYING EXERCISE

This exercise encourages you to remain in the present as you try to imagine your own death. As well, it helps you to think about how you presently deal with issues related to communicating your feelings about these matters.

1. What is the first thought that comes into your mind when you hear the word death?
2. What are the modalities of the death you imagine? What does it taste, smell, feel and look like? What are the colour and shape? What sound does it make?
3. Can you imagine your own death? If you had a choice, what kind of death would you prefer, at what age, and why?
4. Do you fear dying? Discuss.
5. Have you discussed dying and death with your family? With others? Tell about some views they have shared with you.
6. If you were told you were terminally ill with less than a year to live, how would you want to spend your time?
7. What are the qualities that make life worth living?
8. Do you believe in life after death? If yes, what do you think that life might be like after death?
9. Has anyone you know experienced what you would define as a "good death," and how did it come about?
10. Has anyone you know experienced what you would define as a "bad death," and how did it come about?

FEARS OF DYING EXERCISE

Completing this exercise encourages us to identify our fears and thus be able to confront them. How we respond is affected by our previous experiences and knowledge of death.

Rank the following from greatest fear (10) to least fear (1) and explain the reasons for your choices:

___ pain or mental health issues associated with dying
___ leaving loved ones behind
___ being buried alive
___ being put in a jail to die alone
___ going to hell
___ dying alone and lonely
___ abandoning others who depend on me
___ dying as the result of a murder or other horrific crime
___ dying as the result of a natural disaster or accident
___ dying of an overdose

LOSS AWARENESS EXERCISE

Loss, like beauty, is in the eye of the beholder. Its ubiquitous nature acknowledges no boundaries of age, sex, ethnic background or religious preference. Loss has been a part of your life since early childhood. The purpose of this list is to raise your personal level of awareness about the large number of events that you may have experienced and responded to as a loss in your life. It is important to note that when an event occurs, individual members of a family may or may not describe that event as a loss. When you examine these losses, how did you deal with them at the time, would you do anything differently now and why?

Loss Inventory

Make a loss inventory based on your own experiences and take the opportunity to recognize and be comforted by the ways you dealt with them at the time. All losses teach us about our abilities to deal with life's challenges, no matter how difficult and as a result, these losses are learning tools.

Responding to World Events that Impact Our Lives

Reflect on and write about the impacts some of the most recent events in the past five years have had on your thoughts and feelings about death and dying. Examples: COVID-19, the finding of the mass graves of children who lived in Indian residential schools in Canada, the opioid crisis, wars, school shootings in the US, teenage suicide, and anything else which has an impact on your daily life.

CONCLUSION

In this chapter we invited you to reflect on your own attitudes and experiences with death and dying, rather than examine the research and opinions of others. It is important that we situate ourselves in our assumptions and expectations and to think about how they are shaped by our cultural and social circumstances.

Chapter Three

KEY CONCEPTS IN THE MAZE OF DEATH AND DYING

What more chilling commentary on the modern world could there be than that most people die unprepared for death, as they have lived, unprepared for life? (Rinpoche 1993: 47)

DEATH IS A MARKER OF SOCIAL CHANGE in any given culture and acts as a barometer of societal values, personal interests, social and legal policies and spiritual values and rituals for dealing with the dying and their loved ones. The main causes of death in Canada have changed from tuberculosis in the 1950s to cancers of all types, heart disease and strokes, drug and opioid addiction and Alzheimer's disease in the new millennium.

After-death arrangements have moved predominantly from the private sphere of the home and community to the public arena of the funeral home or crematorium. Now, when a death occurs in a community, rather than receive the news at the local level from family, friends, acquaintances and through religious organizations when funerals or other services are being planned, the news of a death is often presented through social media platforms and online newsfeeds. On the website Modern Loss, participants discuss finding out about the deaths of loved ones, not from other family members, but from Facebook, X (Twitter) and other sites. As some point out, this is not the way you want to receive such terrible news. Given changes to social media in 2025, it is uncertain how or if this trend will continue, as some people limit their online presence.

The work of care of the dead has shifted from intimate loved ones in our own homes to complete strangers in institutions such as hospitals, residential care facilities and palliative care and hospice settings. As life expectancy in Canada rises, the age at death generally increases so that most of us will die in old age. Whereas burial was once our only choice of final disposition, according to the Cremation Association of North America (2024), cremation is increasingly becoming the option for Canadians, with a cremation rate of more than 75.3 percent in 2023. These social changes have altered our perspective regarding the role of important practices and carers in our own and loved ones' death and dying, from hands-on caregivers to unknown caregivers, to spectators. Increasingly, we are seeing the strong wish for more environmentally friendly practices, such as green burials and funeral practices. The Green Burial Society of Canada provides a list of certified green burial sites in Canada on its website.

In another area of social change, cryonic suspension promises life after death, while, theoretically, elective prosthetics suggest that with the replacement of healthy limbs with robotic or bionic ones, life can be extended indefinitely, at a high price for those able to afford it. The field of body modification implants also offers increased abilities; these procedures are discussed more fully in other chapters of this book. Media images and presentations of death-oriented topics proliferate, and the internet provides a forum for every conceivable issue, with websites providing online obituaries, funerary products including casket furniture, photo and crystal urns, including ones for pets, burial plots, memorial stationery, keepsake jewellery, which includes the ashes of the deceased, and a great deal of information on the buying and selling of body parts and organs. This also means that almost anyone can have access to information and services which, a hundred years ago, would either not be available at all, be seen as fringe or simply be inaccessible to the general population. We might ask: has this numbed us to the everyday real talk of death, has it made us more aware and conscientious of how others experience dying, or has it simply overwhelmed us with so many options and new approaches?

In any sociological enterprise, we examine, observe and analyze a total phenomenon, in this case death and dying, by breaking it down into its separate issues or concepts. We call this *deconstructing death*. If we imagine receiving a box labelled "Death and Dying," what might be in it? From a complex whole to a set of constituent parts that are interconnected and make up the whole, we recognize that death and dying have many layers of meaning.

As our working definitions, let's agree that:

> Death is the final stage of our physical and embodied life. Dying is a process rich in many ways, and one which leads to a very real physical subsequent death. We are all currently involved in this process through senescence — the physiological mechanism through which all humans are born, live our lives

and subsequently die. Death is viewed differently in religions and cultures around the world, and we can learn about other people and their beliefs by educating ourselves and engaging in this topic.

DEFINITIONS AND THE DIAGNOSIS OF DEATH

To declare a person dead so that a death certificate can officially be produced, a medical diagnosis is necessary. Without one, in most countries around the world, no decisions can be made by family, friends or health professionals about the removal and disposal of the body. The classic indicators of death are the permanent cessation of the functions of the brain, heart and lungs, measured by the absence of circulation (blood flow), respiration (breathing) and neurological activity (responsiveness). Sam D. Shemie and colleagues at the McGill University Health Centre Research Institute (2023) define death as the permanent cessation of brain function and provide corresponding circulatory and neurologic criteria to ascertain that. They state that a brain-based definition of death is now central to our Canadian understanding of what constitutes dying.

Brain death is the irreversible cessation of all functions of the brain, including and especially the brain stem. The upper brain, called the cerebrum, is the most highly evolved portion of the brain and is responsible for the complex processes of thinking and reasoning associated with being human. The brain stem contains the control centre, which is responsible for the "vegetative" functions of the body, like breathing and swallowing. The brain cells, called neurons, make up the cerebrum and its outer covering, the cerebral cortex, and are especially sensitive to oxygen deprivation. The brain dies from the top down, so the death of the brain stem is what is generally referred to as brain death (Leming and Dickinson 1988: 34).

Historically, Manitoba was the only province to have a law defining what constituted death:

> For all purposes within the legislative competence of the legislature of Manitoba, the death of a person was understood to take place at the time at which irreversible cessation of that person's brain function occurs, and when it appears that withdrawal, if already instituted, of any artificial support of that person's vital functions causes or will cause the immediate onset of tissue disintegration throughout that person's body (Manitoba Law Reform Commission 1974: 28).

In the 1960s, medical technological advances, through intensive care settings, provided machine-assisted maintenance of breathing and heartbeat in patients whose brains had irretrievably ceased to function. As well, with the advent of organ transplantation and the necessity that these organs come from otherwise healthy individuals who died from traumatic brain injury, came the necessary development of new criteria for the diagnosis of brain death.

Death does not "just happen" but must be legally certified and medically diagnosed by a physician. If we die in a hospital, a nurse cannot declare us dead until this state has been certified by a physician. In cases of terminal illness, either at home or in palliative care units and hospices, the death certificate may have already been written and signed by a physician prior to death, with date and time being added when death actually occurs.

THE NON-HEART-BEATING DONOR CONTROVERSY

Because of a shortage of suitable organs for transplantation and the growing numbers of individuals requiring them, the controversial topic of the use of the non-heart-beating donor (NHBD) continues. The NHBD is an individual whose heart has stopped beating but who has not been declared dead due to the continuing functioning of their brain. The inventor of the NHBD protocol, Dr. Michael DeVita, has admitted, however, that "the possibility of brain function recovery exists for at least 15 minutes" (DeVita 2001: 179). In his article "Non-Heart-Beating Organ Donation," John B. Shea (2003) suggests that when the criteria for death concerning those in irreversible comas and not technically dead was adopted, it was done so by people promoting organ harvesting and transplantation as an attempt to morally justify these procedures. The quandary faced by both professionals and family members when loved ones are diagnosed as being in a "persistent vegetative state" (PVS) throws the question of when a person is alive or dead into further debate.

There are several reasons why it matters precisely when we die. Legal issues around legacies with estates may be affected by the time of death. Organ donations and transplants rely heavily on time and type of death, and in criminal cases of murder or assisted suicide, time and cause of death are crucial pieces of information. As the Manitoba Law Reform Commission noted in 1974:

A living person, while life endures, is a vessel of civil and human rights, not the least of which is the right to life itself. In identifying the time of death as the occurrence of brain death, we manage to avoid the temptation of killing one patient to provide organs for another. (1974: 15)

The clinical definitions for death are the following:

Necrobiosis refers to the process by which individual cells continually die and are replaced throughout our lifetime.

Necrosis refers to the death of tissue or even entire organs, for example, when a blood clot cuts off the circulation to the heart and as a result an individual experiences a heart attack yet is still alive (unless there is severe damage to the heart).

Somatic death is the end of all life in an organism. (Leming and Dickinson 1988: 11)

When a person's heart and lungs stop functioning, the person can be declared clinically dead, but individual cells can continue to live for several minutes. After about three minutes, the brain cells die. The last cells to die are bone, hair and skin.

Health Canada legislates which organs, tissues and blood products can be donated. In Canada, donors are not paid for their contributions of these products. Organs that can be donated include heart, lungs, pancreas, liver, kidneys, stomach and small bowels. Donatable tissues include corneas, sclera, skin, heart valves, bone and tendons (Sherry and Tremblay n.d.). Fewer than 25 percent of people living in Canada have signed organ donation cards and there is a huge need for more to do so (Government of Canada 2025c).

Bone tissue is used in treating cancerous defects of the extremities and face, disabling spinal problems, scoliosis, birth defects and reconstructive surgery of major joints. Bone marrow is used for research and for the treatment of leukaemia (especially in children) and nuclear radiation injuries. Skin is used in the treatment of severely burned patients. Soft tissue (dura, fascia, tendons and ligaments) is used to treat defects caused by tumours and trauma, to repair tendons and ligaments and to treat sports injuries.

Blood products such as plasma, platelets, vessels and valves are also marketable commodities. Journalist Sean Cate (2024) notes that the human body may be worth more dead than alive, and due to a shortage of organs, blood and bone products and tissue donations, an underground market has emerged in the procurement and trade of these commodities. Many websites provide the amounts of money a person could receive for selling body parts; in this way, human bodies are commodities available on the open market. According to Cate, body parts are worth the following in US dollars:

- kidneys: $200,000
- liver: $157,000
- heart: $119,000
- corneas: $30,000.

Jana Kasperkevic (2014) reports that human reproductive products such as eggs, sperm, wombs, placentas and breast milk can all be sold, and although the rhetoric provided by the companies intent on the purchase of such products is that to do so helps infertile couples and women unable to breastfeed, which it may well do, there is however still a capitalist element to all of these sales, as such companies also profit from them

Numerous websites can be found using the search words "cadaver for sale," which allow you to see what your worth may be after death and also the price of synthetic cadavers for research and study. Because of a shortage of cadavers for medical research, some scientists, especially in the US and China, are producing synthetic ones. Dr. Christopher Sakezles, a scientist in Tampa, Florida, invented a synthetic human cadaver at his SynDaver Labs. "It's made of salt, water and fiber and mimics properties of human tissue. It can even pump heated synthetic blood and can be used to simulate procedures with ventilation." This product, along with other "synthetic humans," is similar to plastinated cadavers, which scientists in China and other countries are working on. China Organ Harvest Research Center states: "Body plastination technology uses silicon, epoxy, and other polymer mixtures to replace fluids in the human body. Other than the plastination technology itself, the barrier to creating specimens is the availability of fresh human corpses. According to forensic medicine, the 'fresh period' for a human body is just two days" (China Organ Harvest Research Center n.d.). Clearly this is a field of technology which will change the way that organ and cadaver donations are dealt with globally. Rather than humans donating such body items for altruistic reasons, scientists will be able to sell them for profit.

Authors Brian Grow and John Shiffman (2017) suggest that

in the US market for human bodies almost anyone can dissect and sell the dead ... [and] when Americans leave their bodies to science, they are also donating to commerce: Cadavers and body parts, especially those of the poor, are sold in a thriving and largely unregulated market. ... Each year, thousands of Americans donate their bodies in the belief they are contributing to science. In fact, many are also unwittingly contributing to commerce, their bodies traded as raw material in a largely unregulated national market.

As noted earlier, donors in Canada are not financially compensated for donating body products.

ORGAN DONATION, BODY BROKERS AND THE TRANSPLANT TOURIST INDUSTRY

As the population ages, globally and within Canada, the need for organ donations continues to grow. One organ donor may be able to save up to eight lives. Health Canada states that there are 2,200 organ transplants every year (Government of Canada n.d.). This excellent record is because,

> from 2018 to 2024, Health Canada and [our] partners led and successfully completed the Organ Donation and Transplantation Collaborative, with implementation of the Pan-Canadian Governance Body for Organ Donation and Transplantation. This new initiative will continue to make improvements to system performance for better patient outcomes.

Understanding the value of organ donation in extending the lives of others is important, and to this end the Canadian Donation and Transplant Research Program, a national research network founded in 2013, is key in helping promote organ donation as a way to "enhance the survival and quality of life" of Canadians. This network is invaluable in shaping healthy and positive choices, as well as improved knowledge for users, developing new policy and legislation and promoting the legal use of organs through research, with the benefit of not being vulnerable to the abuses of an illegal market. Its website hosts up-to-date and interesting talks and webinars so that Canadians can find resources on these topics.

Because of the lack of available body parts for those who need them, an underground market has arisen in which the human body is seen as a commodity. For those with the financial resources, life extension is possible by buying an organ from someone whose life is seen as less valuable. As a result, a new profession of organ brokers has emerged. An organ broker buys organs from (predominantly) poor and disadvantaged people, mostly in the Global South, and sells them to wealthy people living in the Global North, mainly North America and Europe. The broker may also arrange for organ retrieval and transplantation to take place within the country of origin of the organ seller, and seldom is backup care provided to the sellers, who are predominantly males under thirty.

Human trafficking is a lucrative crime and violation of human rights that exploits women, men, transgender people and children. It includes trafficking for forced labour, sexual exploitation, forced begging and military conscription. (World Health Organization 2023). In 2018, around the world, roughly twelve thousand illegal organs are transplanted with a revenue of approximately $1.5 billion each year. Also in 2018, roughly 40 million people were victims of human trafficking, with a majority of them either sexually exploited or forced into labour (Twist 2022). In a November 13, 2013, article, Dr. Dale Archer noted that there are "'broker-friendly' US hospitals, complete with surgeons who either don't know or don't care where the organs come from" and as a result, "this is a multi-million-dollar industry, and as the wealth gap continues to widen, it's only expected to get worse."

Dr. Nancy Scheper-Hughes is a founding member of Organs Watch, a human rights group that monitors the trade in organs. Its website enables viewers to click on any part of the world where the illegal buying and selling of organs takes place to see what the current status is for these practices. In an article written in May 2014 for the *New Internationalist*, Dr. Scheper-Hughes noted that transplant tourism is on the rise, especially among citizens in wealthier countries, where those needing organs travel to countries where organs are being harvested from the poor for transplant purposes:

> For now, transplant tours are more usual. They can bring together actors from as many as four or five different countries, with a buyer from one place, the brokers from two other countries, the mobile surgeons travelling from one nation to another where the kidney operations actually take place. In these instances, the case of a private clinic in Kosovo is perhaps the best example since the participants appear and disappear quickly, with the

guilty parties (including the surgeons) taking with them any incriminating data. When the police finally arrive at the scene, they discover the bloody remains of a black-market clinic, with traces of forensic evidence, but the key players long since disappeared.

Scheper-Hughes also suggests that organ trafficking is now in the hands of organized crime, which sees a tremendous source of profit in the market for body parts:

> Over the course of more than 17 years of dogged field research, my Organs Watch colleagues and I realized that we were not dealing with a question of medical ethics. Rather, we had gained entry into the world of international organized crime. Following fieldwork in Turkey, Moldova, the US, Israel, Brazil, Argentina, the Philippines and South Africa, it became apparent that organ brokers were human traffickers involved in cutthroat deals that were enforced with violence, if needed. Many of the "kidney hunters" who seek out new candidates in poor localities are former sellers, recruited by crime bosses.

Another issue identified in the management of organ donation was that the death certificate could be falsified regarding the deceased's age and cause of death, potentially leading to unsuitable body parts being inserted into living patients and causing more harm than good.

While many of these activities take place within the realm of illegality, there is also a legal venue for the retrieval and transplantation of organs and body parts. In the US and some European countries, organ procurement has become big business and costly, too. To retrieve fresh organs from the nearly dead, individuals are often kept alive using expensive medical technology so that their organs can be harvested as quickly and efficiently as possible and transplanted where they are most needed. Sadly, they are also often available for sale.

What these practices show, whether legal or illegal, is that there is a huge social change in the ways in which the human body, either alive or dead, is viewed, from a private and respected entity to a marketable commodity. Such practices also reveal the continuing trend in the oppression of the poor for the benefit of the rich; they display the enormous threat to social justice and equality for all on a global level.

TYPES OF DEATH

There are many ways to die. As we have discussed, we can speak of people as "clinically" dead even though they have a heartbeat. People are said to be "brain dead" if they are without consciousness for an extended period of time and don't respond to neurological stimuli. After a trauma or life-shattering event befalls an individual, they may say that they feel "emotionally dead." Individuals who feel unable to cope with life's challenges speak of a death of the self or "psychological death." Likewise, when a trauma challenges someone's faith or belief system, they speak of a "spiritual death." "Social death" may occur before "biological death" when some people, such as those suffering from drug or alcohol addiction, are socially ostracized because of their illness. The concept of "sudden death" refers to one where it is unexpected, unanticipated and with no obvious symptoms for its cause; in such cases, those who are grieving have had no opportunity to prepare for it or say goodbye to the person who has died. Examples of sudden loss could include road and other fatal accidents, murder, suicide, war or terrorism, drowning and so on. Accidental death refers to the process where the death is unexpected, or unforeseen, and occurs as the result of the unintended consequences of an individual's behaviours.

SOCIAL RULES OF DEATH

In most cultures, there are social expectations of death whereby we determine that some deaths are more acceptable to a community or individual than others. An obvious example of an acceptable death in Canadian culture and in most cultures of the world is for someone to die in old age when they are "ready to go" after living a full, productive life. On the other hand, the death of a child is seen as unnatural, especially to parents, and not in the "proper" order of things. All cultures share an unwritten idea (or wish) that parents are supposed to die before their children.

In the case of female infanticide, the unacceptability of the deliberate killing of girl babies is obviously culturally defined. While Westerners may find this practice totally unacceptable, in some cultures parents may prefer to kill their infant daughters rather than see them die in poverty or because they will not be able to afford a dowry for them.

NEARLY DEAD

Individuals who have been in a coma for a prolonged period, diagnosed as being in a persistent vegetative state (PVS), are regarded as the nearly dead. The concept of "nearly dead" is also invoked in the literature when "nearing death awareness" is discussed. Nurses Maggie Callanan and Patricia Kelley (1992) suggest that prior to death, many persons, especially those in health-care facilities, communicate both an awareness of their impending death and a description of how the process of dying is being experienced by them. In their book *Final Gifts*, the authors provide examples and narratives of some of their patients; two major themes that palliative patients expressed were preparing for a journey or getting to leave and seeing people and places they used to know. The authors note that patients often "include visions of loved ones or spiritual beings, although they don't necessarily signal death's imminence" (45).

PROCESS OF DYING

Other than the gradual shutting down of all body functions as the result of death, where we die, whether at home or in a hospital, nursing home or hospice, has an impact on our dying experience. Whether we are in pain or pain free and conscious or not also have an impact on the ways in which we experience death. How we die and the legal and medical resources available to us also affect our dying process. If we choose to die for a cause, such as in war or due to a particular religious or political belief, this too will determine how we feel about our death experience.

AFTER DEATH

After we die, discussions are held by others (or perhaps by ourselves prior to death) about the final disposition of our bodies and possessions. Grief and bereavement will be experienced by those who care about us. Counselling services may be required to help our important ones deal with our loss. Funeral, burial and/or memorial services will need to be arranged. Death ends a life but not the social relationships that make us who we are.

CONCLUSION

In this chapter we examined many topics related to death and dying, ranging from a historical overview of the ways in which death and dying are defined, to the prominent causes of death and how care of the dead was and is presently dealt with in the industries to which we have assigned these tasks. Organ donation and transplants were also dealt with in this chapter, and a key issue we discuss is the illegal selling of organs and other body parts.

SELF-REFLECTION AND THOUGHTFUL CONVERSATIONS

1. How would you define death, considering spiritual realms or your own personal thoughts on this?
2. What criteria would you use to measure that a death has really occurred?
3. Would you sell body parts to assist others? Why or why not? Consider this from a personal standpoint and then from a professional or institutional and organizational view. Do you think the government should regulate organ donations?
4. What are your views on the global trafficking of body parts and the sale of organs by poor families and communities to the wealthy?

IN-CLASS ASSIGNMENTS

1. What social, ethical, political and religious issues do the practices mentioned in this chapter evoke? Consider whether each one is negative, positive or neutral? Why?
2. Find out about the medical criteria used to determine death in your province. Discuss and analyze them.
3. Share the types of death and dying that are common in your community and then make your own list of the social rules of death.

Chapter Four

HISTORICAL ATTITUDES TOWARD DEATH AND DYING

Death is sometimes a punishment, often a gift; to many it has been a favour (*Inteeim paena est mori, sed saepe donum; ploeibos veniae fuit*). (Seneca, c.4 BCE–65 CE, cited in Curl 1993)

IMAGINE SENECA SAYING THIS QUOTE such a long time ago — even then societies and cultures tried to understand death and its meaning and purpose. Since time immemorial, people have looked to the stars for answers, to religion and spirituality for a larger-than-us framework and to each other for consolation, rituals and rites. Because death and dying are social events, it is important to look at how societies create practices and rituals related to death and dying. Associated events involve not only individuals but also their families and friends. Social institutions like medicine and law, the funeral and burial industries, religious and spiritual institutions, special interest groups and so on are also involved in these events.

Many elements in social life display how we as a society deal with death. These behaviours include how we *speak* of death. The euphemisms we use to describe it — "passed away," "deceased," "gone to a better place" and so on — help create distance between death itself and the reactions and feelings of individuals to that death. As well, we categorize death by how long people have lived, so it is common to hear how tragic is the death of a young person, who had their whole lives "ahead of them," implying that older people don't and that their deaths are somehow less important and not as sad. Instead we hear that older people "had a good, long life" or something similar. While age creates a baseline for such comments, many people grieve their older family members as deeply or as much as they might grieve the death of younger people. Age doesn't define how we value that person in our lives. These comments and expectations are part of the categorization process we use to differentiate one type of death from another.

Whether or not we are able to and how we express our feelings about death in terms of our cultural, physical and emotional reactions is another measure of how our society deals with death. While some North Americans and Northern Europeans are expected to be more stoic in terms of their expressions of sorrow and loss due to death, other cultures are historically known to make their grief much more visible, with communal sobbing, chest beating and loud wailing, which Marcia Carteret (2010) says is

> expected of mourners because the more torment displayed and the more people crying, the more the person was loved. In other cultures, restraint is expected. Rules in Egypt and Bali, both Islamic countries, are opposite; in Bali, women may be strongly discouraged from crying, while in Egypt, women are considered abnormal if they don't nearly incapacitate themselves with demonstrative weeping. In Japan, it is extremely important not to show one's grief for several reasons. Death should be seen as a time of liberation and not sorrow, and one should bear up under misfortune with strength and acceptance. One never does anything to make someone else uncomfortable. In Latino cultures, it may be appropriate for women to wail, but men are not expected to show overt emotion due to "machismo." In China, hiring professional wailers may be customary in funerals, which may sound odd, but this was also a common practice in Victorian England.

How we choose to die also tells us how we feel about death as a society. For example, in which settings do we die? In North America and Europe, this is often in a hospital, nursing home, at home in a house or apartment or in a hospice or palliative care setting. Historically, though, this was not always the case. In Canada and elsewhere over a century ago, death was a public event, with the deathbed acting as one of the central and social features of community life. People in communities would come together to support the dying and their loved ones, providing in-home care, food and emotional support. Burials and grieving would be shared events with loved ones being cared for by those who lived close. But, with modern medical advances, death stopped being a social event and became a more private one, mostly involving health professionals. As a result death has become invisible and remote, shifting from the social to the private.

With whose help do we die? Palliative care physicians and nurses, volunteers, family, friends and death doulas can all be involved in assisting those who are dying. Some societies and cultures value dying alone in nature, and others prefer dying with family and friends surrounding them. These institutional settings and personal choices are an important reflection of how we as a society also feel about and view life.

From a symbolic interaction perspective (see Goffman 1959, 1961, 1963, 1967), death is a symbol or metaphor for the loss of all the things, people and events that help shape our shared expectations, interactions and experiences. Death represents the ultimate loss of everything and everyone we hold dear. Like all social activity, death is interpreted by the meanings that we, as a culture, bring to it. In this way, we speak of some deaths as tragic and others as predictable or expected. Symbols of death are common in our culture, from the skull and crossbones warning on hazardous materials to crucifixes and crosses in Christian churches. Linguistic metaphors, as we have seen, also abound; we speak of "gone to a better place," "at rest," "sleeping," "kicked the bucket" and so on, when what we really mean is "dead." The word "dead" seems too final, too absolute, so we try to soften the image. These social processes enable us to incorporate death into human existence and, at the same time, help us to alienate ourselves from it.

Death is the converse of birth, a state of the absence of life. As human beings, we cannot imagine life before or without us. We know that we will die, that indeed we must die, yet we often refuse to recognize or deal with the inevitable reality of this endpoint. In other chapters, we discuss the idea of being a "death-denying" society, especially in the West.

Because most of our experiences of death come into our homes via the media, we might ask why newspapers, magazines, websites, movies, TV, radio and other forms of media tell us only about "famous" people's deaths or about the deaths of the "fallen heroes" of war and terrorism or those who take their own lives for a cause. Why are some lives seen as more special and precious? How can it be that millions of people around the world were able to grieve the deaths of celebrities like Michael Jackson and Prince and royalty like the Queen and Princess Diana, yet are ashamed to display grief over the loss of an intimate family member or friend? One way to see celebrity deaths and the ways in which they are publicized is that they may give us all permission to grieve. They may allow us to feel things together with a great number of unknown other people in a way that opens our own grief in our personal lives. Have you ever found yourself crying deeply in a movie or book about a fictional character's death? As a society, we may benefit from these public examples to open our more private grief.

The famous Canadian scientist David Suzuki (1989) recounted the death of his elderly father on a CBC Television program on euthanasia. His mother called for an ambulance and had trouble articulating what had happened, not just because of her panic but because of a language barrier. The ambulance team rushed her husband to the hospital and, on the way, used a defibrillation machine to resuscitate him. He died a few days later. The question Suzuki asked was, what was the point of reviving him? Had he died a natural death, it would have been peaceful and at home. Instead, he died a painful, frightening death in a strange place. Suzuki felt this was because the ambulance team could not accept "losing anyone."

This example highlights the reluctance of some medical professionals to "let go" or to accept what they see as defeat when all medical treatment options of preventing death are depleted. In this sense, death has become medicalized and represents one of the institutional factors of the professions. We can talk about the medicalization of death, and through a social construction lens, analyze how historic and social practices shape an idea that we should always choose life and living forever. We argue that there should be a high quality to dying, just as there is to living. The irony of this situation is that although we may be able to choose the quality of our lives, we don't seem to have many choices about the quality of our dying. Canadians could at least choose to die in a hospice if there were enough of them available. And, unlike so many other countries in the world, medical assistance in dying is available to those who are eligible and choose this option. We certainly don't have enough choices at present, but we hope this will change.

HISTORICAL PERCEPTIONS OF DEATH AND DYING

Philippe Ariès suggested that there were three distinct periods of development concerning understandings of death in post-antiquity and Western culture. The first was between the sixth and early twelfth centuries, the second between the late twelfth and early seventeenth, and the third stage was subdivided between the late seventeenth and nineteenth centuries and the twentieth century (1974: 23). In the first stage, death was seen as a universal process which all living things shared. At this time in Western history there was little medical knowledge information about health protection in terms of accident awareness, nutrition, sanitation and so on; as a result death was seen as inevitable. What awareness and knowledge did exist was based predominantly on the teachings of the church and as such were used to promote and support religious ideologies of good and evil, in that those who led righteous lives went to Heaven, those who did not went to Hell. In this historical period, death was a social event in that families and communities cared for the dying within their own homes, and when they died, buried them within church grounds in plots that were dug by family and friends. In the second stage of development, with the beginning of scientific reasoning and the influence of the Renaissance, when there was less focus on religious thought and teachings, especially among the aristocracy, death was experienced as more of a personal loss rather than a community one. In the late seventeenth and early nineteenth centuries, with the rise of the Romantics in poetry and other forms of literature and art, death was presented as a tragic muse inspiring poets and others to see it as a beautiful and transpiring experience. In the twentieth century, death became something to be feared and dreaded, a process which medical science could "cure" and prevent, and individuals could make lifestyle choices to enhance mortality (23–25). The third phase continues in this century, and death in Western cultures is predominantly presented as the enemy, and we see this most clearly in obituaries where we read that an individual "lost the fight/battle against cancer" or "succumbed to heart disease," "didn't make it due to the spread of the disease" or "was taken away by drug abuse."

During the Victorian era, in the time frame between 1837 and 1901, Western customs surrounding death changed dramatically. During the time of the Industrial Revolution (1760–1840), more families in many parts of Europe became affluent due to technological and health-related advances. Under the reign of Queen Victoria, who lost her husband Albert at a relatively young age for that time (he was forty-two), strict rules were enforced regarding mourning rituals, such a clothing (black) and length of time to mourn (at least one year, depending on one's relationship to the deceased). The Victorians also favoured extravagant burial plots, cemeteries, columbaria, marble memorials, death masks and so on. As well, cemeteries were built not only on private estates, but also in park-style settings in villages and towns. It was during this timeframe that funeral directors (known in Britain as "undertakers") became the sole providers of after-death arrangements (Rawlinson 2012).

In a publication for the Vanier Institute on the Family, Dr. Katherine Arnup (2013) provides an overview of the history of care for the dead in this country, at the same time recognizing that Canada was and is a diverse country comprised of many different racial and ethnic groups. She notes that the experiences faced by Canadians have changed dramatically since the early 1900s:

> In contrast to Britain, Europe and the United States, industrialization came rather late to Canada and its arrival in the mid-nineteenth century led to rapid urban population growth. Lacking adequate sanitation, sewage disposal systems and clean water supplies, cities soon became centres of disease. Babies died from contaminated milk supplies, and adults and children alike were victims of epidemics of smallpox, diphtheria, typhoid, tuberculosis, and other contagious diseases. By the 1930s, medical advances (such as immunization) and public health efforts had resulted in the reduction of deaths from infectious diseases and a shift from infection to chronic illnesses as the number one cause of death. (7)

Arnup notes that, apart from deaths due to wars and accidents, most white Canadians died at home during this period, being cared for by family and friends, who also arranged funeral and burial rituals. As well, many after-burial arrangements took place in the home of the deceased or other relatives. She notes: "While community support no doubt eased the burden of loss for family members, we ought not to romanticize this period, as death was often painful and abrupt. But the approach and attitudes toward dying meant that people were acquainted with death from an early age, as it was not shrouded in silence or mystery" (7). Arnup goes on to say that in Canada in the 1950s, both the general public and medical professionals believed in the power of science to cure or delay death in the case of many illnesses, and it was during this timeframe that death became viewed as a medical failure. It was during this time too, that most deaths occurred in hospital or nursing home settings:

> Modern healthcare facilities in the affluent post-war years was invested in saving lives, not in improving end-of-life care. Most people, however, died in hospitals (often after receiving "pointless, often stressful, heroic measures to prevent death"). Furthermore, with increased life expectancy, people were increasingly living longer with chronic, long-term illnesses, eventually dying in a hospital (perhaps after a stay in a nursing home). Yet little thought was given to dignity, pain relief or quality of care. (9)

Given the tragic reality of hundreds of years of colonization and its impacts, contemporary Indigenous communities in Canada, to their own credit, are experiencing a renaissance. The Truth and Reconciliation Commission asks all Canadians to take to heart what each person can do to work with its Calls to Action and counter that colonizing history. This includes working towards prevention of deaths in all Indigenous communities, urban, Northern and rural.

CARE OF THE DEAD

James Stevens Curl (1993) elaborates the many significant, cultural, religious and social turns care of the dead has taken throughout history. Cremation appears to have been practised first in the Neolithic period and was sometimes "communal in character" (4), with bodies being burned together in a community fire pit. In the Bronze Age, cremation was individual rather than communal, and clothes and personal belongings were also consumed by the fire. The ancient Egyptians had an organized system of care for the dead based on an extensive division of labour. There were embalmers and undertakers who removed the body from homes and prepared them for burial. They embalmed the dead (treated a dead body with chemicals to delay decay and mask odour) because they believed that after death the soul left the body to travel through time and eventually returned and inhabited the body. In other words, they practised embalming because of their belief in a life after death.

> [In Egypt,] many objects were placed with the mummified corpse in the tombs, and several cultures appear to have buried or burned their dead with clothes and other objects for use in life after death (5).

Greek culture profoundly influenced the development of European funerary customs, and care of the dead was a family affair. Although embalming was not practised, perfumes and spices were rubbed on the body to cover up odours. Flowers for burial were provided by friends and family, who chose special colours and types of flowers as a way of exhibiting their unique relationship to the deceased. Later in Greek history, cremation was practised as it was believed to set the soul free. Ashes were placed in burial urns, and the burial spot was marked by small mounds. "Athens developed a series of roads that linked settlements in Attica, and burials were near these roads, with concentrations near city gates" (24).

Death and the disposal of the dead were important aspects of social life for peoples who lived under Roman rule or were under the influence of Rome. Greek architecture, in its purest form, was to influence the designers of tombs in the eighteenth and nineteenth centuries, but it was Rome that led that field in example for two millennia.

The Romans practised both burial and cremation. In either case the body lay in state for public viewing. The wealthy were cared for by professional undertakers, *libitinarii*, who took care of anointing and embalming, supplying professional mourners and mourning clothes and assisting the bereaved. The *libitinarii* were the forerunners of modern funeral directors in that they formalized care of the dead into an occupational model (40). An important aspect of Roman practice was the cult of the dead, similar to that still practised in Mexico. Roses, food and drink were offered at the tombs on family occasions, such as the birthday of the deceased person, and festivities were celebrated at the graves. Lamps were lit at the grave on the "Kalends, ides and nones of each month, a practice that has been transmogrified into common use at Roman Catholic cemeteries in southern Europe today" (41).

The early Hebrews believed that humans were composed of two elements, flesh and breath, and that upon death, flesh returned to dust but breath persisted. Cremation was considered an indignity to the body, and burial, with or without a coffin, was practised. Family members washed and perfumed the body, which was usually buried on the evening of the day of death, for reasons of hygiene (Habenstein and Lamers 1960: 553). Funeral tasks were completed by experienced members of the family, who were responsible for all funerary details and care of the dead. Early Christian burial practices were arranged by family and friends, who commonly viewed the dead. In about the fourth century, the organized church established feast days to commemorate publicly and solemnly the death anniversaries of martyrs. Although most of the death work was carried on by relatives, it was done under the direction of the clergy (Curl 1993: 61–84).

During the Middle Ages, burial took place directly in the ground, in sarcophagi or in vaults. Corpses were "wrapped in shrouds that were knotted at the top and bottom" (72). As the Christian church emerged from persecution, it became increasingly institutionalized and took over many funeral and burial duties from family and friends of the deceased. During this time, embalming was supervised by the clergy and involved removing some body organs, washing the body with alcohol and pleasant-smelling oils and chemically drying and preserving the flesh, as well as wrapping the body in layers of cloth sealed with tar or oak soup, mummifying in a way that was like the methods of the Egyptians.

Leonardo da Vinci developed a system of injections to preserve cadavers so that he could draw anatomical plates. His method served as inspiration to the early embalmers, whose practices continue today (Habenstein and Lamers 1960: 427). By the end of the seventeenth century embalming was used by medical anatomists to preserve the dead for anatomical dissection and exploration, as well as by funeral directors in burial procedures. At this time chemists were developing preserving fluids that allowed the body to be viewed for longer periods of time.

By the eighteenth century, especially in Great Britain and Europe, the funeral director had fully emerged as the most appropriate caretaker of the dead. In urban, industrialized Western countries, care of the dead is performed by undertakers; in rural regions and the Global South, this work is carried out by family and friends. Prior to the Middle Ages people were aware of and responsible for their own after-death arrangements, and then it became a medical and religious responsibility.

In nineteenth-century United States, post-mortem photography became socially acceptable (Ruby 1988: 1). Images of the dead, especially infants, were publicly displayed in wall frames and albums. Initially, Ruby asserts,

> death pictures were portraits which attempted to deny death by displaying the body as if asleep, or even conscious. Today, families take their own photographs, circulating them in a private manner so that many people assume the custom has been abandoned. (1)

Not only are photographs taken of the dead, but today some funeral directors in Canada offer videotaped services and podcasts so that an entire funeral can be screened later (see advertisements in any issue of Canadian Funeral News). As one of our reviewers noted, historically, death pictures/memento mori photography were more than just the denial of death, especially for the Victorians; for example, they commemorated the dead, especially children. Also photography was a new and expensive technology, so it may have been the only opportunity to take pictures of the deceased as if they were alive. Victorians had elaborate mourning rituals because the death rate was so high, religious traditions, and so on. In medieval and Victorian times, especially after the death of Prince Albert, the husband of Queen Victoria, black was chosen as the mourning colour because it was believed it made the mourners invisible. In China white is the preferred colour (Pernick 1988: 27).

The "news" of death is presented in various ways: in England, white sheets hang in windows and one minute of silence is observed on the day of the funeral, while the hearse drives by. In some African countries, drums are used to signal a death. In Hindu countries, families wail to open the heavens and notify gods of the death so the soul can begin its journey back to the circle of life and reincarnation. In Canada, most often the news of death, besides to close family and friends, is presented through obituaries in local and national newspapers, church bulletins and services, funeral homes' websites and, as noted previously, on social media. In smaller, mainly rural communities, the news of death is spread through the local grapevine, with neighbours and friends telephoning or visiting to announce the news and to offer support to the bereaved. This also occurs in Indigenous communities, where people are often related and well-known to each other.

To satisfy our obsession with immortality, which seemingly has always existed, humans created symbolic forms of dialogue between the living and the dead. Tombstones, obituaries, coffins, mausoleums and epitaphs do the work of providing histories, warnings, prayers and comfort to the living (Curl 1993). As Curl notes, "The knowledge that every human being must die has undoubtedly contributed to man's [sic] desire to commemorate his existence by building monuments, erecting funerary architecture, and otherwise celebrating death" (1).

The ancient Egyptians built tombs and pyramids to honour their dead and preserved bodies through mummification both to record the histories of the deceased and to remind the living of their own immortality. Many pharaohs, clergy and people from upper classes may have had lavish tombs built, but even lower classes could have simple tombs. Very poor people may have just been buried deeply in the earth or sand and away from main cities and towns. The Greeks wrote epitaphs in verse to remind readers of the universality of death. The Romans buried their dead alongside major highways, so they would be a constant reminder to the living. They immortalized their dead with a portrait and an inscription, which included the person's name, their position and the names of those who buried the deceased and paid for the tombstone. This form of *memento mori*, which translated means "remember you must die," is still prevalent in one form or another in our culture today.

HISTORICAL DEFINITIONS OF DEATH

Up until around the sixteenth century, death was thought to occur when the heartbeat and breathing stopped. The ancient Greeks believed that the brain served a vital role, especially insofar as reason, logic, sensation and motion were concerned. Philosophers such as Plato, Aristotle and Pliny attempted to identify the brain's role in "life." The notion of the soul as either part of a body or separate from it was as controversial then as it is today.

With an increase in medical knowledge from around 1740 to 1850 in Europe, there were changes in people's definitions of death. During this time, there was a general panic among the public about premature burial or being buried alive. This fear came about in part because of two key medical breakthroughs: resuscitation, which means to bring back alive by artificial respiration techniques; and suspended animation, a deathlike condition like trance, brought about by hypnosis, drugs or biofeedback (Ariès 1975: 1541).

In 1774 in Italy, the first case of electric shock was used to resuscitate a "dead" man, further alarming the general public as to whether or not they had buried "live" friends and relatives. Failure to respond to resuscitation became an acceptable diagnosis of death, as well as other more primitive tests, such as holding a mirror, candle or feather to the nose, submerging the body and watching for bubbles, putting a bowl of liquid on the chest or severing an artery to see if blood flowed. Also, in the Enlightenment era, as it was called because of so many technological discoveries, vivisection played a crucial role in understanding whether or not a person could live without a particular body organ, such as a kidney, spleen, liver, etc. Prior to this work, it was generally believed that all body parts were needed to maintain life. Because of the fear of premature burial and the many grave robbers seeking bodies to sell to doctors and medical schools, legislation was adopted requiring some sort of death certificate to be provided prior to burial.

During the late nineteenth century, doubts about a doctor's ability to define and diagnose death gradually subsided, due to a growing dependence on medical expertise and technology. The stethoscope was first used in 1819 to diagnose death by the absence of a heartbeat, followed by the invention of electrical tests for neuromuscular functions and the thermometer to measure body heat. In the mid-nineteenth century, the hypodermic syringe was produced and used to inject chemicals into bodies to detect reactions (Fulton and Metress 1995).

Today, the debate about defining and diagnosing death continues and has done so since the first heart transplants in the 1960s, especially regarding the whole-brain/higher-brain controversy and the non-heart-beating donor controversy, discussed earlier. In relation to the former, Martin Pernick (1988: 59) notes, "The underlying controversy at issue between 'whole brain' and 'higher brain' ... is the question of whether mental consciousness or psychological integration is the basis of individual human life." The notion of the "higher brain" implies that there are functions specific to humans, such as thinking, reasoning and logic, that comprise human life. Most whole-brain advocates assert that an individual is these things plus a set of measurable neurological stimuli that affect basic responses to pain, hunger, light, touch and so on.

Death, then, is not a timeless and permanently definable term. Its meaning has changed over time, in response to changing technology, social structures and values. Defining death is complicated now due to two advances in biomedical technology: (1) artificial devices to sustain respiration and heartbeat indefinitely, even when there is no brain activity, and (2) transplantations, which require people to be declared dead at the earliest possible moment to make their organs available to others.

CONTEMPORARY WESTERN VIEWS OF DEATH

Today we see many examples of publicly visible mass deaths: deaths from the wars in Ukraine/Russia, Israel/Palestine and elsewhere, airplane-crash related deaths, COVID-19 deaths and deaths from extreme events, like wildfires and hurricanes. Death is a familiar, visible reality, and we all may know one or more people linked to one of these events.

Philippe Ariès (1982, 1985) described the following five dominant patterns of death in contemporary Western societies: tame death; death of the self; remote and imminent death; death of the other; and invisible death or death denied. Let's explore those patterns and see how they apply to our society today.

Ariès defines tame death as one that is regarded as the opposite of a wild force beyond our control and not subject to human domination. People who believe in a tame death know that they are dying and do not evade it. Instead, they calmly accept that death is coming, and they prepare themselves for death by dealing with unfinished business. Those dying in hospices and palliative care units are more likely to have a tame death. In Jeanette's experiences of visiting hospices in the UK, several patients spoke of "coming to terms" with their impending death. They also wanted to say goodbyes to family and loved ones and to put their personal affairs in order. Those who follow the Buddhist tradition can also be said to prefer a tame death as, through the teachings of Buddha and the *Tibetan Book of the Dead* (Rinpoche 1993), they formally prepare themselves through meditation, chanting and other rituals to leave this life and enter the next.

When speaking of "death of the self," Ariès (1985) is referring to the process through which individuals experience anxiety about what happens after death in terms of eternal judgement. Much of Ariès' assumptions deal with the notion of humans as essentially religious, especially Judeo-Christian, with fears of hell and the afterlife. According to Ariès, individuals dwell on their biography and look to past events to ensure that their past deeds are honourable ones. Indeed, some Christian religions, most notably Roman Catholicism, have specific rituals, such as the sacrament of anointing the sick (formerly extreme unction), to cleanse the soul of sin before death so that it can enter heaven.

Ariès also noted that there is a social fascination with the dead body. Throughout history, bodies have been placed in shrouds, or today in body bags, en route to mortuaries or funeral homes. In some funeral ceremonies, coffins are covered by cloth, in others they are layered with funeral wreaths and in the case of military personnel, with the flag of their country. Ariès contends that in the West, in addition to a fascination with dead bodies there is also dread or fear. In 2014, in Michigan, the Paradise Funeral Home began to advertise its services via a drive-thru viewing window. Each week, a corpse lies in a coffin in an enclosed glass window so that would-be consumers can observe the layout and design of both body and final resting place. According to a *Global News* story written by Elton Hobson (2014), funeral director Ivan Phillips says he is "hailing his innovation as a step forward for making funerals more accessible. Previously, he had allowed funerals and visitations to be streamed over the internet, so that those with physical disabilities or social anxiety can still participate." Phillips also commented that he believes "the drive-thru visitation may be a step forward for the funeral industry. The funeral industry is changing rapidly. So, my intent was to bring something here that was accessible to the community."

As any edition of *Canadian Funeral News* or *Canadian Funeral Director* will show, the funeral industry, in its publications and educational programming, emphasizes the notion of "presenting the dead." The idea is to prepare the corpse in such a way as to have it appear life-like and healthy. Clearly the perpetuation and maintenance of some of these modern-day funeral rituals expresses our ambivalence about death and dead people.

According to Ariès (1982), during the sixteenth to eighteenth centuries, important transitions took place with regards to Western attitudes toward death. He asserts that as the topic of death became a common site of discourse, it was viewed with great ambivalence. On the one hand death was regarded as beautiful and "edifying"; on the other hand, it was seen as frightening and untamed. In this sense death is viewed as remote and imminent. Ariès notes, "These attitudes are associated with a struggle to keep death-related feelings and behaviours under tight control, but that control is very fragile" (68). Even though Ariès was writing about the past, we can still see that anxiety, fear and frustration about death are common in Canadian cultures today.

"Death of the other," as Ariès uses the term, relates to the loss of relationships, social and professional, which occurs when someone dies. Death is thus seen as an intolerable separation of not only the body from the soul but the individual from all the social relationships and networks of which they were a part. Although death does end a life, it does not end the relationships we have had with others, who, through collective and individual memories, keep our sense of "self" and "other" alive. Memorial markers, tombstones, photographs, videos, shared stories and discussions of the past also enable us to continue living in the collective consciousness of others.

Ariès suggests that in the twentieth century a new attitude towards dying emerged, which he terms invisible, or death denied. Part of this denial of death for Ariès is structured around the medicalization of Western society in general. Rather than die at home, most North Americans and Europeans die in hospitals. In these cultures, hospices and especially palliative care units are located within medical bureaucracies. Because dying is removed from the community, death is hidden, and care of the dead moves from the private realm of home, relatives and friends to the public domain of health-care professionals. For Ariès, the denial of death also distances the dying person from their own death process. It denies prolonged community mourning, and it creates a new set of funerary rites, which emphasize consumer capitalism rather than thoughtful loss.

Certainly, in the UK, the US and Canada we see much more discussion about dying and being buried the "right way," and urban consumers seem to have more choices as to their final disposition than those who live in rural areas. Once again, the processes of dying and after-death arrangements change through historical time and space, and according to shifting cultural values.

CRITICAL MOMENTS IN CANADA — HIV/AIDS AND COVID-19

One of the most challenging medical conditions historically, which has also caused its sufferers to experience social death, discrimination and stigma, is HIV/AIDS. This is true especially in communities and countries where religious beliefs and cultural values around sexuality and sexual behaviour impact the ways in which individuals are perceived. In Canada, another tragic historical moment in health care led to related stigmatization, as reported by Márcia Martinho Costa (2019):

> When the HIV/AIDS epidemic started in the early 1980s little was known about how it was transmitted. The disease was initially associated with minorities (i.e., the gay community, Haitians, and injectable drug users), and generally stigmatised and downplayed in the medical community. Stigma, along with the scarcity of knowledge, permitted the accidental contamination of blood products. The risk of infection for people regularly treated with blood products rose sharply and the haemophiliac community suffered. Their condition, which affects the body's ability to clot and makes them more susceptible to bleeding and bruising, meant that taking blood products (to supply clotting factors) was their only option for survival. Unfortunately, for thousands of them, this treatment also led to an early death.

In countries where women's sexuality is controlled by the men in their lives or where there is a lack of education, contraception and limited healthcare resources, women's ability to refuse sexual contact or request safe sex practices may be non-existent. In countries where homosexuality is illegal and/or frowned upon, individuals who engage in same-sex relationships are less likely to seek medical attention, where it is available, for fear of going to prison and being ostracized by family, friends and their communities. Since the HIV/AIDS epidemic was diagnosed in 1981, 88.4 million people worldwide have acquired the disease. As of 2023, according to the WHO (2024a), 42.3 million died.

In 2020, the COVID-19 pandemic was declared a Public Health Emergency of International Concern (PHEIC) by the United Nations and the WHO. According to the WHO, as of August 2025 7.1 million people worldwide died from the pandemic. Because of reporting anomalies, the true death toll of COVID-19 is estimated to be much higher (World Health Organization n.d.).

Mass deaths due to mysterious diseases and infections globally have always been part of our lived experience on Earth. Cultural and religious differences, rural and urban divides and technical and medical advances change the way we understand these from century to century.

CONCLUSION

In this chapter we dealt in depth with the differences between historical notions of death and dying and how those expectations, assumptions, rituals and beliefs compare with contemporary, predominantly Western views. We also focused on some of the recent events, such as HIV/AIDS and the COVID-19 pandemic, which caused so many deaths worldwide. As well we discussed how gender and sexual orientation stereotypes played a role in attitudes towards those who contracted HIV/AIDS especially.

SELF-REFLECTION AND THOUGHTFUL CONVERSATIONS

1. How have attitudes towards death changed since your grandparents' time?
2. How are present-day funeral/celebration-of-life rites practised in your community and by whom?
3. How do you know when a death has occurred in your community?
4. How do you experience and relate to the many events and deaths visible in contemporary social media today?

IN-CLASS ASSIGNMENTS

1. Look up obituaries for the past week in any local newspaper or on the internet. How many people died, of what, at what ages, and what can you tell about them?
2. Find out what choices for final disposition of bodies exist in your local community and share this information with your classmates. What have been the final disposition choices of members of your family over the past fifty years? Find out what social, religious, economic, geographic, cultural or other factors contributed to these choices.
3. What are some well-known pandemics that have historically impacted our globe and mortality? How many people died, and how did we make sense of these deaths across time?

Chapter Five

TYPES OF DEATH AND DYING

WHEN WE EXAMINE SOME OF THE TYPES OF DEATH and ways of dying, especially in a highly industrialized and medicalized Western context, we discover that conflicts abound about what constitutes death. Let us look at some sociological, biomedical and historical developments surrounding the struggle to define death and then discuss how we might want to operationalize these concepts. According to an article in the *Huffington Post* by Rachael Rettner (2014), "Today, with ventilators, blood-pressure augmentation and hormones, the body of a brain-dead person could, in theory, be kept functioning for a long time, perhaps indefinitely. But with time, the body of a brain-dead person becomes increasingly difficult to maintain, and the tissue is at high risk for infection."

CLINICAL/BRAIN DEATH

In May 2012, a two-day meeting was hosted in Montreal, Canada, by the WHO and Canadian Blood Services. The conference was convened to determine an internationally agreed-upon definition of death, especially considering the need for standardized criteria in relation to organ donations. Those in attendance recognized that there are three medical definitions of death: 1) irreversible loss of function of the organism; 2) irreversible loss of capacity for consciousness; and 3) a combination of the two. Those present arrived at the following definition: "Death occurs when there is permanent loss of capacity for consciousness and loss of all brainstem functions. This may result from permanent cessation of circulation and/ or after catastrophic brain injury. In the context of death determination, 'permanent' refers to loss of function that cannot resume spontaneously and will not be restored through intervention" (Canadian Blood Services and World Health Organization 2012: 31).

Definitions of death are important when an individual and/or her important ones have agreed to donate their organs or to keep them alive or put them on a life-support system for some reason, for example, to bring a pregnancy to term.

EMOTIONAL/PSYCHOLOGICAL DEATH

When an individual has been painfully rejected, hurt, disappointed or injured emotionally or psychologically, they may experience a situation in which their feelings are, in a sense, "turned off," so while their body continues to maintain its "normal" routine, their emotions no longer function as they used to. These experiences are known as emotional or psychological death. Although death ends a life, as we have seen, it does not end the relationships that the living have with the deceased. As the British novelist Julian Barnes wrote after the death of his wife Pat, "The fact that someone is dead may mean that they are not alive, but doesn't mean that they do not exist" (2010: 12). In this sense, the dead do live on in the hearts and minds of others as they are remembered and what they said or did is incorporated into ongoing lives. When immigrants come to Canada, they bring with them specific rituals from their countries of origin, which they incorporate into their lives here. These sorts of activities help them remember not only the old country, but also those people who helped shape their lives when they lived there. We are learning more about people who transition from one sex or gender to another, and for some people, their old self dies, and a new self and identity begin.

SPIRITUAL DEATH

Spiritual death refers to the experience of losing faith or belief, often of a religious nature, after the death of a loved one or after receiving a personal terminal diagnosis or some other profound loss. Some formerly religious individuals, when learning of their impending death, lose their faith in a "higher being." Also involved in the notion of spiritual death are attempts at understanding the meaning of life and coming to terms with the loss of self. Some Indigenous Peoples speak of spiritual death in terms of a lack of recognition of their spirituality through colonialism, but also in regard to a contemporary lack of resources and support from governments at all levels, to recognize and celebrate spiritual diversity. As well, they may use this term when speaking about the destruction of the environment and our continuing lack of care for the land, sea and air upon which our lives depend.

SOCIAL DEATH

The causes of human death, the social distribution of death and the ways in which death are now socially organized have all changed drastically during the last century in industrialized societies like Canada. In sociology and some of the other social sciences, we increasingly speak about "social death." In their book *Social Death: Questioning the Life-Death Boundary*, editors Jana Králová and Tony Walter suggest that this concept has three components, all associated with social exclusion: loss of social identity, loss of social connectedness and losses associated with disintegration of the body or mind (2018:4). Using this definition of social death, experiences such as slavery, dementia, solitary confinement, genocide, dying alone, terminal illness and suicide are examples of undergoing social death. In these contexts, many people die socially before they die clinically or biologically. This can also be seen when dying patients are moved out of communal wards and into private ones to "die in peace," isolated from wardmates.

Whereas biological death can be determined to some extent via medical technology, social death remains difficult to define because individuals are not always aware of its occurrence in their lives. In the words of Barney Glaser and Anselm Strauss (1965), "Our intent was, above all, to ask whether people can die socially before they die biologically, and what this means for human relationships." Erving Goffman invoked the notion of "non-persons" to discuss individuals suffering from social death, noting that non-persons are "standard categories of persons who are sometimes treated in their presence as if they were not there" (1959: 152). Daniel Baum (1977) argues that nursing homes are warehouses for death and that the institutionalized elderly often suffer from social death.

STAGES OF DEATH AND DYING

As a result of interviews with thousands of patients, the late Elizabeth Kübler-Ross (1969) described the following six stages of dying: 1) denial: "not me"; 2) anger: "why me?" 3) bargaining, usually with God; 4) depression; 5) acceptance; and 6) hope. Kübler-Ross's work was first published in the late 1960s, and she was a pioneer in the field of working with the dying. Partially due to her work in the US and the late Dame Cicely Saunders' work in the UK, care for the dying has become more sensitive and patient-centred. Even though there has been much debate about the validity of Kübler-Ross's six stages (their order and the flow, as well as whether other stages exist), everyone agrees that her contribution to openness about how the dying are treated, especially in hospital settings, is important.

The language surrounding death has also changed our experiences of it. We may have read about and heard people speak of "life after death," not meaning heaven, hell or reincarnation, but referring to those who claim to have revived after having clinically died. In 1975, Raymond Moody published the book *Life after Life*, in which he relates experiences of those who claim to have returned from the dead. The US-based website The Near-Death Experience Research Foundation invites those who have had such experiences to share them; as well they provide a vast array of resources for people interested in this topic. There is a great deal of controversy as to whether individuals who believe they have had near-death experiences were actually dead. As Charles Corr, Clyde Nabe and Donna Corr (1997: 526) state, "To be near death is not the same as being dead. So, it is not certain that near-death experiences tell us anything about what happens after death."

PERSONAL/STRUCTURAL ELEMENTS

There are both personal elements of how individuals experience emotional and psychological responses to death and structural or societal elements. When we lose a loved one, we experience that loss within the personal realm; we grieve, feel sad, reflect on the relationship and so on. These internal and personal reactions to loss are diverse because each person experiences loss in their own unique way, based on their cultural, ethnic and spiritual beliefs and social expectations. Even though we experience loss primarily at the personal level, we also interact with the societal/structural level when we make end-of-life decisions and deal with wills, death certificates, obituaries, etc. The personal/structural elements of death also come into play when we examine pre- and post-death requirements. What may take place in the privacy of our own homes becomes public after death, when funeral and burial practices are adhered to.

GOOD DEATHS VERSUS BAD DEATHS

For many people, a "good" death comes in old age after a full, productive life. The individual has had time to say goodbye and to come to terms with their demise. Whenever we ask students when they want to die, this is the response that 95 percent give. The other 5 percent say they want to die suddenly in their sleep, but in old age. This fits our cultural notions of what it means to die a good death. Those who are supportive of the goals and philosophy of palliative care would add that the good death is pain-free, with symptoms under control and the dying person in charge of their own dying. Normally, a good death includes being surrounded by loved ones and being able to say goodbye. Tony Walter (2003), among others, argues that a good death is one in which the dying person is autonomous and able to make decisions as to how they want their end to be. The way that people die is particularly important to those who are left behind, and this concern is not limited to the moment of death but encompasses the entire end-of-life phase. A good death depends on one's culture, and its characteristics may change over historical time. Increasingly in Canada and elsewhere, the concept of a good death is expressed most fully by those who adhere to the principles of the hospice and palliative care movements, which "allow patients to gain more control over their lives, manage pain and symptoms more effectively, and provide support to family caregivers" (Canadian Hospice Palliative Care Association 2017: 12)

In contrast, a "bad death" is one that society sees as unacceptable and not sanctioned; examples include death following prolonged unnecessary pain and suffering, death following a persistent vegetative state, dying as a suicide bomber or for a political or religious cause, keeping a terminally ill individual alive against their written wish to die, death from torture and death from prolonged hunger. Such deaths might include suicide and, for some, euthanasia. The deaths of young people, especially young children, are often seen as "bad." As parents related while Jeanette was visiting children's hospices in the UK in 1997, "children should not die before their parents, it's not natural, this kind of death is just bad," and "I wanted my son to get married and have his own kids. I was going to die first with his kids at my bedside. If there's such a thing as a bad death, this is it." Some people think dying alone is bad, but for others, dying alone might be peaceful and quite alright.

As well as cultural notions of good and bad deaths, we also speak of natural and unnatural types of death. A good death or a natural one occurs in our beds, at home, in old age, either suddenly or because of a terminal illness. Unnatural deaths, like bad ones, see us hooked up to lifesaving and maintaining machines and in hospitals being cared for by strangers. One of the reasons COVID-19 was so tragic was that some people who lived in long-term care homes could not have loved ones visit as they approached end of life, and those who went to the hospital unexpectedly could not easily see their own family during the health crisis. The concepts of good and bad, natural and unnatural are related to cultural values of how it is best to die. These notions also define where, how and when it is preferable to die and in what condition, namely pain-free but conscious. Much of the discourse on the good/natural death versus bad/unnatural death is played out in the fields of hospice and palliative care, where not only are criteria established to create and enhance the good/natural death, but this rhetoric is also used to suggest that this is the best way to die. In many ways, there are similarities between the palliative care/hospice movement and the midwifery movement, where the goal is to establish the best way to enter the world rather than to exit. In both arenas of professionalization, the goal is to assist clients to do it their way with guidance from experts.

In his article "Natural Death and the Noble Savage," Tony Walter notes that in modern society, there is the belief that dying and grieving should be regarded as natural processes. Walter argues that the natural death myth is predicated on the following four assumptions: "1) that most primitive cultures deal with death in an accepting way, 2) that this way is different than our own, 3) that it is a good and noble way and 4) that traditional societies see death as natural" (1994–95: 237). Walter suggests that none of these assumptions is clearly supported by empirical evidence and that the concept of a natural death is culturally defined and socially constructed in settings, especially hospice and palliative care settings, where the intentional goal is to promote a "good" or "natural" death. The notion of the "good old days," when people died at home of "natural causes" surrounded by loved ones, is, for Walter, pure rhetoric. He concludes, "The myth of the thanatologically noble savage is one that bears a price of a most deliberate falsification" (247).

Natural death is culturally defined by actors living in specific times and places who engage in cultural rituals around death, which they socially construct out of the fabric of their lives as they are being lived. Discussions of natural/unnatural deaths are not fixed, but alter as circumstances, social and health policies and attitudes towards death make themselves visible.

Since this book was originally written, world events have occurred that emphasize the idea of a bad death. Since the bombing of the World Trade Centre in New York on September 11, 2001, the US and other countries have been engaged in a "war on terrorism." Canada has played a role in these events, and many young soldiers have given their lives. As well, Canadian forces have been involved in peacekeeping efforts in the Middle East and elsewhere. When catastrophic events such as wars, terrorism, tsunamis, famines, droughts and pandemics occur, the sense of the bad death becomes prominent, so that we speak of people "dying for the cause," "giving their lives to serve their country," "dying for democracy" and other such platitudes intended to assist people make sense of essentially senseless deaths. In some countries, death is a more daily occurrence and one which everyone witnesses on a regular basis. As well, private grief once again becomes a cause for public scrutiny and political manipulation as was the case when then prime minister of Canada, Stephen Harper, decreed that the media could not film, or otherwise record, the return of the bodies of Canadians killed in military actions in Afghanistan and elsewhere. Later, after an outcry from family members and the public, who felt that such public acts were ways of recognizing the country's communal loss, the prime minister rescinded this rule.

DEATH EDUCATION

The first Canadian course about death and bereavement was taught by Dr. John Morgan at what was then Loyola College in Montreal in 1976. Since then, a vast number of similar courses have sprung up in medical schools, universities, seminaries, palliative care programs, schools of nursing, social work and pastoral care, and a small number of high schools (Morgan 1986).

Our own experiences of teaching courses in death and dying for many years concur with Richard Kalish's (1989: 75) suggestions that there are several concerns that create an interest in education in the field of death and dying:

> Some people are interested in death education because of (1) personal concerns because of some previous experience that has not been resolved; (2) personal concerns because of ongoing experiences, such as the critical illness or recent death of a close family member; (3) involvement with a relevant field of work, the ministry, or volunteer services; or (4) a wish to understand better what death means and how to cope more effectively with one's own death or the death or grief of others.

Our students also speak of a fascination with learning more about how other cultures and religions deal with death and dying within and outside of Canada, as well as having the opportunity to explore and reflect upon their own experiences and fears about the dying process.

Another goal of death education is to teach and inform students about the infrastructure of goods, services, programs and professionals that makes up the death care system and to educate them, and us as teachers, as to how to become more critical and self-reflective consumers of these services.

CONCLUSION

The types of death and dying were introduced in this chapter, where we examined and discussed the differences between how as a society we define a good death and a bad one. We also looked at different types of death, such as spiritual and social death, as well as the stages we may go through when we die. Death education and some of the key social issues surrounding this controversial subject were also discussed.

SELF-REFLECTION AND THOUGHTFUL CONVERSATIONS

1. How do you feel about death education? When should it be offered?
2. What do you think is important for people to know about death and dying?
3. Where have most of your family members died?
4. Where would you prefer to die: at home, in a hospital or in some other institution, and why?

IN-CLASS ASSIGNMENTS

1. Make a list of the words associated with death. What kinds of emotions or images do the words evoke?
2. Make a list of the personal and structural elements that occur around death in your community.
3. What do you think about Kübler-Ross's six stages? Would you add or subtract any? Discuss.

Chapter Six

HOSPICE PALLIATIVE CARE

Spiritual care lies at the heart of hospice. It says we are here. We will be with you in your living and your dying. We will free you from pain and give you the freedom to find your own meaning in your life — your way. We will comfort you and those you love — not always with words, often with a touch or a glance. We will bring you hope — not for tomorrow but for this day. We will not leave you. We will watch with you. We will be there. (Ley and van Bommel 1994)

DYING, LIKE BIRTHING, IS A PROCESS that can be improved with assistance. Hospice and palliative care programs provide help and support for dying persons and their important ones so that the terminally ill may live fully and comfortably until they die. Palliative care is a neglected area of medicine in the global community, but advances and awareness of the benefits of such care are increasing dramatically worldwide. In Canada, there were 142 such program sites as of 2023 (Government of Canada 2023b). The WHO (2020a) notes, "Each year, an estimated 56.8 million people, including 25.7 million in the last year of life, need palliative care. Worldwide, only about 14 percent of people who need palliative care currently receive it. Unnecessarily restrictive regulations for morphine and other essential controlled palliative medicines deny access to adequate palliative care." In Canada it is also the case that many, especially those in remote and rural areas of the country, are less likely to be able to receive palliative care at the end of their lives. In a report conducted by the Canadian Institute for Health Information (2023), the authors note that some progress has been made in the delivery of such programs:

> More people are receiving some form of palliative care compared with 5 years ago. More people are dying at home with palliative support compared with 5 years ago. Some people experience

greater barriers to accessing palliative care because of their age, where they live or their disease diagnosis. Things have improved in the last 5 years but there are still signs of poor-quality palliative care, including people not getting palliative care until just before they die, and people dying in hospital even when they have community supports such as long-term care or home care.

Research articles on many facets of palliative care are abundant in Canada, particularly because the *Journal of Palliative Care* is published out of the Centre for Bioethics at the Clinical Research Institute of Montreal, thereby allowing Canadian scholars and practitioners a forum for discussion of their work. As well, the Canadian Virtual Hospice website provides a vast array of information and material on this topic, as does the Canadian Hospice Palliative Care Association. The Canadian Network of Palliative Care for Children provides information and resources for parents and others who are dealing with children with terminal illnesses. Professional organizations which represent some of the individuals who work in these areas include the Canadian Society of Palliative Medicine, the Palliative Care Coalition of Canada and the Canadian Palliative Care Nursing Association, and at McGill University there is a program for social workers engaged in hospice palliative care work. Most provinces in this country also have provincial palliative care associations. As well, most provincial branches of the Victorian Order of Nurses have some form of in-home hospice palliative care program, as do many provincial home-care associations.

The Government of Canada defined palliative care in the following way in 2024:

> Palliative care is a holistic approach that treats a person with serious illness of any age, and in any setting. It involves a range of care providers and includes the person's unpaid caregivers. (Government of Canada n.d. "Palliative Care: Overview")

If you have a serious illness, palliative care can help improve the quality of your life, reduce and relieve your symptoms, and help you grieve.

Palliative care can be provided at home, in a hospital, in a residential care facility or in a hospice. Ideally, care is provided by primary health-care providers, such as family doctors, nurses and nurse practitioners, volunteers, caregivers, social workers, personal support workers and others in the community. Health Canada (n.d.) produced an interesting infographic entitled "Explore the Full Spectrum of Palliative Care," and a printed copy can be ordered through their website.

HOSPICE PALLIATIVE CARE: AN OVERVIEW

If you were told that you or someone you love was going to die from a terminal illness soon, there would, in the industrialized parts of the world, be four places where your death might occur. One possible setting is a hospital, where most Canadians die. Hospitals are designed to meet acute care needs, which are usually short in duration, even if severe. People go into hospitals to have tests and surgical procedures performed and rarely "stay" for more than a week to ten days. Because hospitals are geared towards cure, rehabilitation and short-term stays, they are inadequate places to die.

Another setting in which we might die is an institution like a nursing home or some other long-term residential care facility. These institutions, like homes for the elderly, provide chronic care over prolonged periods of time, perhaps years. Some have called nursing homes the setting of last resort for the old and infirm — a stepping stone to death. Many nursing homes are not equipped to deal with dying residents, so those residents are often moved into hospitals when more advanced terminal care is needed. Because most chronic-care settings are structured around the assumed needs of the old, infirm and mentally or physically challenged, they too are inadequate settings for those with terminal diagnoses.

We could also die at home, if we have the necessary resources and people who feel comfortable dealing with the death of a loved one and possibly providing twenty-four-hour care to us. However, even the most loving families and friends are often overwhelmed by the magnitude of the task of caring for an important one at home; as a result, dying at home is not an option for many.

The fourth option in terms of where and how we die might be within a palliative care program or unit or in a hospice. The term "hospice" is used most frequently in Europe, where the movement towards alternative (to hospital) care for the dying originated. In European countries, especially the United Kingdom, most hospices are community-based and predominantly funded by charitable donations and governments at the national level. In North America, the term "palliative care" is more prominent because most of the programs are provided through hospitals, long-term care facilities and consultation teams attached to hospitals.

Hospice was a medieval concept that meant a place of shelter, usually for travellers, the sick and the poor. Today, hospice means the provision of symptom control and management, as well as a wide range of therapies, treatments and services, either in a free-standing structure, within individuals' own homes, or a combination of these options as the patient and care providers see fit.

Palliative, from the verb palliate, means to lessen pain without hope of cure. Palliative care is a philosophy of care that combines active and compassionate therapies intended to provide comfort and support to individuals and their important ones who are living with a life-threatening illness. Palliative care strives to meet psychological, social and spiritual expectations while remaining sensitive to cultural and religious values, beliefs and practices (Canadian Hospice Palliative Care Association 2005).

Both concepts — palliative care and hospice settings — in thought and practice, aim to care without cure by emphasizing the improvement of the quality of life until death. They are not places to go to die; rather, their focus is on how to help us live until we die.

HOSPICE CHRONOLOGY: EUROPE

Hospices were originally begun and maintained by religious orders. The word hospice was used from the fourth century onwards, when Christian orders welcomed the sick and those in need (Jackson and Eve 1997: 146). The modern European hospice movement began in 1842 in Lyon, France, when Jeanne Garnier founded the Dames du Calvaire, a hospice for the mortally ill in. In 1879, the Irish Sisters of Charity opened Our Lady's Hospice in Dublin for the poor, elderly and sick. In 1905, St. Joseph's Hospice was opened by the Irish Sisters of Charity in London's East End to care for those dying from tuberculosis. Today, patients with a variety of terminal conditions may receive care at the hospice. In 1967, St. Christopher's Hospice was opened in Sydenham, London, by Dame Cicely Saunders. It has become the pre-eminent model for hospice care throughout Europe, North America and other countries around the world (Jackson and Eve 1997: 148).

In Canada, palliative care programs began in 1975 at the St. Boniface General Hospital in Winnipeg and in 1976 at the Royal Victoria in Montreal. In 1988, Casey House HIV/AIDS hospice opened. This was Canada's first free-standing hospice. Canada's first residential hospice, La Maison Michel-Sarrazin, opened in 1985 in Sillery, Quebec.

In this country, there are two types of palliative care programs offered within hospital settings. One is a system of designated units, usually on a particular floor of the hospital, where all the patients in the unit have terminal diagnoses. The other type of palliative care system is called the scattered-bed approach. In this case, a palliative care nurse or other members of the palliative care team will visit patients throughout the hospital. The scattered-bed approach is preferred by some palliative care nurses because there are reduced "territorial wars" over who can use palliative care beds. In the case of designated units with a limited number of beds, there are usually waiting lists and specific catchment areas. In the scattered-bed approach, the dying are not segregated from the living as they are in a palliative care unit.

Ideally, there would be numerous accessible programs located throughout Canada, but this is not the case. Some programs, for example, in urban settings, offer a wide variety of services, while other programs, for example, in rural settings, might only involve one service, such as in-home volunteers who provide friendly visiting. In the Canadian palliative care community, concern has long been expressed about what Elizabeth J. Latimer (1995: 107) calls the ethics of "partial" palliative care. She asks whether partial care is "meeting the need of patients and families in a comprehensive way, or is it merely better than nothing — a compromise between a costlier program and no program at all?" Across the country, different provinces offer more or less comprehensive programs of care based on funding, resources and personnel. In rural areas, there are likely to be fewer necessary components; in these communities, care of the dying often relies on the voluntary sector, with professional guidance and backup support.

Although volunteers are undoubtedly a crucial component of the delivery of palliative care services to Canadians, additional training, funds for transportation to clients' homes and increased resources are also required. Latimer calls for vigilance in these areas and a renewed commitment from governments at all levels to enhance the quality of new and proposed palliative care programs. She notes, "We must not allow evolving programs to distort palliative care so that it is watered down or technocratized into just another health care system" (110).

Balfour Mount (1992: 64), a pioneer in the Canadian palliative care movement, noted that volunteers have been integrated into multidisciplinary care teams since the inception of such programs. He, too, suggests that the effective use of volunteers in hospices is a means of "facilitating improved care in other clinical settings. A successful volunteer program depends on strong leadership, skilled volunteer selection, training, role definition, continuing education, feedback and support."

There are unique elements of hospice palliative care that make it different from other types of services for the dying. The Canadian Hospice Palliative Care Association (2024) outlines the following essential components of palliative care:

- Total care will be provided to both the patient and their important ones. This care would meet physical, psychological, social, cultural, and spiritual needs. The unit(s) of care would be the dying person and their important ones.
- Services are provided twenty-four hours a day, seven days a week, and all who need such care would have access to it.
- Patients will have access to an interdisciplinary team of professionals and service providers who transmit information and education about the illness and its treatment options in an easy-to-understand manner. This team could include physicians, nurses, social workers, spiritual counsellors like clergy, volunteers, physiotherapists, and a wide range of complementary therapists, where available.
- There will be a seamless, coordinated plan of care so that wherever the patient chooses to die, in a unit or at home, service is continuous.

When receiving palliative care individuals are provided with the following: 1) symptom control and pain management; 2) comfort care, including, where available, complementary therapies; 3) respite care; 4) terminal care; and 5) bereavement care and follow up. Hospice palliative care, then, attempts to provide a total package of care to the whole person, and not just to the dying patient but also their important ones. In this sense, the unit of care is all the individuals connected to the dying person who may be impacted by the death. People of all ages may receive palliative care; no distinctions are made based on age, sex, sexual orientation, race, ability, income, religion, etc. In Canada, the most prominent diseases of those utilizing the palliative care approach are cancer and heart-, liver- and lung-related diseases.

In the last ten years, it has been recognized by Canadian researchers and those who provide hospice palliative care that these services must be provided at the community level and offer culturally sensitive care. The

Canadian Cancer Society, in its report *Analyzing Hospice Palliative Care Across Canada,* commented on this:

> From what we were able to determine, Canada still lacks the capacity to consistently deliver palliative care in the community, particularly in hospice. While best practices identified by the Auditor General of Ontario and others would suggest that Canada should have 7 hospice beds per 100,000 people, by our count, as of May 31, 2022, Canada only has 3.97 hospice beds per 100,000 people. Only British Columbia and Yukon exceed the 7 beds per 100,000 people target. All jurisdictions noted that more could be done to improve culturally safe palliative care, including grief and bereavement. (2023: 9)

One of the groups most affected by the lack of hospice palliative care is Indigenous communities. In their research examining the availability of hospice palliative care to Indigenous people in rural and remote areas of British Columbia, authors Heather Castleden, Valorie A. Crooks, Vanessa Sloan Morgan, Nadine Schuurman and Neil Hanlon, in partnership with Inter Tribal Health Authority, noted:

> Aboriginal peoples in Canada represent many distinct cultures. Approximately 170,000 Aboriginal peoples live in BC alone, with over 200 separate First Nations and a strong Métis presence throughout the province. Yet they share a common history through the colonial experience of marginalization, exploitation, and maltreatment. Shortly after contact with white settlers and up to the present, Aboriginal peoples have also shared significant health inequalities relative to the non-Aboriginal Canadian population. (2009: 6)

Because many Indigenous Peoples in British Columbia and other provinces often live in rural areas, it was noted further:

> Access to hospice palliative care services is often limited in rural and remote communities. For Aboriginal peoples living in BC, rurality and a lack of cultural sensitivity can create barriers to accessing and receiving quality palliative care. In 2008, a study focused on palliative care in the BC interior demonstrated that

issues of cultural visibility, contradictions in the provision of palliative care and a lack of culturally sensitive training creates additional obstacles for Aboriginal people in terms of accessing formalized palliative care. (6)

Because of their extensive dialogues with groups of Indigenous people in BC, the authors concluded, "Aboriginal people living in rural and remote communities may have a strong desire to provide formal and informal local hospice palliative care. However, accessing the necessary human and material resources, such as training and supplies, and upholding the need for choice often make this goal difficult to achieve" (12).

In a similar research project conducted in Northern Ontario with Cree and Ojibway bereaved individuals, authors Len Kelly, Barb Linkewich, Helen Cromarty et al. (2009) also concluded that "cross-cultural care at the time of death is always challenging. Service delivery and communication strategies must meet cultural and family needs. Respect, communication, appropriate environments and caregiving were important to participants for culturally appropriate palliative care" (2009:394).

Sociologists are interested in hospice palliative care for the following four major reasons:

1. Hospices are seen as part of a reform movement to change mainstream Western medical systems, their management, pain management, communication skills and symptom assessment.
2. Hospice palliative care is part of a social movement away from institutionalized care towards a more holistic approach for dealing with the dying. Another framework that sociologists have used to view hospice palliative care is from the perspective of organizational dynamics. Organizations play a critical role in our society by providing collective achievements that would otherwise be beyond the reach of the individual. When speaking of health care, organizations ensure that a complex of services can be efficiently delivered to many individuals. Yet, as the Canadian Hospice Palliative Care Association points out in their "Fact Sheet: Hospice Palliative Care in Canada," using data from the Canadian Institute for Health Information:

    - Data from an international survey of primary care physicians shows that Canadian doctors feel less prepared to manage care for palliative patients than do their peers in 10 other countries.

- Although 90% of medical curricula have lectures related to palliative care, there is little mentorship and just 12% of students were required to participate in mandatory clinical rotations in palliative care.
- Few residents are exposed to hands-on palliative care training — 18% in acute care facilities, 16% in palliative care units within an acute care setting, 18% in cancer centres and 11% in a community or outpatient environment.
- There are few faculty positions in Canadian universities to address undergraduate and postgraduate needs for education in palliative care. (2024: 8)

3. Sociologists are also concerned with the sociopsychological aspects in how care is provided, to whom, by whom, how theory differs from practice and how consumers perceive the services they receive.
4. Access to palliative care resources is an area of interest for sociologists concerned with the provision of health care to Canadians. In Jeanette's own work in the early and late 1990s on palliative care in both Nova Scotia and the United Kingdom, she noted that most recipients of palliative and hospice programs were white people from middle-class backgrounds. The absence of lower-income persons and people of colour caused some health-care professionals to suggest that palliative care is "Cadillac service for a few." With patient/nurse ratios, on average, at one-to-one, palliative care in the hospital setting is clearly an expensive form of care.

THE IMPACT OF THE COVID-19 PANDEMIC ON HOSPICE PALLIATIVE CARE

The COVID-19 pandemic had a tremendous impact on people around the world, including severe effects on hospice and palliative care programs. Tania Pastrana, Liliana De Lima, Katherine Pettus et al. interviewed seventy-one palliative care workers from forty-one countries about their experiences of attempting to provide this service during the COVID-19 pandemic, and the authors, themselves from several countries, conclude that the pandemic had

> a huge impact on palliative care workers including their ability to work and their financial status. It has generated increased workloads and placed them in vulnerable positions that affect their emotional well-being, resulting in distress and burnout.

Counseling and support networks provide important resilience-building buffers. Coping strategies such as team and family support are important factors in workers' capacity to adapt and respond. The pandemic is changing the concept and praxis of palliative care. Government officials, academia, providers, and affected populations need to work together to develop, and implement steps to ensure palliative care integration into response preparedness plans so as not to leave anyone behind, including health workers. (2021)

Throughout the first waves of the pandemic, restrictions were placed on visitors, and some families were unable to spend final moments with dying loved ones or attend funeral services after their death. This was especially the case in government-run hospitals, residential care facilities and nursing homes. Volunteers were unable to spend time with persons they had been caring for prior to the pandemic and, as result, were not able to adequately share their grief. As well, volunteers could not provide their skills and services to people dying at home with the assistance of hospice palliative care. Daniel Vincent, Hailey Moore, Judy Miller and Pamela Grassau spoke with caregiver volunteers at two residential hospices in Quebec. The volunteers "identified several factors that impacted the quality of care in residential hospice, including the impact of the COVID-19 pandemic itself. The findings are presented in three main themes: 1) quality of residential hospice end-of-life care; 2) caregiver perceptions of their grief and bereavement; and 3) impact of the COVID-19 pandemic on hospice quality of care and caregiver bereavement" (2024: 1156). In their conclusions the authors note, "The COVID-19 pandemic had a significant impact on the patient and caregivers experience of hospice, including perception of quality of care and caregiver experience of grief and bereavement" (1162).

While some facilities were able to provide virtual care to persons dying in their own homes, usually through telephone assistance and in some cases other forms of digital technology, a lack of skills on the part of care receivers hindered their effectiveness. Many medical professionals also came down with the disease, so staff at all levels were working shorthanded and often without the necessary personal protective equipment (PPE). Staff were often unable to provide the skills they were trained to use in such circumstances. For example, restrictions when using PPE, like being unable to have face-to-face conversations, presented challenges for both patients and staff. In facilities with outside meeting spaces, it was sometimes possible for family and friends, volunteers and staff to sit with hospice palliative patients, but only when staff were able to help take the patients outside. Because volunteers are a crucial component of the provision of hospice and palliative care, their absence due to COVID created an even higher workload for staff.

One of the conclusions arrived at from the challenges faced by hospices and palliative care facilities during the COVID-19 pandemic was presented by the above authors in the following statement:

> The COVID-19 pandemic impacted palliative and end-of-life care programs and services across Canada and provided a timely opportunity to explore the perceptions of bereaved caregivers of patients in residential hospice on quality of care, grief and bereavement, and the impact of the covid -19 pandemic in residential hospice. Given high rates of severe grief symptoms during the COVID-19 pandemic, bereaved caregivers may have benefited from participation in hospice bereavement support programs. Our study findings address a gap in the literature by exploring perspectives of bereaved caregivers on the impact of the COVID-19 pandemic on grief and bereavement and help guide bereavement support programs. Decision makers must continuously evaluate and carefully consider the impact of pandemic policies and procedures in residential hospice on patient care, as well as caregiver grief and bereavement. (1161)

THE IMPACT OF MEDICAL ASSISTANCE IN DYING ON VOLUNTEERS IN HOSPICE PALLIATIVE CARE

The introduction of medical assistance in dying (MAID) legislation in Canada on June 17, 2016, created challenges for those providing care in hospice and palliative care programs, especially in government-run facilities, and created the need for additional education and training on both the process of applying for such services and receiving them. It also necessitated that volunteers be supplied with additional bereavement support and communication skills when dealing with patients and their important ones who chose this method of ending their lives.

Some members of the palliative and hospice care movement hold a diametrically opposed position to those who support MAID; each takes the idea of death and dignity seriously but from deeply different belief systems and moral positions. The differences may be faith-based, but they can also emerge through complex discussions related to institutions. In situations where palliative care units and hospices exist within hospitals and government-run facilities, staff and volunteers have to sort through their personal views, their political stance, and the way in which their views might affect their employment. Some health-care clinicians refuse to offer support for those who choose MAID, and in those cases, another staff member provides it or the patient is moved to a location which offers the service. Other clinicians promote the choice and support those who wish to access MAID. The palliative and hospice care movement contains a wide range of views, both personal and institutional, many of which still need reflection and consideration as we move forward.

Stephen Claxton-Oldfield and Sophie Beaudette (2021) conducted research into the attitudes and experiences related to MAID of forty-eight volunteers working in a hospice in Atlantic Canada. The authors noted that the majority of respondents were supportive of and agreed that advance requests to receive these services should be permitted. The authors also stated that 15 percent

> of the volunteers reported that a patient of theirs had tried to initiate a conversation with them about MAID. Nearly all (96%) of the volunteers indicated that it was not appropriate for them to bring up the topic of MAID with their patients or patients' family members/caregivers. Seventy percent of the volunteers reported that if a patient of theirs chose to pursue MAID that they would be comfortable with being present (if asked) when it was being administered. (1283)

These experiences are a graphic example of the kind of communication which hospice palliative care volunteers share with their patients and families.

Because the number of Canadians requesting MAID has increased by almost 30 percent since its inception, according to the fourth annual report on the topic published by the Government of Canada (2023a), it is likely that volunteers will continue to play vital roles in hospice and palliative care program delivery, and it is crucial that they are adequately trained and educated in the governmental rules and procedures for this service.

THE WORK OF A PALLIATIVE CARE VOLUNTEER

> The work we do is specialized. You never know whether a person is going to be joyous or down. You must be prepared for anything. (Margaret, palliative care volunteer, (unpublished work Jeanette did for the VON)

Palliative care volunteers try to meet the physical, cultural, emotional and sometimes spiritual needs of their clients. They also provide a complete range of services to the dying. They are not just "hand-holders" but personal care workers, homemakers and house cleaners, cooks, counsellors, advocates, readers and card players, confidantes and comforters. Those who work with the dying are prepared to do anything to make the lives of their clients more manageable and meaningful. Listening is a major component of the work done by palliative care volunteers. Just "being there" and actively listening is one way they value the life and the dying of their clients.

Dealing with the inevitable death is a very personal event for the dying person, their family and the palliative care worker. Intimacies have been shared, perhaps for years, or perhaps for only a few days or moments. Whatever the degree of connection, it is often deeper than much of the interaction that characterizes our culture. Palliative care is also family care. Again, volunteers are informed by their own experiences of what they felt they needed — and perhaps didn't get — while their own loved one was dying.

Volunteers sometimes experience frustration at being powerless to effect change in medical care for their clients or when observing family dynamics they felt were harming the dying person. Some volunteers said they could not generally make this known to family members or medical staff, but they agreed it was important to have a place to talk about the difficulties they were having and to discuss their feelings.

Hospice palliative care is a process, not a single event. During that process, individuals may influence each other's lives in profound ways. Learning how to value life is a major factor in the work that volunteers participate in with the dying. Dying people teach volunteers to recognize the benefits and joys of their own lives and to appreciate their family and friends in a more conscious way. Ultimately, life and death may both become more conscious acts. Most importantly, some volunteers told Jeanette that they learn that there are no second chances. Working with people who have little time left to deal with unfinished business helps them deal with theirs now, while they do have the time.

CONCLUSION

The connection between birthing and dying is seen not only in the social movements to reclaim these greatest of life events from medical control. Birthing and dying are both events where the presence of human comfort can help to surpass pain and fear and render the experience to be one of learning and even joy. Providing human comfort to the dying must happen with a celebration of life, and women are at the forefront of this celebration. They are the pioneers on the journey of accepting death.

SELF-REFLECTION AND THOUGHTFUL CONVERSATIONS

1. What are the components of hospice palliative care which appeal to you and why?
2. Do you think hospice palliative care programs will expand in Canada, why and when?
3. Why is there a cultural expectation in Canada that caregiving is primarily women's work?
4. In your family, or amongst those you know, who in the family has cared for the ill and dying?

IN-CLASS ASSIGNMENTS

1. Find out about palliative care or hospices in your community. How many such services are there, and how many patients are cared for?
2. Find out how many volunteers work in the hospice palliative care programs in your area. What are the age and gender breakdowns?
3. Make a list and discuss the differences between dying in a hospital and dying at home.

Chapter Seven

MEDICAL ASSISTANCE IN DYING AND EUTHANASIA

> If I can choose between a death of torture and one that is simple and easy, why should I not choose the latter? (Seneca c. 4 BCE–65 CE, cited in Curl 1993)
>
> I want to be in charge of my life. … And my death. Whose life is it, anyway? (Sue Rodriguez, in her appeal to the British Columbia Supreme Court in December 1992, quoted in Downie 2004: 113)

SELDOM HAS A TOPIC TOUCHED the hearts and minds of Canadians and others around the world in the way that medical assistance in dying and euthanasia have. In 2016, the federal government enacted Bill C-14, allowing Canadians to request and possibly receive this service, given specific conditions. According to the *Fifth Annual Report on Medical Assistance in Dying in Canada*, produced for the Government of Canada (2024a),

> Medical assistance in dying (MAID) is a health service that allows someone who is found to be eligible to receive assistance from a medical practitioner to end their life. The Criminal Code sets out strict eligibility criteria to determine who can receive MAID, and robust safeguards to ensure that MAID is safely provided. MAID is only available to persons who freely choose it and only under very specific circumstances and rules. *To be eligible for MAID, an individual must:*
>
> - be at least 18 years old and mentally competent
> - have a *grievous and irremediable medical condition*, specifically:
>   » have a serious illness, disease or disability;
>   » be in an advanced state of decline that *cannot* be reversed; and

» experience unbearable physical or mental suffering from the illness, disease, disability, or state of decline that *cannot* be relieved under conditions that the person considers acceptable
- make a voluntary request for MAID
- give informed consent to receive MAID
- be eligible for health services funded by the province or territory, or the federal government.

In addition, there are a *number of safeguards that must* be met before MAID can be administered. Where an individual's death is not "reasonably foreseeable," additional safeguards have been put in place.

The initial 2016 legislation came about due to what is known as the *Carter v. Canada* decision. As Stuart Chambers (2016), writing in *Impact Ethics,* a forum for the discussion of Canadian bioethics in the Faculty of Medicine at Dalhousie University in Halifax, Nova Scotia, notes:

> In 2012, British Columbia's Supreme Court "unsanctified" human life by permitting the intentional hastening of death for a terminally ill woman named Gloria Taylor. In this decision, Justice Lynn Smith endorsed the quality of life principle. In her decision, she allowed that Taylor's death could be intentionally hastened based on quality-of-life considerations. Three years later, the Supreme Court of Canada upheld this decision. Consequently, any remaining traces of the traditional sanctity of life doctrine in law all but disappeared.

Under this legislation, those who can provide MAID are "physicians and nurse practitioners (in provinces where this is allowed)," and this may include pharmacists and other professionals that you ask to help, as well as health-care providers who help physicians or nurse practitioners. These people can assist in the process without being charged under criminal law. However, physicians, nurse practitioners and others who are directly involved must follow the rules set out in the Criminal Code of Canada and the applicable provincial and territorial health-related laws, rules and policies. It is important to note that individual health-care practitioners who can legally perform MAID who are opposed to medical assistance in dying due to reasons of faith are not obligated to perform MAID if requested.

Key is that they will not face retribution regarding their employment if they say no.

The 2016 law continues to change and evolve, and it also continues to come under scrutiny due to aspects of both expansion and regulation and protection of vulnerable groups. In October 2024, Quebec began to move ahead with allowing advance requests for assisted dying. The fifth annual MAID report (Government of Canada 2024a) delineates some of the findings related to the progress of MAID since it began in 2016. According to the Department of Justice (Government of Canada 2021),

> The changes are the result of over five years of experience with MAID in Canada. The new law responds to feedback from over 300,000 Canadians, experts, practitioners, stakeholders, provinces and territories, provided during the January and February 2020 consultations. It is also informed by the testimony of over 120 expert witnesses heard throughout Bill C-7's study by the House of Commons and the Senate.
>
> Specifically, the new law:
> - removes the requirement for a person's natural death to be reasonably foreseeable in order to be eligible for MAID, in response to the 2019 Superior Court of Québec's *Truchon* ruling
> - introduces a two-track approach to procedural safeguards based on whether or not a person's natural death is reasonably foreseeable
>   » existing safeguards are maintained and, in some cases, eased for eligible persons whose natural death is reasonably foreseeable
>   » new and strengthened safeguards are introduced for eligible persons whose natural death is not reasonably foreseeable
> - temporarily excludes eligibility for individuals suffering solely from mental illness for twenty-four months, and requires the Ministers of Justice and Health to initiate an expert review tasked with making recommendations within the next year on protocols, guidance, and safeguards for MAID for persons suffering from mental illness

- allows eligible persons whose natural death is reasonably foreseeable, and who have a set date to receive MAID, to waive final consent if they are at risk of losing capacity in the interim
- allows for expanded data collection and analysis through the federal monitoring regime to provide a more complete and inclusive picture of MAID in Canada

The Government of Canada recognizes that other important outstanding issues related to MAID must still be explored. Areas such as the eligibility of mature minors, advance requests, mental illness, palliative care, and the protection of Canadians living with disabilities will be considered during a parliamentary review of the MAID legislation. The committee responsible for the parliamentary review process will be required to submit its report to Parliament no later than one year after the start of the review.

CANADIAN HOSPICE AND PALLIATIVE CARE ASSOCIATION

A key body involved in developing resources and support for Canadians seeking information on medical assistance in dying is the Canadian Hospice and Palliative Care Association. On Friday, September 22, 2017, the association presented a workshop entitled "Hospice Palliative Care in the MAID Environment: Practically How Do We Co-Exist in the New Environment?" The workshop was based on a survey of its membership between July 19 and August 16, 2017, to get feedback on their experiences with MAID. Almost five hundred responses were received from all ten provinces (there were no responses from any of the three territories). Among the respondents, 36 percent were nurses, 17 percent were administrators, and 12 percent were physicians (2017: 6). Some of the biggest challenges invoked by those who responded to the survey were the following: 1) public and professional confusion about the difference between palliative care and MAID; 2) local public backlash against MAID; and 3) public backlash against our position to not allow MAID to be performed. The conclusions to this workshop and the survey arrived at by those in attendance were, first, "MAID is here to stay, we need to figure out how to co-exist keeping patient-centred care front of mind"; second, "We need to promote universal access to HPC [home-based palliative care]"; and third, "More funding is needed to expand HPC services and programs, we need to better articulate gaps in care, among others" (16). This discussion is relevant today as we come to understand better what options are available for those at the end of life.

Clearly, there is a need for new and continuing resources to be put into palliative care services of all kinds, at the same time as understanding how to best apply MAID for those who want it. Canadians need to be more informed about the role hospice palliative care can play. While Canadians are legally allowed to request MAID, the important and crucial element now becomes whether they have a real choice in fairly having access to other options (e.g., hospice palliative care).

CURRENT CONTROVERSIES

(This section was written by Dr. Kerstin Roger and co-authored by Dr. Mary Shariff [Law], Dr. Genevieve Thompson [Nursing] and Dr. Karen Duncan [Community Health Sciences] at the University of Manitoba.)

Vital questions and controversies about the expansion and development of MAID continue, and their foundations remain a sobering account of what we as Canadians need to consider, especially as the law ends its first decade of existence in 2026. Globally, Canada has become one of the nations with the highest numbers of people requesting MAID (Buchholz 2022). The eligibility requirement of a "foreseeable" natural death was removed in March 2021, and there was an anticipated extension for March 2024, which would permit those with only mental illness as the underlying condition to access MAID. This expansion is under parliamentary review and may continue to be delayed due to, amongst other things, concerns such as those expressed by members of a Special Joint Committee on MAID and other community stakeholders regarding competing values and safeguards and a perceived lack of preparedness (Campbell 2024; Phillips 2024). These concerns need to be addressed with a fair ear, discussion of the principles in question and respect for the groups speaking out against the expansion. While many have celebrated MAID as a legal success under the Canadian Charter of Rights and Freedoms, and as a personal choice and reflection of freedom, others to critique Canadian lawmakers for being overly permissive in a context which provides few helpful alternatives (Gaind 2020; Hansen, Janz and Sobsey 2008). In the news, examples are emerging regarding people who felt they did not have any other choice but to select MAID.

In this context, choice can be seen as a rational decision and expression of one's rights and freedoms, but it does not speak to systemic impact and effects when few better options exist. Critics, including the Canadian Association for Community Living, have seen personal choice in this realm as potentially harmful, in effect silently relieving social and health-care systems of having to deal with possible resource-based solutions for core social issues such as overburdened and under-resourced health-care systems and discrimination against people living with chronic illness and disabilities, including aging populations and those living below the poverty line or in substandard housing. Sathya Kovac (2022) said as much on why she chose MAID. The UN Special Rapporteur to Canada expressed concern that there is no protocol in place to demonstrate that persons with disabilities deemed eligible for assisted dying have been provided with viable alternatives (Devandas Aguilar 2019: 13). This is key for other groups as well. Critics have stated clearly that an underfunded and sometimes "broken" health-care system may be seen to benefit when Canadians choose a kind of death that places less of a burden on the system (see, for example, Henderson 2024).

Let us further explore the situation of gender and older women. Care and caregiving remain firmly planted, by and large, in the domain of labour of women, and in this case, impact older women, who have also spent their lives caring and caregiving. Debbie Selby, Brandon Chan and Amy Nolen (2021) point out that even those over age seventy who are not captured by common aging disease groups are being assessed for MAID. Is "high age" a main driver? Should it be normative that we expect older people to consider and request MAID? This could be a big societal shift and one that we as Canadians need to pay attention to: not only protecting those who feel they have no other choice, but also the case in which older people are simply considered "natural" contenders. The "slippery slope" argument applies, where if we begin to see some groups (e.g., older women) as natural contenders for MAID, we might begin to "naturalize" this choice for other groups as well.

TYPES OF EUTHANASIA

The term euthanasia comes from the Greek *eu* (well) and *thanatos* (death), meaning happy or easy death. Literature on euthanasia is vast and covers every academic discipline, profession and area of public discourse, including the popular media. Currently, the topic of MAID and euthanasia is one of the most discussed and studied topics surrounding research on death and dying. Palliative care and euthanasia are frequently presented as mutually exclusive entities, with arguments positing that if more palliative care were available to consumers, euthanasia would not be necessary.

Euthanasia is a deliberate act undertaken by one person with the intention of ending the life of another to relieve that person's suffering, where that act is the cause of death. It is also viewed in conjunction with the concepts of the right-to-die and the death-with-dignity movements; the right to choose and self-determination. Leading up to the 2016 legislation on MAID, the Canadian courts had been dealing with the issue of euthanasia since 1972, when suicide was decriminalized in Canada, and someone who now attempts suicide is not liable to sanction under the Criminal Code. On February 6, 2015, the court voted unanimously (9–0) to allow physician-assisted suicide for "a competent adult person who: 1) clearly consents to the termination of life; and 2) has a grievous and irremediable medical condition (including an illness, disease or disability) that causes enduring suffering that is intolerable to the individual in the circumstances of his or her condition." The court reasoned that the Criminal Code prohibition was unconstitutional because it breached the rights to life, liberty and security of the person as enshrined in section 7 of the Charter (Health Law Institute n.d.).

There are two main types of euthanasia: active and passive. Active euthanasia involves the deliberate act of providing a lethal dose of medication, either via injection or orally, to another person. Passive euthanasia is to withhold medical treatment from a dying person, even when doing so may hasten death. Harvey Chochinov and Keith Wilson (1995: 593) state the difference between euthanasia and assisted suicide: "Euthanasia refers to a positive act of commission, such as lethal injections, which are undertaken deliberately by physicians to end the lives of patients who have asked to die. 'Assisted suicide' refers to the provision of advice or the means for an individual to commit suicide."

A CANADIAN LEADER: DR. JOCELYN DOWNIE

One of the most prominent Canadians to be involved in the debates around MAID is Dr. Jocelyn Downie, who besides being a retired faculty member at the Health Law Institute at Dalhousie University is also a member of the Canadian Council of Academies Expert Panel on Medical Assistance in Dying, the Royal Society of Canada Expert Panel on Physician Assisted

Dying, the Provincial-Territorial Expert Advisory Group on Physician Assisted Dying and the pro bono legal team for the plaintiffs in Carter v. Canada. In January 2018, she was given the Order of Canada. In collaboration with her colleague Jennifer A. Chandler, also a member of the Canadian Council of Academies Expert Panel on Medical Assistance in Dying and a research chair at the Centre for Health Law, Policy and Ethics at Dalhousie University, Downie produced a report for the Institute for Research on Public Policy entitled *Interpreting Canada's Medical Assistance in Dying Legislation* (2018). In their opening remarks to this report, Downie and Chandler state, "Uncertainty about the meanings of specific terms in the Canadian MAID legislation put Canadians at risk in a number of ways. Eligibility for MAID may be determined too broadly or too narrowly, and there may be arbitrary inequality of access when the various MAID assessors and providers interpret the law differently" (4). The authors sought to propose interpretations of key phrases in the law that urgently needed clarification. To start, they talked to a wide range of experts and MAID providers: "We then posted it on the Social Sciences Research Network (Downie and Chandler 2018) and sought feedback through an open call (Twitter networks and e-mails to various people we know are interested in the topic) and direct contact with MAID assessors and providers. In-person conversations with key experts from legal or regulatory entities led to further refinements" (2018:7). On August 2017, they held a meeting with fifteen key experts on the topic was held in Halifax, Nova Scotia, with participants ranging from persons representing the fields of medicine, law, ethics and nursing, the Canadian Medical Association and other agencies. Those in attendance discussed the ways in which the legislation needs more definitive interpretations; their opinions and expertise mirror those of many others who agree with these concerns, especially the organization Dying with Dignity Canada (n.d.).

The six main areas of concern in the current legislation are those dealing with what constitutes a "reasonably foreseeable natural death," a "serious and incurable condition," "intolerable suffering," "irreversible decline in capability," "imminent loss of capacity to provide informed consent" and the "exclusion of mental illness" (2). Below we explore some of those six.

The first area of concern explored in the Downie report deals with what constitutes a "reasonably foreseeable natural death." The concept here typically depends on a medical diagnosis and understanding how and when illnesses have a trajectory which can lead to a natural death. Some conditions are understood in a specific medical context, specifically whether treatment can alleviate symptoms and/or the illness trajectory altogether. Concerns arise when we think about the nature of a brain tumour or dementia, in which a long-term trajectory may be understood, but at which time, capacity may no longer be possible. We might also question what "foreseeable" means in terms of timelines — is an event likely to occur in ten years foreseeable?

Another concern is that the person has "a serious and incurable illness, disease or disability." The individual should also be in such a state of decline that it "causes them to endure physical or psychological suffering that is unbearable to them," and finally, a natural death has "become reasonably foreseeable, taking into account all of their medical circumstances, without a prognosis necessarily having been made as to the specific length of time they have remaining" (9). Clearly, each of these criteria is open to many interpretations, and some individuals could meet some of the criteria and not others.

One might also ask, what is a serious and incurable condition? "Does 'incurable' mean incurable by any means? If so, as long as there is any chance of a cure from any available treatment, the patient would not be considered incurable" (2018: 12). The authors of the report ask who would determine whether or not the patient can decide if their disease is "incurable," and especially in terms of the potential side effects of the treatment available to them? An example that raises concern is when a teenage girl with a serious eating disorder, having tried all treatments, requests MAID as soon as she is eighteen, saying her condition is incurable. It is crucial that such interpretations and understanding of the present law are clarified.

The third area discussed in the report asks who defines "intolerable suffering"? The authors point out that opinions about what constitutes "intolerable suffering" are extremely subjective, not just for patients, but also for those providing care to them. What is intolerable for one person (e.g., starting tube feeding at a late stage in life) may be experienced by another as tolerable (e.g., someone who has lived with this most of their life and says they have quality of life). A related question is how we define suffering and whether this should be seen as a subjective state? Is my suffering the same as yours? How can we determine which kind and type of suffering qualifies under a legal definition? Again, the dilemma is to have clear and precise definitions of what this term means, and to whom.

The fourth area of concern is that of "irreversible decline in capability." The authors ask, "Is 'capability' limited to physical function or does it also include cognitive function?" Do the terms "advanced state" and "decline" mean that the loss of capability must be a gradual, protracted process? Or could it be a sudden event, or one that has stabilized, or may be continuing? With the aging population in Canada and globally, asking tough questions about what decline means in a legal sense is important. Would it be appropriate to say that all aging individuals are in decline, and if so, at what age do we suggest that they are eligible for MAID? For example, the term senescence suggests that we begin aging physically at age thirty, and as such, are in decline. Many questions emerge over the processing of this law, which require us to consider our interpretation and subjectivities related to matters of death and dying.

CONCLUSION

Clearly, there are many voices for and against the promotion of MAID in Canada. This book takes the stance that having MAID be a legal and viable option in Canada, and given specific criteria for eligibility, is key and fundamentally positive for Canadians. Legally, individuals should be able to choose medically assisted dying if they fit the criteria. There is no contest for the value of that freedom. However, we also need to consider the less visible impacts of regulating and providing this service in a society which includes systemic issues of marginalization, poverty and lack of resources and services in some health-care areas. Many argue that Canadians also deserve more options for better health care (e.g., mental health resources) and end-of-life care (e.g., palliative and hospice care) before MAID becomes their first choice for dying. With all the academic, professional, community-based and media-driven debates taking place in Canada on the topic of MAID/euthanasia and assisted suicide, as a society, we need to continue to grapple with this issue by educating ourselves and speaking out.

SELF-REFLECTION AND THOUGHTFUL CONVERSATIONS

1. List the main controversies surrounding MAID today in Canada. Do these vary by province, and if so, how?
2. In your own opinion, what is the main issue concerning MAID today in Canada? How do you see those issues presented by your local media — is this a fair or biased presentation?
3. If you were put in charge of developing MAID in Canada, given what you now know, what are the changes or allowances, protections or regulations you would like to see? Why?

IN-CLASS ASSIGNMENTS

1. Make a list of all the relevant arguments you can think of for and against MAID. Who gains from these, and who is at risk?
2. Look up written media accounts of MAID/euthanasia over the past ten years, starting in 2016. Do these stories seem to be pro or con MAID? How are their arguments made visible?
3. How are the issues of abortion and euthanasia related? List the similarities and differences.
4. According to the *Fifth Annual Report on Medical Assistance in Dying in Canada* (Government of Canada 2024a), the age group most likely to request MAID is 75 years and older, with the average being 75 and a high percentage being over 80. Besides an aging population, why that age group? What could be the social factors?

Chapter Eight

DEATH EDUCATION AND THE ARTS

Rita Giancola

(This chapter was written by Rita Giancola, a master's student in Interdisciplinary Studies at York University whose research interests include the cultural aspects of death and dying.)

"I paint flowers so I will not die." (Frida Kahlo)

DEATH AND DYING ARE USED AS ENTERTAINMENT throughout the arts, as well as to express, process and overcome our feelings about mortality. Why do we use art forms to experience death and dying? Emotions around death and dying are complicated, and the arts' inherent connection to the human experience makes them a powerful tool to deal with this difficulty.

Participating in art therapy makes us feel safe and protected (Rankanen 2016). Sandra Bertman, a pioneer in utilizing the arts to support death education, argues, "Since grief is not a cerebral problem but a subjective experience, we understand grief only and entirely as we filter and interpret it through our own experience. ... The expressive arts and therapies function beautifully as vehicles to help us reshape grief" (1999: 15). Art lecturer Mimmu Rankanen (2016) measured how art therapy impacted participants' physical health, mental health and social relationships. Her results demonstrated the power of art therapy: 67 percent, 98 percent and 82 precent of participants, respectively, stated that their physical health, mental health and social relationships were positively affected.

Many studies explore the efficacy of death education through the arts, whether through visual arts, music, media, theatre or literature. These mediums improved individuals' psychological wellness and appreciation of life by allowing them to explore and express their emotions around death and dying (Chang 2005; Cummins 2004; Ginicola, Smith and Trzaska 2012; Harrawood, Doughty and Wilde 2011; Kim, E.H., and Lee 2009; McClatchey and King 2015; Nan et al. 2020; Ordal 1980; Orkibi 2011; Pentaris and Yerosimou 2020; Pfaffenwimmer 2014; Ronconi et al. 2023; Skye et al. 2014; Stack 2002; Testoni, Tronca et al. 2020a; Guy 1993; Tsiris et al. 2012; Walter 2012b). The arts are necessary in our daily lives, especially during difficult times. In their book *Talking Through Death*, authors Christine Davis and Deborah Breede argue, "Death and dying are such personal, confusing, mysterious, painful and mystical experiences, sometimes poetry and artwork, literature and mediated stories are the only ways we can communicate about it" (2018: 21). Likewise, Tony Walter, at the Centre for Death and Society at the University of Bath, writes, "Mortality and grief provide a motor for artistic practice" (2012a: 76), and Christine Davis and Jan Warren-Findlow state, "People have always coped with trauma through creating" (2011: 570). In our times of stress and need, we turn to the arts for support. Lewis Aiken explains, "To the creative person, even greater than the fear of death is the fear of living an incomplete life — life seems too short or rapid to do the things the person is capable of doing" (2001: 166). Understanding and accepting that life is limited gives us the motivation and courage to accomplish our dreams so that when faced with the end of our lives, we have fewer regrets.

VISUAL ARTS

The creative process of art-making — art therapy — is known to be effective in reducing anxiety toward death, loss and the end of one's life (Dunphy et al. 2019; de Guzman et al. 2011; Testoni, Tronca et al. 2020). The practice of making visual art, whether painting, sculpture, photography or another art form, improves end-of-life experiences. It helps individuals overcome their fears and anxieties of death and dying by providing an outlet to express and process their emotions.

Painting

Nineteenth-century Norwegian painter Edvard Munch (best known for *The Scream*) was six when his mother died and eight when his sister died. These events triggered his obsession with death and illness, making it a predominant and expressively graphic theme in his work (Aiken 2001). Paintings such as *The Sick Child*, *The Death Chamber*, *By the Death Bed* and

The Dead Mother are narratives of his anguish and anxieties. These paintings predominantly feature "death beds" and sorrowful figures crowded around them. Munch is considered the exception to the romanticized and symbolic way artists from the Middle Ages to the twentieth century encapsulated death in their work (Aiken 2001). In contrast, Munch used art personally to express his grief.

Whether a piece of art has been created by a professional or an amateur, art speaks to us personally (Cardany 2018). The painting *The Last Supper* by Leonardo da Vinci focuses on the emotional aspects surrounding Jesus's impending death announcement. This well-known painting can spark conversation around death and dying. I cannot look at this painting without asking, "How did he feel?" or "What would my last meal be?"

Photography

Another medium used in art therapy is photography, specifically PhotoVoice, which involves photography around a social issue, usually followed by a written or verbal discussion of the photos taken. Ines Testoni, Elisa Tronca, Gianmarco Biancalani et al. (2020) used photovoice in a study to initiate death education. After watching a film, the participants were asked to take photos that answered the prompt "In my life I would like to" and afterwards elaborate on the significance of the photos. The deliberations promoted positive life wishes which are directly related to positive end-of-life views.

According to the Oxford English Dictionary, the Latin phrase "*memento mori*" translates to "remember that you must die," and "*memento vivere*" translates to "remember you must live." In 2011, artist Candy Chang created the *Before I Die* wall in New Orleans as a *memento mori* to help Chang through her grief. The wall was a public and interactive installation with the phrase "Before I die I want to ____" painted multiple times across the wall for the public to complete with chalk. It was a locus where community members could contribute their own "bucket list" items. The installation promoted personal and community well-being and discussion. This aroused interest in the topic of death, and as a result, over five thousand Before I Die walls have been created in over seventy countries (Testoni, Iacona et al. 2018).

Sculpture

American sculptor Richard Serra is known for his minimalist but large-scale steel sculptures. The death of his mother played a key role in his work. It inspired him to create larger and more immersive pieces that reflected his personal grief and his interpretation of the meaning of life. Serra's installations, like *Torqued Ellipses* and *The Matter of Time,* focus on the viewer's relationship with the sculptures as they walk in and around each massive piece, engaging their senses and states of mind (Solomon R. Guggenheim Museum). Historian and curator Leah Dickerman (2024) states that Serra's last works surrounded the theme of death, calling attention to Serra's own feelings of mortality and the fragility of life. The installation *Grief and Reason,* one of Serra's last, consisted of four forged-steel rectangular blocks, stacked in two that lay parallel to each other. They resembled large, stacked coffins and captured stillness instead of his usual themes of movement.

Other artists, such as Susan Hiller and Judit Hersko, produced immersive art installations that reflect loss, mourning and traumas experienced from the Holocaust. They used sculpture, photography, artifacts and projections in combination with factual and fictional narratives to help heal wounded souls (Bloom 2024).

Munch, Chang, Serra, Hiller and Hersko are only a few of the many artists who create original work with themes of grief, loss, death and dying. The visual arts are a powerful way for individuals to reflect on and deal with end-of-life anxieties. Following is a list of art therapy organizations and studios in Canada that offer specialized workshops and programs that help individuals cope with grief, loss, death and dying:

- Art Can Heal (<artcanheal.ca>)
- Beyond Words Art Therapy (<beyondwordsarttherapy.com>)
- Kristen Roberts The Art of Healing (<kirstenroberts.ca>).

MUSIC

Songs tell alluring stories. Scientists have discovered that listening to and creating music triggers more parts of the brain than any other activity (Holford 2021). Music about death, grieving and our mortality helps us deal with our fears, leading to a deeper outlook on life. From Verdi to gospel to funeral music, music is celebrated around the world, with different melodic phrasing evoking different emotions and reflecting different cultures.

Classical Music

Schubert's classic song *Ave Maria* was sung at my mother's funeral — I cannot listen to it without thinking about her. The song transports me back to a time when I believed that without my mom by my side, I could no longer continue living. Audrey Cardany, professor of music and director of music education at the University of Rhode Island, succinctly wrote, "Music and the arts mediate between life and death by giving form to death while we live — an essential role for the arts given that the dead cannot describe their experiences for others" (2018). Today Schubert's *Ave Maria* gives me strength to face my sadness and anxieties while helping me realize that the memory of my mom lives on within me.

Contemporary Music

Metallica, a heavy metal band, dedicated their 2008 album, *Death Magnetic*, to the theme of death. James Alan Hetfield, original songwriter and lead singer of Metallica, said, "Just like the poles of a magnet, some people are drawn to death and others are repulsed by it, but we all have to deal with it." Despite its more aggressive nature, heavy metal music helps fans deal with death anxiety passionately — validating music as an "anxiety buffer" (Kneer and Rieger 2016).

After the death of his four-year-old son, Eric Clapton was inspired to write *Tears in Heaven* about his loss. For a year, Clapton wrote emotional and sorrowful songs to help himself heal — sharing his grief through music was Clapton's way of dealing with the pain (Leerhsen and Peyser 1992). Music has a way of healing the soul.

In the 1920s and 1930s, German composer and music teacher Carl Orff, in collaboration with Gunild Keetman, developed the Orff Methodology at the Günther School in Munich. Nearly a hundred years later, the Orff Methodology continues to be used by teachers, therapists and counsellors. It uses music, movement and drama to teach music and other topics. This holistic approach to learning has shown to be an effective tool for all ages (He et al. 2024; Kim, S.H., and Lee 2023; Paolino and Lummis 2015; Shamrock 1997).

Through the use of the Orff Methodology, threshold singing (bedside singing) and songwriting circles, Gina Burgess, a Canadian musician, music teacher and internationally known advocate of death education, helps young students benefit from exploring themes of death and grief through music to eliminate their fears around dying. She writes: "Not every student will go on to be a mathematician or musician, but every student *will* encounter death. Students deserve to have preparation and necessary tools for the inevitable. Like other sensitive issues, we owe it to ourselves and our students to bring in these realities of life" (2024: 8).

According to Youth Music (2024), young people believe it is more important to listen and make music rather than participate in sports, social media or gaming, and 84 percent of those surveyed say that "music makes their world better." Understanding, discussing and reflecting on death through music at a young age is a gateway to help students cope with and manage their death-related concerns and questions. Starting death education at an early age will change the way we see death and dying in the future.

Cultural

Palliative care cancer patients frequently struggle to control pain and often turn to pharmaceutical drugs to manage it. Gönül Düzgün and Ayfer Karadakovan (2024) conducted a study measuring levels of pain, comfort and anxiety with sixty palliative cancer patients. All sixty patients continued to receive their medical treatments, but half of the patients also received music sessions in their preferred genre. The group that received music therapy reported lower pain and anxiety levels as well as improved comfort during treatments.

Music plays an important role in helping the sick and those that mourn a loved one. Following is a list of certified music therapy organizations in Canada that assist with grief, loss, death and dying:

- Canadian Association of Music Therapists (<musictherapy.ca>)
- JB Music Therapy (<jbmusictherapy.com>)
- MacMillian Therapy (<macmillantherapy.com>).

MEDIA

Media is powerful and influential. It often depicts death and dying as synonymous with fear and anxiety and imparts these thoughts (Walter 1991). As viewers, we have become detached from death scenes in film and television; we see vicious deaths as casual occurrences with very little grief responses from the actors on the screen. "Death is distorted into a sensational stream of violent attacks" (Schultz and Huet 2001, 137). In entertainment, death is almost never represented as we experience it in reality. Are we trying to escape reality? Are we aware of the mortality shown in the media? The effect movies and television have on society should be a concern (Schultz and Huet 2001). When we engage in media of any form, we need to be aware of the stories we are being shown and untangle the truth from interpretation.

Film

Ned Schultz and Lisa Huet (2001) analyzed death representations in several American films. They found frequent conversations about death but noted that crying and grief in a response to death were portrayed more often than scenes showing illnesses, treatments, deaths, funerals and burials — death happens off-camera. The authors also found that euphemisms for death were used more often than the word "death" itself. Among the dozens of euphemisms used, the most common were "passed on," "departed," "resting in peace" and "was called home." Scripts even went so far as to include phrases such as "expired," "kicked the bucket," "their number was up," "dirt nap" and "pushing up daisies." Avoiding the word "death" does not change the reality that a person has died. The use and vast number of euphemisms for death confirms that modern society is in denial of it (Corr 2014).

Death is the essence of horror films. These fictional narratives are a tool for us to use to confront death. Horror films explore connections between the living and dead that spark conversation about mortality among viewers, which, in turn, unravels worries about life and death (Davis and Crane 2015). By directly confronting death, as is done in horror films, viewers overcome death avoidance.

Roger Ebert was a film critic for forty-six years before dying of cancer. He critiqued many films about death, stating that movies about people dying are not for the dying but for the living to "provide a way for [them] to deal with [their] fears" (2011). Several studies demonstrate that discussing one's own mortality — prior or following a movie about death — dismantles death anxiety (Hofer 2013; Rieger and Hofer 2017). Once again, we see that creative narratives about death and dying are a means of death education.

Tim Burton's 1988 film *Beetlejuice,* its 2024 sequel, and Scott Brown and Anthony King's 2018 Broadway musical adaption have a cult following. After thirty years, because of a strong fanbase — over two million tagged posts on Instagram — *Beetlejuice* is again loved by multiple generations, all laughing at the same death-related jokes, while dressed up in costume to go see the live performance (Thomas 2023). *Beetlejuice* is about a deceased couple who, with a trickster ghost, haunt their home's new dwellers, the Deetz family, made up of Charles Deetz, his second wife Delia and his teenage daughter Lydia, from his first marriage. A funny storyline, steeped in horror iconography with the theme of death is woven throughout. In this way, *Beetlejuice* frequently transitions from horror to humour. For example, the gruesome appearance of the deceased couple, which should frighten audiences, is comical and compassionate, consequently making it amusing, establishing horror and humour to be similar (Carroll 2001). As Schultz and Huet point out, "by pairing humour with death-related behaviours and conversations, [stories] distort psychological reactions to death," which can evoke more positive emotions (2001: 147).

Television

The Cultural Indicators Project, created by researcher George Gerbner in the late 1960s, introduced cultivation theory, which analyzes the long-term effects of how viewers interpret themes from television and how they are perceived as real. For decades, topics such as homosexuality, gender roles, mental health, dietary health risks, violence and death have been researched using cultivation theory (Calzo and Ward 2009; Diefenbach and West 2007; Kahlor and Eastin 2011; Netzley 2010; Russell and Buhrau 2015). The prominent topic of research is whether exposure to violence on television contributes to higher rates of hostility and violent actions (Hermann, Morgan and Shanahan 2021; Al-Ibrahim 2023; Riddle and Martins 2022; Schiappa, Gregg and Hewes 2004). Cultivation research shows that extensive amounts of television watching alters a viewer's perspectives and beliefs about the world around them, making what is seen on television their understood reality (Gerbner 1970).

The HBO drama series *Six Feet Under* premiered in June 2001. The series' five seasons, written by Alan Ball, are about the dysfunctional Fisher family, who own and operate a funeral home on the main floor of their home. At the beginning of each of the sixty-three episodes, a death occurs; some are realistic, but often the deaths are improbable; yet we, the audience, believe in the story. The episodes explore realistic questions about loss, grieving, death and dying and go into detail about the necessary paperwork that must be completed after a death; what to expect when visiting a morgue, crematorium or funeral home; the preparation required for a body before a funeral viewing; and the way a body is embalmed.

Edward Schiappa, Peter Gregg and Dean Hewes (2004) conducted research on death attitudes associated with television. Over the course of five weeks, 174 participants viewed ten episodes of *Six Feet Under*. The authors found that the show was a successful death education tool and helped participants explore and overcome their negative attitudes associated with death and dying. While the narratives in *Six Feet Under* are filled with thought-provoking information about death and dying, the episodes are equally about the meaning of life. Each episode makes viewers laugh and cry and think about mortality, yet it also makes us appreciate the amazing experiences shared in life. More than twenty years after the first episode aired, the subject matter remains relevant, given that we are still living and thus, we are still dying. *Six Feet Under* is fundamentally death education.

Animation

Disney Entertainment chooses to confront mortality in many of its animated films. While the subject of death is usually avoided with children, Disney embraces it, placing death as a primary theme in films such as *The Lion King*, *Up*, *Soul* and *Coco*. These films, specifically Disney Pixar's *Coco*, give children a way to communicate their feelings, especially when confronted with loss, thus generating fewer fears. *Coco* takes place in Mexico during Día de los Muertos (Day of the Dead), where a twelve-year-old boy named Miguel journeys to the Land of the Dead in search of his great-great-grandfather. *Coco* faces the subject of death "dead-on," framing death as playful and as a tradition of remembering one's ancestors. Films such as *Coco* reflect a broader demand for fictional films to allow us to "reflect upon our life as it is lived ... not as it has been lived, or even as it might be lived" (Crosthwait 2020). *Coco* is an effective conversation starter to introduce children to the concept of death, where they can face death as a celebration (Castillo 2017). Meredith Cox, Erin Garrett and James Graham (2005) analyzed how death was portrayed in animated Disney films and how children conceptualized death after viewing such movies. They discovered that Disney movies are an influential means to teach children about death and facilitate conversations with each other, parents, teachers and counsellors.

Theatre

Theatre is a way to share stories. Straight theatre and musical theatre address countless themes: love, religion, war, being different, animals, social challenges, mental illness, poverty, wealth, family and death. For over four thousand years, theatre has been used to demonstrate, articulate and illuminate knowledge to spectators. Theatre is vital for humanity. This art form physically brings people together to share an experience and spark communication. Storytelling, a form of theatre, can be used as a healing tool for individuals coping with grief and bereavement (Bosticco and Thompson 2005). Specifically, stories that have themes of death and loss have proven to be effective in stimulating conversations about mortality (Ordal 1980; Guy 1993).

As a means to expand health research, Kate Rossiter, Pia Kontos, Angela Colantonio et al. (2008) examined the advantages and disadvantages of using four theatre genres: non-theatrical performances, ethnodramas, theatrical research-based performances and fictional theatrical performances. They conclude, "Theatre has the potential to enhance health care practitioners' understanding of the complex emotional, interpersonal and psychological dynamics that arise in medical practice, many of which are difficult to fully convey in more traditional forms of dissemination" (145).

Erin Michalak, James Livingston, Victoria Maxwell et al. (2014) studied the power of theatrical performances in mental health spaces. The play they used was about a woman coping with the struggles and stigmas associated with bipolar disorder. The study was designed specifically for patients with bipolar disorder and for health-care providers working with them. They were asked to view the theatrical performance and afterwards communicate the insights and emotions they experienced. The authors conclude, "Theatrical traditions clearly hold the potential to impact audience members, both at affective and cognitive levels and to foster insight and deepened understanding" (10). This theatre-based exploration shows the power of a live performance on audiences.

Theatre motivates discussions while creating awareness. It allows the audience to be cognitively and emotionally engaged. Theatre performances with realistic characters focusing on addressing social issues promote beneficial discussions among audiences (Blignault et al. 2010; Cheechov 2016; Rossiter et al. 2008; Szostak 2022).

Margaret Edson's play *Wit* is about the struggles Vivian Bearing, a cancer patient, encounters at the end of her life. The connecting and disconnecting qualities of life, death and life-everlasting are presented throughout the play to promote end-of-life discussions. The scenes are thought-provoking, demonstrating the empathy and compassion that can be found in human relationships in the final days of life. Researchers Karl Lorenz, M. Jillisa Steckart and Kenneth Rosenfeld started the Wit Educational Initiative to help medical students assist dying patients by boosting their empathy, understanding and kindness (Rossiter et al. 2008). This is death education presented in the form of straight theatre.

Ilse Blignault, Sally Smith, Lisa Woodland et al. (2010) explored how to promote mental health and well-being for the Australian Macedonian community utilizing a play in Macedonian titled *Fear and Shame*, which depicts the emotional collapse of a young man and the negative encounters he faces. Strategies of dealing with his distress unfold throughout the play, ending with a positive outcome. More than 1600 Macedonians went to see the performance, and 236 were later interviewed by telephone to discuss if the play was successful in supporting mental health. The authors report, "Theatre was an effective means of disseminating information and reducing stigma around mental illness in the target community" (120).

Susan Neilson and Alison Reeves (2019) discuss the importance of successful conversations between medical professionals and their dying patients. Theatre influences audiences by allowing them to reflect on their personal attitudes toward topics. Neilson and Reeves' exploration of good and bad communication was demonstrated using live theatre performances. Seven scenarios with challenging conversations about end-of-life care were developed by undergraduate drama students into a performance for student nurses. The performances were successful in assisting the medical professionals in real-life situations, where delicate communication and empathy were essential.

Recreating biblical stories is called bibliodrama. As the performers in a bibliodrama interact with each other, they explore the characters through fictional interviews as they investigate the deeper meaning of the text. A study using death education with bibliodrama proved it to be an effective approach to helping participants express their emotions and encourage a positive mindset around their fears and avoidance-of-death discussions (Testoni, Biancalani et al. 2021).

Dr. Jacob L. Moreno developed psychodrama in the 1920s. Psychodrama is a technique where psychologists have their patients roleplay their personal issues to help them understand and initiate new ways of dealing with their emotions and anxieties. Intermodal psychodrama expands psychodrama by letting patients use characters from written plays. Individuals who engage in psychodrama are more able to identify and describe their feelings of adversity toward death and dying, confirming this to be a beneficial form of death education (Orkibi 2011; Testoni, Ronconi et al. 2018; Testoni, Ronconi et al. 2021). Psychodrama's greatest appeal is that it allows the participant to act out what is in their imagination and personal reality (Testoni et al. 2019; Testoni, Ronconi et al. 2018). This is called "surplus reality," a term Moreno coined for what is considered to be the "magic ingredient" in psychodrama (Watersong 2008). Psychodrama and artistic activities were successfully used among teenagers in Southern Italy and with Italian university students in two death education studies. Students were encouraged to communicate about death, dying and immortality, which subsequently diminished their death anxiety and promoted emotional competence while encouraging creative thought (Ronconi et al. 2023; Testoni, Ronconi et al. 2018).

Musicals

Theatre is a valuable tool to inform people and reduce stigmas (Faigin and Stein 2010, Michalak et al. 2014, Blignault et al. 2010). Musical theatre is a genre of theatre that includes song and dance and has been around since Ancient Greek and Roman times — even Shakespeare included songs in his plays (Atkey 2006). Showtunes (songs from musicals) are educational — they reveal personal and other information through lyrics accompanied by music. Professor of economics Matthew Rousu (2018) argues that showtunes are a powerful tool to familiarize people with topics. In fact, he taught economics by using eleven songs from musicals. The idea of watching a musical about death and dying may feel uncomfortable, but death is already a prominent topic in musicals. In fact, 68 percent of the hundred top-grossing Broadway shows and 63 percent of the longest-running Broadway shows involve death in some manner. Still, death remains an avoided subject, and Broadway musicals can help us through difficult conversations and emotions. Sondheim, the acclaimed American composer and songwriter, states that, "death is a swell curtain for a story, you know, quote, 'the final curtain.' It's a natural ending, a logical ending to a story" (Ann Reynolds 2021, 1).

Michelle Sherman, Jessica Larsen and Robert Levy (2021) used musical theatre to stimulate discussions around mental illness for actors, audiences and behavioural health consultants. Participants were asked to share their thoughts after watching a musical. The following five themes emerged from the interviews: 1) the influence of musical theatre on the audience; 2) the actors' exposure to issues of mental illness; 3) the intensity of character development; 4) the function of behavioural health consultants; and 5) the positive support behavioural health consultants can deliver to both the audience and actors. Participants reduced their stigma around mental illness through discussing sensitive themes. The following are only a few of the thoughts shared by the participants about the power of watching musical theatre:

- "Telling human stories that others can see themselves in are like, 'Oh, my God. That's exactly what I think.'"
- "Musical theatre in particular has a sort of doorway into the soul."
- "People can see themselves and the incredible buoyancy and resilience of the human spirit."
- "Thank God for musical theatre, it has a way of shining a light and it just creates a different kind of conversation."

While there are pages of positive insights from the inquiry, a few are somewhat negative:

- "Musical theatre is so potent, it seeps in … it can do beautiful things, but it can also do damage."
- "Theatre can be hard."
- "Why the hell did I come and see this show today?" (584)

As the study recommends, these negative feelings can be reduced by distributing resources and offering question-and-answer sessions after the show for actors and audience members.

Actor Ben Platt, who played the protagonist Evan on Broadway in *Dear Evan Hansen*, written by Steven Levenson, speaks of the positive reactions audience members had after seeing the performance: "It seemed to be such a powerful icebreaker. There were just consistent tears and sharing of real difficult emotional conversations afterward" (Topel 2021). Actor Julianne Moore, who played Heidi, Evan's mom, in the film adaptation of *Dear Evan Hansen*, hopes the movie will spark conversations with families — "giving people a place to find their shared humanity is a wonderful thing."

Fascinatingly, a study from University College London discovered that audience members' hearts literally beat together while watching a live musical performance — for this study, they were watching *Dreamgirls*. Joe Devlin, Daniel Richardson, John Hogan and Jill Nuttall (2017) conclude, "This clearly demonstrates that the physiological synchrony observed during the performance was strong enough to overcome social group differences and engage the audience as a whole."

In the musical *Rent* (Act 1 Scene 16), written and composed by Jonathan Larson, the whole cast, whether healthy or critically sick with HIV/AIDS, sing "Will I?." This song is about their fears of facing death. The title words are repeated throughout the entire song — "Will I lose my dignity, will someone care, will I wake tomorrow, from this nightmare?" I have seen this musical at least ten times on Broadway and in Toronto and twice at Stratford, Ontario, and every time the cast sings "Will I?," I reflect on my mortality, having similar fears about dying. The characters in *Rent* lean on each other for encouragement, gathering at life-support groups to talk and help them cope with life and death. The audience recognizes how this helps the characters and can use similar coping mechanisms to assist themselves with their fears and anxieties about death and dying.

Many musicals portray serious issues; here are a few examples:

- *Hair* depicted youth protests in the 1960s about the Vietnam War and their struggles with drugs and sexuality;
- *West Side Story* showed the challenges of racial intolerance and gang violence;
- *Showboat* embodied interracial relationships;
- *Les Misérables* confronted the unjust class system and the treatment of women;
- *Come From Away* recounted the true story of 9/11 emergency landings in Newfoundland.

The actors were ready and willing to perform the difficult moments, and audiences were ready to engage in the experience. These musicals gave way to discussions about their subject matter. For example, *Rent* raised awareness about HIV/AIDS, and *Dear Evan Hansen* jumpstarted conversations about anxiety, depression and suicide. Musical theatre reflects the human experience, which fosters awareness and discussion about social and cultural issues.

In opera, characters do not die instantly (as in movies and television) but rather they "sing a death song that may last a half hour" (Stack 2002: 432). Characters in musical theatre productions also sing death songs, although not such long ones. These death songs, referred to as "swan songs," are a character's final performance before they die. They are filled with heartbreaking and authentic emotion, eliciting the audience's senses. Uta Hagen, a pioneer in acting pedagogy, affirms that "theater is an experience that should provoke, challenge and enlighten" (Bookey n.d.). The following are a few of examples of swan songs found in Broadway musicals:

- "Eva's Final Broadcast," from *Evita*;
- "Somewhere That's Green (Reprise)," from *Little Shop of Horrors*;
- "One Last Time," from *Hamilton*;
- "Judas' Death," from *Jesus Christ Superstar*.

Even though the main theme of the above musicals is not death, these swan songs add emotional tension and lead audiences to a moment of truth.

People around the world have attended musical theatre performances about difficult topics — HIV/AIDS, religion, politics, gender identity, racism, inequality, social justice, politics, mental health, sexual violence and drug addiction. When these sensitive and important themes are depicted on stage, the door opens for audiences to have meaningful and impactful conversations.

Dance

Trudi Schoop was a pioneer of dance/movement therapy (DMT), as well as a dance therapist, educator and researcher. Her 1974 book *Won't You Join the Dance? — A Dancer's Essay into the Treatment of Psychosis* explains how she used dance, drama and performance to assist patients with expressing a richer understanding of their feelings and emotions through physical movement. Schoop has been an inspiration to many dance therapists since 1947 (Chodorow et al. 1999: 116). Although DMT has been used for over seventy years, there is limited research on its benefits; however, it is widely documented that "creativity can cultivate a sense of meaning and serve as a means for emotional processing" (Allred 2023: 165).

Dance therapist Alexandria Callahan engaged with a group of bereaved parents for seven weeks to learn how they physically internalized their grief, each week focusing on a new activity. Sitting in a circle, Callahan began each gathering with time for the parents to share and discuss their children's memories. The activities the parents engaged in included

- guided meditation that led parents through the memories of their lost child and how these events affected their physical well-being;
- writing and sharing letters written to their deceased child to continue connection and empathy; and
- drawing and walking personal bereavement journeys to create a visual presentation of their loss.

Callahan concluded that, after the seven weeks of DMT, the parents were able to physically and emotionally release built-up tension, communicating sincere thoughts and feelings attributed to their pain (192). In turn, Callahan learned how the life-altering grief of a child's death affects the body. McKenna Allred's literature review of DMT and death suggests that DMT offers meaningful emotional and physical support for individuals in the final stages of life and that further research will only reinforce its benefits (2023: 166). The Dance Movement Therapy Association in Canada is a non-profit organization that builds recognition of dance therapy throughout Canada. It has as members many therapists who specialize in bereavement and loss, offer peer-reviewed journal articles and provide resource ideas for patients and therapists. DMT is yet another art form that can be used to express and cope with feelings of loss and dying. As Trudi Shcoop would say, "Won't you join the dance?"

Literature

Stories transport us to different worlds. Regardless of whether these worlds resemble our own, we, with the characters, can discover more about ourselves and learn strategies to overcome obstacles. Connecting with characters "helps us relate to trauma and lets us rewrite our stories as people who can overcome and cope with real-world traumas" (Davis and Warren-Findlow 2011: 568). Reading stories about dying, loss and grief makes death less frightening. Knowing that others have similar feelings makes the reader feel "normal." Literature provides useful vocabulary to promote discussion and a place to explore feelings, especially when faced with the death of a loved one. Narratives "give voice to stories that are difficult to tell and understand and open spaces to reflect alternative ways of knowing" (563).

Bibliotherapy is the use of literature and stories to promote healing in therapeutic environments (Oxford English Dictionary n.d.). It is helpful for patients of all ages, their families and their caregivers, as well as social workers, therapists, counsellors and support groups. Rachel Rusch, Jennifer Greenman, Caitlin Scanlon et al. (2020) suggest that reading stories that delve into loss, bereavement, grief, end of life and the dying process improves coping mechanisms by providing vocabulary for real-life conversations and by allowing readers to identify with characters and their situations. Books and stories can open lines of communication while validating emotions and reducing stress.

Writing helps with emotional healing, release and stress, especially during difficult times. Therapeutic writing involves two types of writing: first, creative writing, which is writing that originates from imagination, and second, expressive writing, which emerges from emotions after a painful event (Costa and Abreu 2018). Christina Thatcher, creative writer and professor at Cardiff University, conducted a study consisting of thirteen bereaved participants who answered ten creative and expressive writing prompts about grief. Afterwards, twelve participants reported having improved self-awareness, and eleven participants found that the writing opened up new perspectives on understanding loss and grief. Thatcher concludes that writing is as valuable as therapeutic counselling (2022).

Clinical psychologist and professor Margaret Stroebe (2018) believes that poetry can help us to understand and process grief: "The poets not only put grief into eloquent words for us but they also write ardently ... of the impact of giving words to grief" (68).

Whether reading or engaging in writing, literature, short stories, longer narratives and poetry reflecting grief, loss, death or dying are beneficial in healing and understanding and validates the emotions we experience.

CONCLUSION

We are surrounded by death. We see it in hospitals, funeral homes, cemeteries, social media and the arts. Each contributes to the lessening of the death taboo, and, during the past decades, death is slowly being discussed more (Aiken 2001; Neimeyer 1998). This is a step in the right direction. Would it not be wonderful to have your dying wishes known and become a reality? Still, there is more work to be done. The arts — whether visual arts, music, media, theatre or literature — are powerful tools to dismantle death anxiety.

We all have different views about death. I do not know what is going to happen to me after I die, no one does, and we struggle with this unknown. Gradually, the more we communicate about our mortality, the less afraid we will become. I only came to this realization when my mother suddenly passed away. These discussions were missing from our lives, and through the arts, they become easier. Death and dying are inevitable. They loom over our everyday existence. Expressing ourselves creatively or engaging with existing art helps us become comfortable with this truth — we can deconstruct our anxieties, take control of our fears and live more enriched lives. Iconic actor Alan Rickman said, "Actors are agents of change; a film, a piece of theatre, a piece of music or a book can make a difference ... it can change the world" (Vibes 2016).

SELF-REFLECTION AND THOUGHTFUL CONVERSATIONS

1. When you speak of someone who died, do you use euphemisms or just say "died"? Why? If you use euphemisms, what is your favourite one to use?
2. Look up the following paintings: *The Sick Child*, *The Death Chamber*, *By the Death Be*, and *The Dead Mother* by Edvard Munch. How would you describe the stories depicted in the paintings?

IN-CLASS ASSIGNMENTS

1. In a small group or as a whole class, create a Before I Die wall.
2. Draw — using any medium — what your idea of an afterlife looks like (if you think one exists at all).
3. Using the camera on your phone, take ten photos that represent life and ten photos that represent death to you. Share and discuss your pictures with the group.
4. Choose a song that you would want played at your funeral celebration. How does the song make you feel? Why did you choose this song? What are your favourite lines?
5. Write a poem about how you felt when you lost a loved one or how you would feel if you were to lose a loved one.

Chapter Nine

DRUG AND OPIOID DEATHS IN CANADA

THE TOPIC OF DRUG AND OPIOID DEATHS is a global phenomenon with many facets, which range from the increased production of synthetic opioids and the huge increase in drug trafficking to over-prescribing of opioids and the controversy over safe injection sites in Canada. The United Nations' *World Drug Report* states:

> Drug production, trafficking, and use continue to exacerbate instability and inequality, while causing untold harm to people's health, safety and well-being. We need to provide evidence-based treatment and support to all people affected by drug use, while targeting the illicit drug market and investing much more in prevention. (2024:1)

The report also addresses the alarming reality of synthetic opioid production, especially in Asian and Middle Eastern countries, where, "since 2008, more than 1,000 new psychoactive substances have been reported to the UNODC [UN Office on Drugs and Crime]" (16). The UNODC is also concerned that gender plays a role in whether an individual receives treatment for their addiction: "Though an estimated 64 million people worldwide suffer from drug use disorders, only one in 11 is in treatment. Women receive less access to treatment than men, with only one in 18 women with drug use disorders in treatment versus one in seven men." (1)

While the drug and opioid crisis is global, it also has a severe impact on Canada. According to the Public Health Agency of Canada,

> The overdose crisis is one of the most serious public health crises our country has ever faced. It is driven by a dangerous illegal synthetic drug supply that is unpredictable and increasingly toxic. Powerful drugs like fentanyl, and other emerging synthetic opioids are flooding the illegal drug supply and resulting in an

increase in harms and deaths. No community has been left untouched. The tragic impacts are seen and felt among our friends, our families, and our neighbours. (2024a: 1)

In Canada, between 2016 and 2024, there were 52,544 apparent opioid-related deaths. Despite ongoing efforts at all levels of government and with partners across the country, 6,601 people lost their lives to opioids from April 2024 to March 2025. That is an average of 18 people dying each day. Most accidental opioid deaths in Canada occurred amongst males (73 percent). The majority of these deaths (63 percent) were as a result of a fentanyl overdose (Health Canada 2025).

Drug, alcohol and tobacco use is not recent phenomenon. Indeed, throughout history, everywhere in the world, people have used stimulants derived from opium, tobacco, cannabis, mushrooms and an assortment of alcoholic spirits from corn and other plants for religious rituals and ceremonies, as medicines, for personal and community enjoyment and for the treatment of pain. These can also be used for confronting trauma, fear of death, ego death, psycho-spiritual, cultural and health reasons. When used outside of community- and culture- sanctioned protocols or therapeutic settings, adverse events and risks increase.

Opioids are psychoactive substances derived from the opium poppy, or their synthetic analogues. Examples are morphine and heroin. There are effective treatments for managing and tapering opioid dependence, yet only 10 percent of people who need such treatment were receiving it, according to the WHO in 2020: "Due to their pharmacological effects, opioids in high doses can cause respiratory depression and death. The inexpensive medication naloxone can completely reverse the effects of opioid overdose and prevent deaths due to opioid overdose" (2020b).

The breakdown of the number of deaths according to the provinces and territories shows Ontario with the highest number of deaths, followed by British Columbia, Alberta, Quebec, Manitoba, Saskatchewan, New Brunswick, Nova Scotia, Newfoundland and Labrador, Yukon, Prince Edwards Island and the North West Territories. Nunavut had zero, according to a report by Statista (2025b).

The issues presently, in Canada and globally, are three-fold. First, there is concern that opioids and other narcotics are being over-prescribed to patients by physicians. Another concern is with the illegal acquisition of opioids and other drugs. Traffickers exploit the most vulnerable addicted individuals, and this has an impact on global economies, especially when it comes to health-care costs. The third, interrelated concern is the role which pharmaceutical companies play in promoting and selling these drugs. In the case of fentanyl, which is produced primarily by Purdue Pharma Canada, it is prescribed for pain management, leading to thousands of new addictions. On June 29, 2022, the Government of British Columbia, on behalf of all Canadian governments, brought a class action suit against Purdue Pharma for the role they played in the production and marketing of OxyContin. While they won the case and were awarded $150 million in damages, this is to be shared amongst those who had become addicted to this substance, and the consensus across the country then was that this was an insufficient amount to compensate those affected. At the time of writing (2025), fentanyl has become a new political football thrown between the US president and the Canadian government, as an issue relating to border control and increased tariffs.

Opioid addiction is also a serious concern in many Indigenous communities in this country. In a report entitled *Opioid Crisis Devastates Indigenous Communities in Canada,* produced by the Yellowhead Institute with ICT (formerly Indian Country Today) and Indigenous Services Canada on October 3, 2024, Miles Morrisseau states that Indigenous communities are hit hardest:

> Canada is among the largest consumers in the world of prescription opioids and was ranked as the second-largest consumer of any country, second only to the United States, in a 2018 report released by the Canadian government. The volume of opioids distributed by hospitals and pharmacies for prescriptions by then had increased by nearly 3,000 percent since the early 1980s, with prescriptions for First Nations and Inuit paid for by the Canadian health-care system. In 2016, nearly 20 million prescriptions for opioids were dispensed, the equivalent to nearly one prescription for every adult over the age of 18, the report found. (Morrisseau 2024: 2)

Another group concerned about the over-prescribing of opioids is the Canadian Association of Retired Persons. In November 2017, the association noted, "Almost a quarter of all Canadian hospitalizations for opioid poisoning over the past eight years were for people over the age of 65. Seniors were hospitalized at higher rates than Canadians in any other age bracket." The

Canadian Coalition for Seniors' Mental Health (2019) is also concerned about opioid addiction in older adults: "There is a growing population of older adults developing opioid use disorder (OUD). In addition to this, there are older adults with longstanding OUD (including people who use illicit opioids) who require treatment for their addiction and related health problems."

In Canada, 43.9 percent of adults over 55 have used a prescription opioid and 1.1 percent of that group have done so daily (or almost daily) in the last year (Flint, Merali and Vaccarino 2018). Most of these opioids are a result of prescriptions provided by health-care practitioners to deal with chronic pain and other conditions, such as fall injuries and trauma. This issue is discussed in a *Canadian Medical Association Journal* article titled "Recent Opioid Use and Fall-Related Injury among Older Patients with Trauma," written by Raoul Daoust, Jean Paquet, Lynne Moore et al. (2018). The authors of this research-based paper discuss their work, which was conducted in Quebec with elderly patients (the average age was 81) in fifty-seven trauma centres who were hospitalized due to falls. The researchers conclude, "Recent opioid use is associated with an increased risk of fall and an increased likelihood of death with fall-related injuries in older adults" (190).

Clearly, this is an issue of great concern for older persons living in Canada and those who care for them. The Canadian Coalition for Seniors' Mental Health (2019) propose a series of guidelines to assist with the prescribing of opioids to people aged 65 and over. The coalition expects that the number of OUDs will decrease with the implementation of these guidelines:

> Older adults are susceptible to adverse health consequences of opioid use, and an increasing number of older adults are presenting with an OUD. There is a growing need for opioid management guidelines for older adults as the population in Canada ages. The current guideline is intended for use to prevent, screen, and assess for an OUD in older adults as well as to help treat those who are already suffering from the disorder. These guidelines are meant to provide evidence-informed, clinically relevant direction and advice on how to manage older adult patients with an OUD. We hope practitioners will find it a practical and useful clinical aide, and that the community at large will find it a helpful educational resource.

Most agencies that discuss the misuse of drugs and opioids differentiate between those that are medically prescribed, such as opioids, and those that are not, known as "street drugs." These illegal drugs come in the form of pills, powders, patches, capsules and injections and are apparently readily available on the streets in all Canadian towns, villages and cities. Opioids are normally prescribed to treat and manage different types of pain. They are also used to control moderate to severe cough, to control diarrhoea and to treat addiction to other opioids, such as heroin. On April 22, 2024, Health Canada proposed a series of treatments to deal with opioid use and addiction, with the title *Opioid Use Disorder and Treatment* (Government of Canada 2024b). The three main strategies the report puts forward are "medication, strong support systems such as family, friends and peer support groups, services like therapy, drug education and harm reduction" (1). The report discusses in detail what each of these strategies might entail.

The Canadian Mental Health Association (CMHA) released a position paper on the opioid crisis in Canada in April 2018, suggesting that this country ought not to treat opioid use as a criminal matter, but instead should view it as a health matter: "Criminalizing people who use drugs stigmatizes substance use, fosters a climate in which they feel unsafe in accessing life-saving interventions and treatment, and further marginalizes those living in poverty or at social disadvantage ... The war on drugs doesn't work, and it's time we lay down our weapons and start getting people help." Further, the CMHA recommends decriminalizing all illegal substances for personal use with the goal of aligning Canadian drug laws with public health. Decriminalization, which is not the same as legalization, means that the possession, use and acquisition of illegal drugs would no longer be criminal offences; however, producing, supplying and selling drugs would remain criminal offences.

Although cannabis was banned as an illegal substance in Canada in 1923, a bill to decriminalize it was introduced in the House of Commons by the presiding Liberal government on April 13, 2017. After various amendments, Bill C-45, the proposed Cannabis Act, as passed on October 17, 2018. The Access to Cannabis for Medical Purposes law came into effect in Canada on August 24, 2016 (Government of Canada 2016a).

One of the strategies recommended across the provinces is that naloxone be provided to everyone involved with dealing with the opioid crisis in this country. According to the Canadian Drug Policy Coalition (2012), naloxone is a safe, highly effective chemical compound that reverses the effects of opiates such as heroin. It has been used in clinical settings as an emergency treatment for opiate overdose for 40 years. Naloxone has been approved for use in Canada for over 40 years and is on the World Health Organization List of Essential Medicines. Naloxone has no potential for abuse — in the absence of narcotics it exhibits essentially no pharmacologic activity. Naloxone will work only for drugs in the opiate/opioid family — it is not effective for overdoses of other drugs such as cocaine.

As part of the strategy for harm reduction and prevention, many provinces across Canada make available take-home naloxone kits, which are provided free of cost from most pharmacies. These kits are also provided to all service providers who work with and for users of opioids, including needle-exchange programs, homeless shelters, the RCMP and other policing agencies, health-care facilities, first responders and drug users themselves. All Canadian provinces have created strategies for dealing with the opioid and drug overdose situation; many include the provision of safe-injection sites, which provide a safe, clean space for people to bring their own drugs to use in the presence of trained staff. As of August 22, 2024, according to the Government of Canada (2025b), there were forty-eight such sites, the majority located in Alberta, British Columbia, Saskatchewan, Ontario and Quebec.

Overall, the federal government has worked closely with the provinces to ensure that funding is available to provide more educational resources to help the public be more informed and aware of the difficulties impacted by these issues. It will be interesting to see if these strategies bring about the benefits we all wish for, but much needs to be done.

CONCLUSION

Clearly the issue of drug and opioids use is multifaceted in Canada. As we discussed in this chapter, all provinces and territories are trying to produce strategies for harm reduction and treatment options for those using these substances, for whatever reasons, and for those who care for them. Doubtless this will be a topic which will be discussed in this country and globally until more support and education is provided.

SELF-REFLECTION AND THOUGHTFUL CONVERSATIONS

1. What do you think can be done about drug and opioid trafficking in Canada, and what are some of the more global issues that connect to Canada?
2. Were you aware that opioid addiction is an issue for older adults? What social factors do you think contribute to this hidden epidemic?

IN-CLASS ASSIGNMENTS

1. In small groups, discuss the reasons why people consume alcohol, tobacco and other drugs.
2. Make a list of the ways in which you hear about drug and opioid addiction and concerns in your community and share these experiences in class.
3. In small groups, discuss some social solutions to the drug addiction issues discussed in this chapter.

Chapter Ten

CROSS-CULTURAL VARIATIONS IN DEATH AND DYING

Zohreh BayatRizi

(This chapter was written by Dr. Zohreh BayatRizi, an associate professor in the Sociology Department, University of Alberta, whose research interests include sociology of death and grief, sociology of Iran, history of sociology, law and society, and medical sociology.)

CULTURE AND DEATH ARE CLOSELY INTERCONNECTED. Social thinkers like Ernest Becker (1973) and Hanna Arendt (1958) argue that culture is a response to our knowledge of mortality. It helps us to cope with our awareness of our end. It does so partly by giving meaning to death and by wrapping it in customs, rituals, language, art and beliefs. Culture provides guidance for the most appropriate and meaningful ways to live and die. Our reactions to death and dying are not merely biological or instinctive. We learn how we are supposed to think, feel and behave in times of loss and grief from the social and cultural values and expectations of those around us. For survivors, these cultural elements can act as a source of familiar comfort. This is evidenced in a research project I carried out among Iranian Canadians in Edmonton, after the Ukrainian Flight PS752 disaster in 2020, which killed many Iranian Canadians. A major public ceremony was held in which dignitaries of all levels of government attended, including the prime minister. Apart from a Persian song, the ceremony mostly included speeches in English. Afterwards, while people of Iranian origin were thankful for the support they received, they felt the ceremony was emotionally lacking because it did not include familiar cultural elements associated with "mourning ceremonies" in Iran. As a result, some in the community held a more private, Persian-language commemorative event afterwards. But culture can feel constraining for some people, and, in some cases, instead of comforting the survivors, cultural beliefs can lead to the dismissal or even aggravation of their sorrow.

The above anecdote gives me an opportunity to situate myself in this chapter. I was born in Iran and lived the first twenty-five years of my life there, after which I came to Canada as a graduate student and stayed as a permanent resident. My interest in death and dying stems from life experiences and cultural observations in Iran and Canada, including living during a devastating eight-year war between Iran and Iraq in the 1980s, losing a beloved uncle to suicide in the prime of his life, witnessing end-of-life cultural practices and doing research on the experience of grief among immigrants in Canada. In this chapter, I occasionally discuss my research or cultural observations on death and grief in Iran.

When people refer to "culture," they often refer to things like shared beliefs, eating practices, clothing, language, symbolic representations of life events and rituals. In a sense, culture is the way of life of a people. Cultural practices include the institutional requirements of dying, such as death certificates and wills, the religious or spiritual aspects, like funeral services and memorials, the kinds and colours of clothes we wear, the types of food we serve, the kinds of music we want played, if any, and the words we use to define death and to comfort the bereaved.

There are two major ways to understand culture. Sometimes we think of culture as a common way of life that is shared among a community, and everyone adheres to it. This is the case when we say things like: "Christians believe in life after death" or "Hindus believe in reincarnation." But culture is often more like a toolkit (Swidler 1986), offering a variety of options that members of a community can pick and choose from. Cultures are also often far from homogeneous. There are internal discord and struggles within every cultural community over the right way of doing things, the right beliefs, rituals, dress, speech, etc. Ask ten different people of Italian heritage in Canada about the "authentic" way to make spaghetti, and you might get ten different answers. Sometimes internal heterogeneity and conflicts within a culture represent power-related, class-based, gendered or generational dynamics. Those who have power and privilege, as well as older generations, might want to maintain the cultural status quo, while others might be more interested in cultural innovation and change. Lastly, cultures are dynamic. They change due to the above-mentioned conflicts and struggles or because of encounters with new ideas and cultures or out of necessity. While this chapter discusses death-related cultural beliefs and practices within various cultural communities in Canada and around the world, it is important to keep in mind that individuals in these communities do not necessarily subscribe to the same beliefs or engage in the same practices.

RELIGION

Religion is a major cultural force which plays a particularly important role in how people make sense of and deal with death and loss. Those who hold strong religious beliefs may take death-related rituals seriously because they are consequential for the dying person. In some religions, the soul's journey to the afterlife depends on proper religious rituals, including proper burial, prayers and emotional expressions among the survivors. For example, in the Roman Catholic Church, the sacrament of anointing the sick (formerly extreme unction), to cleanse the soul of sin before death so it can enter heaven, is given to the dying person prior to their last breath (or after if before is not possible). Among the Kanak People of New Caledonia, rituals are performed after death to revitalize the spiritual body of the deceased in the invisible world. Mourning ceremonies are important in the successful ancestralization of the deceased (Simon 2021: 31–2). In Bali, Indonesia, the main purpose of funeral rituals is to calm the deceased, who are confused at this time, and prevent them from going around and haunting (Djelantik et al. 2021: 776). In many Islamic traditions, for the afterlife of the spirit to begin, it is important to bury the deceased as soon as possible, ideally on the day of death, according to strict rituals for washing and wrapping the body, praying over it and burying it. Sometimes, even those who are not strict believers adhere to religious funeral and grieving rituals either for conformity with community expectations or because these rituals provide a tried-and-tested script for what to do and how to proceed in a time of crisis.

LANGUAGE AND ART

Language is also a cultural element that has significance for death and grief. Language, both oral and written, refers to the verbal and symbolic means used to communicate with one another. Different people not only speak different languages, but they also invoke different symbols to refer to the same things. For instance, different cultural groups might mean different things by the words "death," "illness," "disease" and "the body," as well as the euphemisms for describing death and the metaphors for defying it. The

English language has many words, metaphors and euphemisms for death; some are more direct, such as "death" and "to die." Others are medical and sanitized, such as "expired," "succumbed" and "flatlined." There are also many metaphorical words and phrases: "passed away," "departed," "met their maker," "bit the dust," "made the ultimate sacrifice," "kicked the bucket," "received their wings," etc. In some cultures, people try not to mention death directly. In China, death is an inauspicious topic, and the word 死 sǐ (death) is avoided. Even the number four is avoided because it sounds like sǐ. Instead of saying someone died, many people in China say that the person "left the world" or "departed like an immortal." On the subreddit r/AskEurope, there is a thread discussing euphemisms for death across Europe, which includes the Finnish phrases "to sleep away" or "to go from time to eternity." These metaphors are often thought to be a reflection of taboos and concealment around death (Wachowski and Sullivan, 2021).

Closely connected to language are symbols, as well as art and literature. Many symbols and icons invoke notions of death and dying. They include coffins, black armbands, skull and crossbones, scythes and the red poppies worn on Remembrance Day. In Iran, red tulips symbolize those who have fallen for the country. Graveyards provide a perfect example of the types of symbols and monuments which people use to remember and honour their dead.

The world of art and literature has long served as a space to ponder death and its meaning. Some examples include cemetery plots, plays, novels, opera, popular music, painting and sculpture. The Ancient Mesopotamian poem *The Epic of Gilgamesh*, Shakespeare's play *Hamlet*, Gustav Klimt's painting *Death and Life* and Tolstoy's novella *The Death of Ivan Ilyich* are all striking and enduring examples. One of my students gave a presentation on Pablo Picasso's 1937 painting *Guernica*, which he painted in response to the bombardment of Guernica by Nazi and Fascist forces. It originally received mixed reactions due to its unconventional approach but is now embraced by the people of Spain and is widely considered to be the most powerful anti-war painting in the world. In the world of architecture, the Pyramids of Egypt were built to house the tombs of the dead in much the same way that crypts and mausoleums were built to do so in Europe and North America. The Canadian Centre for Architecture, located in Montreal, has a fascinating photographic essay entitled *The Architecture of Death* on display on its website.

FOOD

In many cultures, food consumption around a person's death is culturally regulated, and there are specific expectations around what, if anything, can be eaten. Some cultures prefer fasting while in other cultures, food is an integral part of death rituals. Many people in Canada offer food to those who attend the wake or celebration of life. Conversely, in many Canadian communities, after an individual dies, neighbours and others come with food, usually casseroles and baked goods to help the bereaved. The assumption is that the family will have many chores to attend to rather than cook for themselves and others who may come to offer condolences. In Iran, certain sweets, such as dates and *halva* (a buttery flour paste), are associated with death. They are offered to visitors and passersby on behalf of the deceased, with the implicit expectation that those who take the offering will say a prayer for the deceased, asking for God's mercy. Those who participate in the funeral are offered a feast afterwards.

CLOTHING

Clothing is another major cultural element in death and grief, including the dressing of the corpse and of mourners. Among most Muslims, the corpse is completely wrapped in plain white, unsewn pieces of cloth, three pieces for men and five for women. In many European traditions, the deceased is dressed in formal clothes or in the outfit chosen by them when alive. Some Tibetan sky burials discourage against clothing because the goal is to return the body to nature.

In many countries, black and other dark colours are seen as appropriate colours for mourners. In China, Tibet and India, white is preferred as the colour of clothing for mourning because it represents rebirth and renewal. In the Hindu religion, mourners ceremonially bathe and wash the clothes they wore to the funeral. The garments worn for sitting shiva in the Jewish tradition are often torn during the mourning period.

GRIEF ACROSS CULTURES

Sociologically speaking, grief is an emotional experience that unfolds in a social and cultural environment. As sociologists of emotions argue, our emotions "are experienced and have meaning in the context of our social relations" (Bericat 2016: 495). Group membership, social background, identity, culture, social structures and power relations play a role in whether and how we experience certain emotions. Culture shapes what we feel when we experience grief, how we express grief and how long we are expected to maintain the public role of grieving. Mourning takes place within cultural frameworks that dictate who can grieve, how grief should be expressed and what constitutes "proper" mourning. Social norms police grief expressions, reinforcing the idea that certain emotional reactions are culturally acceptable while others are discouraged (Silverman et al. 2021: 3). As in any other social experience, not everyone's grief is equally validated and supported in society (Doka 1989).

As a socially situated emotional experience, grief is bound up with social and cultural forces, rules and norms. Across cultures, it is mediated by rituals, traditions and aesthetic experiences that help individuals navigate loss. Many societies see grief not as a problem to be solved, but as a process to be honoured through collective practices that reaffirm social bonds and continuity with the deceased. In some societies, public displays of grief are expected, while in others, grief is meant to be contained and internalized. Below, we examine cultural variations in grief expression, ritual mourning, disenfranchised grief and the social policing of mourning practices, highlighting how cultural norms shape grief responses worldwide.

Cultural Scripts and Ritual Frameworks

Rituals serve as structured mechanisms that facilitate emotional processing, reinforce communal ties and provide meaning to loss. Mourning practices, whether public or private, offer structured ways for individuals to cope with loss and maintain, or break, bonds with the deceased. Rituals serve multiple functions: they reaffirm social connections, regulate emotional expressions and help individuals make sense of their loss. For example, the recitation of Mourner's Kaddish in Jewish traditions is not just an individual act of remembrance but a collective affirmation of continuity and religious identity (Silverman 2021).

Cultures provide "scripts" that dictate how grief should be expressed, including expectations regarding emotional display, duration and appropriate behaviour for mourners. In some cultures, emotional restraint in mourning is highly valued. Many people of Western origins value emotional restraint during funerals. Relatives suppress excessive crying and emotional outbursts. Western norms often conceptualize grief as an individual psychological process requiring emotional resolution. Likewise, in Japan, silence and solemnity are central to the grieving process, with the bereaved expected to demonstrate endurance and inner strength rather than overt emotional distress (Kim 2015: 18). Similarly, widows in Taiwan are expected to suppress outward expressions of grief, as crying in front of the deceased is discouraged (Hsu et al. 2004).

Other cultures embrace and even encourage public mourning. The Dagara People of Burkina Faso believe that grief must be passionately expressed and that suppressed grief can harm both the living and the dead. Funerals include music and drumming to channel sorrow constructively (Tateo 2023: 426). The Ayoreo People of Paraguay engage in ritual mourning through song. Weeping alone is not enough. The grieving must accompany weeping with words, and only then will they be able to fully release their grief. Otherwise, the suppression of grief leads to a potentially dangerous buildup of emotions. The songs also help the Ayoreo community to collectively process loss while reaffirming social cohesion (Otaegui 2021). In Iran, music selection and religious lamentations by hired professionals at funerals create a sombre, poignant and sentimental vibe and act to legitimate (even elicit) public and collective displays of sorrow, such as weeping.

The duration of mourning also varies widely across cultures. Many societies treat grief as a linear, time-bound emotional experience, where people are expected to mourn for a culturally specific period. Other societies see grief as an ongoing process that unfolds and evolves over long durations of time. Among the Lihir People of Papua New Guinea, mourning is divided into two phases: an initial period of intense, public emotional displays followed by a later phase that emphasizes moving forward and remembering the deceased in a structured way (Hemer 2010). In Egyptian society, grief is expected to be long-lasting and highly visible, with extended bereavement and muted depression being socially acceptable (Rosenblatt 2008: 212). Mexican Día de los Muertos challenges Western ideas of detachment by celebrating the deceased as part of the community rather than encouraging people to "move on" (Tateo 2023: 416).

Mediterranean cultures, such as those in Greece, Italy and Spain, have historically allowed for prolonged public mourning, especially for women, who used to be expected to wear black for years and refrain from public celebrations (Doka 1989: 42). Charlotte Hilberdink, Kevin Ghainder, Alexandre Dubanchet et al. (2023: 3) cite multiple examples of the culturally prescribed duration of grief: traditional Chinese mourning for parents and children extends for three years as a sign of filial piety. In Bali, Indonesia, mourning rituals can continue for up to a decade, involving multiple ceremonies to ensure the well-being of the deceased's soul. In contrast, in Germany, mourning typically lasts for a year, aligning with societal expectations that grief should be resolved within a defined period.

In Iran, many people in the mainstream Shia sect wear black for forty days when mourning the death of a family member. After this period, family and friends might bring them new, non-black clothes to change into and signal a return to a measure of normalcy. Traditionally, people refrained from discretionary activities during this period and avoided unnecessary grooming, such as getting a new haircut, hair dye or shaving the face for men. With the ubiquity of office-type jobs, which require certain business-like aesthetics, and the prevalence of middle-class consumerist lifestyles, it is no longer possible or desirable for many people to continue this tradition.

In some societies, grief is viewed as a process that ends in detachment. In fact, in some cultures, grieving is structured to facilitate forgetting rather than remembering the dead. For instance, among the Achuar people of Ecuador, survivors actively distance themselves from the deceased's name, image and memory (Rosenblatt 2008: 213). In contrast, in many societies, people maintain ongoing relationships with the dead and engage in rituals meant to remember and honour them. In some traditions, ancestors are considered active participants in the lives of the living, requiring ongoing rituals and offerings. For the Kanak of New Caledonia, grief is culturally shaped through ritual actions that emphasize the continuing relationship between the living and the deceased through regular offerings, storytelling and spiritual invocations (Simon 2021: 32). My parents in Iran visit their relatives' graves every Thursday afternoon, and I remember as a child my mother instructed me to turn on the lights inside and outside the house on Thursdays after sunset because that is when the spirits of the dead relatives visit us and we want the house to be bright and welcoming. Even though I have doubts about the spirits, I still think this is a nice way to remember our dead relatives on a regular and ongoing basis. Again, modern lifestyles have led to the demise of these traditions among many: Thursday evenings are the beginning of the weekend in Iran, and many people spend this time socializing or resting at home.

Cultural Policing of Grief

In a series of influential works on "disenfranchised grief," published since the 1980s, Doka argues that cultures have rules about *who* is entitled to grieve, *how* grief should be expressed and *what losses* are deemed worthy of public recognition. Grieving within these rules is supported by the community; otherwise, it is "disenfranchised," meaning it lacks social recognition. Disenfranchised grief happens when society does not validate the relationship between the griever and the deceased, does not acknowledge the significance of the loss or questions the legitimacy of the griever's emotions.

Regarding *who* can grieve, Doka (1989) describes cases in which individuals who lose an ex-spouse, an unborn child, a same-sex partner (in certain societies) or a pet may experience grief that is not socially accepted. In Italian and Hispanic cultures, the role of godparents is highly significant. If a godchild or godparent dies, grief is deeply felt and socially recognized, whereas in other cultures, such relationships might hold only symbolic meaning. Regarding *what* losses are worthy of public recognition, Doka argues that certain types of death, such as those resulting from suicide, drug overdose or criminal activity may bring stigma, leading to a lack of communal support for the bereaved.

As for *how* grief can be expressed, each society has distinct grieving rules, which determine acceptable mourning behaviours. In some cultures, stoicism and restraint are expected, while in others, loud lamentation and physical expressions of grief are encouraged. In many Western cultures, grief is seen as a private emotional process, and public expressions of sorrow may be limited. Funerals serve as the primary public ritual to acknowledge a death, but after the funeral, mourners are often expected to return quickly to normal life and work. These grieving rules manifest in laws, workplace bereavement policies and religious doctrines. For example, in some workplaces, bereavement leave is granted only for immediate family members, excluding losses such as close friends or other people considered family.

In an article critical of Doka's "disenfranchised grief," Patricia Robson and Tony Walter (2013) argue that the notion of "disenfranchisement" is binary. In reality, there is a "hierarchy of grief." Their research in the UK aims to illustrate how this hierarchy is formed based on people's relationship with the deceased: the closer you are to the deceased, the higher your grief is in the hierarchy. Whether grief is disenfranchised or merely placed low in a hierarchy, the bereaved are not always supported. While cultures are overall thought to help the bereaved by wrapping the grief experience in rituals, structures and collective empathy, they are not always supportive of all individual grief experiences in all situations.

Grief Pathology and Cultural Considerations for Bereavement Support

Modern psychology emphasizes the universality of emotions. From this perspective, grief is a universal human experience. Modern psychology also distinguishes between healthy/normal and unhealthy/abnormal emotional experiences. Sometimes what is considered normal or healthy depends on the cultural context. In many modern societies, especially those that are individualistic, consumerist and secular, grief is primarily a private experience that is expected to be resolved within a period of time. While the bereaved are given time and space to adjust, they are expected to accept the loss, detach from the lost person and "move on." People who grieve longer than "normal" or who do not properly detach from the lost loved ones are given a psychological diagnosis. The eleventh edition of the *International Classification of Diseases*, published by the WHO (ICD-11), and the latest edition of the *Diagnostic and Statistical Manual of Mental Disorder* (DSM-5-TR) have classifications for prolonged grief disorder (PGD). Most PGD research is based on Western populations and therefore it might not account for cultural differences. For example, while Cambodian refugees in the US view dreams and hallucinations of the deceased as a natural and meaningful part of the grieving process, Western cultures often pathologize these experiences, considering them symptoms of mental illness. Chinese bereaved individuals often report somatic symptoms, such as head, stomach, back pain; functional impairments, depression and emptiness, in response to loss, whereas Swiss parents who lose a child are more likely to experience intrusive thoughts and severe grief-related preoccupation (Hilberdink et al. 2023). These cultural differences suggest that standardized PGD criteria may not accurately reflect grief experiences worldwide.

Grief, while universal, is profoundly shaped by cultural, religious and social contexts. Whether through controlled expressions of sorrow, elaborate public mourning rituals or quiet introspection, societies across the world have developed diverse ways of grieving and making meaning out of loss. Modern grief research increasingly recognizes the importance of these varied perspectives, challenging one-size-fits-all models of bereavement and highlighting the richness of cultural approaches to mourning. Understanding these differences not only deepens our appreciation of global mourning traditions but also informs grief counselling.

MULTICULTURAL DEATH AND GRIEF PRACTICES IN CANADA

There is an incredible amount of diversity both *between* and *within* cultures. Inter- and intra-cultural diversity are a worthy topic to investigate in settings like Canada, which has always been a multicultural, multiethnic, multilingual and multireligious space, both before and after colonization. This book has a separate chapter dedicated to death-related cultural practices among Indigenous Peoples in Canada. In the next section, I focus on two other significant sources of death-related cultural diversity in Canada: immigration and religion.

Religious and Cultural Diversity in Canada

The Government of Canada (2022) produced a special report based on the 2021 Census, with the title *The Canadian Census: A Rich Portrait of the Country's Religious and Ethnocultural Diversity*. According to this report, more than 450 ethnic origins or ancestries were reported by the Canadian population, and more than 35.5 percent of people reported more than one origin. The British and French origins remain among the most common, but the composition of the population continues to evolve. The top five origins reported alone or in combination with other origins were: Canadian (5.7 million people), English (5.3 million), Irish (4.4 million), Scottish (4.4 million) and French (4.0 million). In addition, German (3.0 million), Chinese (1.7 million), Italian (1.5 million), Ukrainian (1.3 million) and East Indian (1.3 million) were each reported by at least a million people. The 2021 Census revealed that approximately 1.8 million people reported Indigenous ancestry. Among First Nations ancestries, the most common were Cree (250,000 people), Mi'kmaq (122,000), Ojibway (92,000) and Algonquin (56,000).

In that year, almost one in four Canadians (23 percent) were foreign-born, marking the highest proportion in over 150 years. Canada had 1.3 million new immigrants who had permanently settled between 2016 and 2021. These recent immigrants represented 3.5 percent of Canada's total population in 2021. Asia (including the Middle East) remains the top source continent of recent immigrants, with 62 percent of newcomers born in Asia. For the first time, Africa ranked second as a source continent of recent immigrants, with a share of 15.6 percent, surpassing Europe (10.1 percent). The report noted that the share of recent immigrants settling in the Prairie Provinces continued to grow: Alberta received 14.3 percent of new immigrants,

Manitoba 5.1 percent and Saskatchewan 4.7 percent. This marks a significant increase compared to previous decades. These findings underscore the ongoing diversification of the Canadian population, driven by immigration but also by evolving self-identification patterns; that is, by the fact that people change the way in which they report their identity over time.

It is important to note that people do not necessarily share the same cultural beliefs and practices with other people of the same national, ethnic or racial origin. A person emigrating from northern Spain will have grown up in a somewhat different cultural milieu than someone emigrating from southern Spain. A young adult emigrating from Colombia might have grown up in a different sub-cultural environment than a middle-aged person from that country. In addition, when people migrate, they adjust to the new setting in different ways. Some people seek the comforting familiarity of their cultural community. Others deliberately distance themselves from their culture of origin. Most engage in hybrid cultural practices, retaining some of their ethnic culture while adopting some mainstream Canadian cultural beliefs and practices.

The 2021 Census results indicate a continued decline in Christian affiliation and an increase in religious diversity as well as secular identification in Canada. Christianity remains the largest faith in Canada, with over 19.3 million people identifying as Christian, representing 53.3 percent of the population. However, this marks a significant decline from 67.3 percent in 2011 and 77.1 percent in 2001. Among Christian groups, Roman Catholics remain the largest, numbering 10.9 million people (29.9 percent). The United Church of Canada and the Anglican Church are the next biggest churches, followed by other Christian groups, including Orthodox Christians, Baptists and Pentecostals, which make up smaller percentages of the population.

The proportion of Canadians identifying as Muslim (4.9 percent), Hindu (2.3 percent) and Sikh (2.1 percent) has more than doubled over the past two decades. The Jewish and Buddhist populations remain relatively stable at 0.9 percent and 1 percent, respectively. In Ontario and British Columbia, the proportion of people adhering to non-Christian religions is the highest in Canada, at 16.3 percent and 13.7 percent, respectively.

One of the most notable trends is the significant rise in the population with no religious affiliation. In 2021, 12.6 million people (34.6 percent) reported having no religious affiliation, more than doubling from 16.5 percent in 2001. This trend is particularly pronounced among younger generations and urban populations. British Columbia and Yukon stand out for having the highest proportion of people reporting no religious affiliation, at 52.1 percent and 59.7 percent, respectively.

Even among those who report religious affiliation, one cannot assume active participation in worship, adherence to specific religious beliefs or engagement in regular prayer. A 2022 poll by Angus Reid Institute categorizes Canadians into four groups: non-believers (19 percent), spiritually uncertain (47 percent), privately faithful (19 percent) and religiously committed (16 percent). The latter category indicates a high level of worship attendance, prayer and belief in God. Except for Evangelical Christians, only a minority of people who self-identify as belonging to one of the other main religious groups (Roman Catholic, mainstream Protestant, Muslim, Hindu, Sikh) classify themselves as religiously committed. Many who identify with these religions are non-believers or spiritually uncertain. A paradoxical finding was that many people who belong to a major religion do not believe in God or a higher power, while 8 percent of those who self-identify as non-believers firmly believe in God or a higher power. Some of the believers said they never pray, while some of the non-believers said they regularly pray. These findings suggest that belonging to a religion does not necessarily mean practising it actively or holding firm doctrinal beliefs. Instead, they reflect a broader trend of individual spiritual expression over institutional religious participation.

Sometimes, diversity of religious practice can stem from personal and individual preferences. In other cases, it can be attributed to the diversity of sects and churches within a religion. Most religions have at least a few sects, so even among firm believers of a religion, there are vast differences in beliefs and practices. For instance, in the Muslim religion, there are two major sects, Sunni and Shia, along with smaller sects. Within the majority of Sunni Muslims, the most conservative schools regard frequent grave visitation with caution because it might lead to excessive veneration of the dead. They also advocate against any form of headstones to prevent reverence of specific burial sites. The more traditional Sunni schools, as well as Shia followers, encourage regular visits to the grave and have no reservations about using headstones to mark graves. When caring for persons from any faith or spirituality, it is important to ask them and their important ones how they use their beliefs at the time leading up to and after death.

End-of-Life Care and Cultural Diversity in Canada

In Canada, a highly multicultural nation, end-of-life care practices can vary across ethnic, religious and linguistic communities. While higher-income countries, including Canada, often delegate death-related tasks to professionals, such as funeral directors, cultural traditions and familial expectations continue to influence end-of-life decision making.

A 2021 scoping review of Canadian palliative care literature emphasizes that cultural competency, sensitivity and accessibility are critical in ensuring effective and inclusive end-of-life care (Monette 2021). Cultural competency is not simply about awareness — it requires active engagement and adaptation. As one hospice care provider noted, "You can't just learn about cultural competency once and be done with it. Each patient brings a different perspective, and it's our job to meet them where they are" (Mian and Rejnö 2024: 11). This is particularly important when addressing deeply personal matters such as death and grief.

Cultural and religious beliefs can influence the dying process and end-of-life care. An enduring and complex issue in end-of-life care is cultural preferences for or against disclosure of terminal illness. Many people of Western origins prefer complete transparency from their health-care team. If they have a terminal diagnosis, they prefer to know. Canadian medical guidelines and rules also require health-care professionals to openly and directly communicate diagnosis and prognosis, as well as treatment options, with the patient. However, not all people and cultures adhere to this rule. In many cultures, discussing death is often seen as a bad omen that invites misfortune. Many cultures see hope as an important factor in prognosis and recovery. In these cultures, families might create a separate channel of communication with the providing physicians to discuss diagnosis and prognosis of a potentially terminal illness, especially cancer. This was the case when my aunt was diagnosed with an aggressive form of cancer in Tehran, and her family withheld information from her regarding how aggressive her cancer was until the end. This is a common practice in Iran, and it aligns with the cultural belief that it is cruel to tell a person they have a potentially fatal illness or that they are dying. Many Iranians believe that devastating health news will shatter the patient's hope and optimism and will lead to worse health outcomes. In contrast, when I told my American husband about this practice, he strongly disapproved and made sure to tell me that in a similar situation, he demands complete transparency. I have lived in Canada for twenty-seven years now, and I understand and respect both sides, and when it comes to myself, I would also prefer full transparency so I can plan accordingly.

Several studies document complexities arising from cultural communication preferences in end-of-life care in Canada. A palliative care social worker in Vancouver notes, "Some Chinese families insist that doctors use softer language when discussing prognosis, avoiding words like 'death' or 'terminal' and instead saying 'serious illness' or 'long recovery'" (Mian and Rejnö 2024: 4). This reluctance to engage in open discussions can sometimes lead to delayed hospice referrals and unnecessary suffering. One poignant example comes from a study on cross-cultural hospice care: a South Asian family requested that doctors not inform their elderly mother of her terminal diagnosis, fearing it would cause unnecessary distress (Nayfeh 2023). This is a practice rooted in the belief that discussing death openly might hasten it. The attending physician struggled with this request, torn between medical ethics and the family's cultural expectations. Such situations illustrate how different worldviews on autonomy and protection play out in medical decision making (Tareen 2024: 15).

Similarly, palliative care services are not always perceived in the same way across cultures. For some patients, faith influences their acceptance of pain management. Some devout Catholics might refuse palliative sedation despite severe pain because they believe suffering can bring them closer to God. Some devout Muslims might also prefer to avoid opioids for pain relief, fearing that such medications may cloud their consciousness and interfere with their final prayers. The US National Library of Medicine provides a summary of how religious beliefs might influence patient preferences in palliative care (Givler et. al. 2018).

Hospice care is also influenced by culture. The hospice movement began in England to stop futile aggressive treatments at the end of life in hospitals and instead provide comforting care to the dying in an institutional setting that accepts death and prepares people for it. While many people in Canada embrace hospice as a compassionate and necessary service, others, particularly immigrant communities, may associate it with giving up on life. A hospice volunteer program in Canada found that many Filipino families strongly preferred to care for dying loved ones at home rather than in a hospice facility, due to the belief that "family care is the highest form of love" (Monette 2021: 156). This cultural belief clashes with the realities of life and work in Canada, especially the scarcity of support for families who take care of the dying. One Filipino caregiver in the same study shares, "My father wanted to die at home, but we had no nurses or home-care support. I had to leave my job to take care of him. It was hard, but it was my duty." Another study examined recruitment for hospice care volunteers among immigrant communities in Southern Ontario and found that a main barrier to volunteer recruitment is that some immigrants see hospice care as formal and structured, while they prefer a more informal and family-based approach to end-of-life care (Cait and Lafreniere 2024).

Ultimately, ensuring compassionate end-of-life care might require moving beyond rigid protocols to engage with individuals and families. We can neither ignore cultural and religious diversity in end-of-life-care nor assume that people are shaped by their cultures in a deterministic way. As one provider put it, "Dying is a universal experience, but the way we approach it is deeply personal. We need to listen more and assume less" (Mian and Rejnö 2024: 11).

CONCLUSION

Culture is a source of meaning and a repertoire of approved actions during times of death and grief. People's relationship to their culture falls within a broad range from strict adherence to individualistic distance. In modern societies, people might draw on some cultural elements and personal beliefs to make sense of mortality and guide themselves and others through grief. As sociologist Norbert Elias (2001) remarks, in modern societies many people might not know how to react in the presence of the dying and the grieving. The usual cultural expressions seem formulaic, and many people feel embarrassed or unable to freely express their own thoughts and feelings.

As many Western societies have culturally diversified, more people might hesitate about how to act in their encounters with the dying and grieving because they do not know about the culture and beliefs of other people and they might be worried about saying or doing something offensive. But ultimately, while it is important to be aware of cultural differences in how people approach death and grief, we cannot assume that people are shaped by their cultures in a determinist way. People are not culturally programmed robots. Instead, each individual finds their own way to internalize and personalize their culture.

SELF-REFLECTION AND THOUGHTFUL CONVERSATIONS

1. What is your ethnicity, and what are some related beliefs and practices?
2. What specifically Canadian rituals and cultural traditions exist around death and disposal in your ethnic and cultural community?
3. How will your ethnicity and culture impact your dying?
4. To what extent are you representative of your cultural and ethnic background?
5. How do you think people's cultural and religious preferences should be treated in end-of-life care?

IN-CLASS ASSIGNMENTS

1. Divide the class into groups of 3–4 students. Each group chooses one of the cultures discussed in the chapter and tries to find as much information about it as possible through a web search or scan of existing academic articles. The task is to imagine how the death- and grief-related rituals of the chosen culture might undergo changes if they adopt a Western, individualistic, consumerist lifestyle or if members of it immigrate to Canada. Would that be a good thing or a bad thing?

Chapter Eleven

INDIGENOUS PERSPECTIVES ON DEATH AND GRIEF

Audrey Medwayosh

(This chapter was written by Audrey Medwayosh, who is Potwatomi, a citizen of the Wasauksing Nation and a PhD student at the University of Alberta in the Faculty of Native Studies. Their research interests include death and grief, Indigenous feminist theory, abolition and decolonization.)

INDIGENOUS PEOPLES WHOSE LANDS ARE now occupied by Canada constitute 1.8 million of Canada's population of about forty million people (Indigenous Services Canada 2023). The Indigenous population consists of people who identify as First Nations, Métis and Inuit and includes a wide variety of culturally distinct groups within each category. There are over 1,100 different Indigenous Nations in Canada, and each nation has its own unique approach to art, song, dance, spirituality, land-based teachings, and death and grief rituals. While Indigenous Peoples make up only 4.6 percent of the population in Canada, they are often overrepresented in statistics on health inequities and have a higher mortality rate than the non-Indigenous population (Reidpath and Allotley 2003; Roy and Marcellus 2019). The disparities in Indigenous health can be explained through an understanding of the processes of colonization, which have had detrimental effects on Indigenous Peoples since it first began.

COLONIAL HISTORY

The implementation of policies and procedures designed to erase Indigenous Peoples in Canada was a strategic move on behalf of the newly developing nation. The success of the colonial project was dependent upon the acquisition of land, which required Indigenous Peoples to be either assimilated into settler colonial society or eradicated altogether. Canada's history of formal Indigenous dispossession began with the Royal Proclamation in 1763 and was further reified with the creation of the North-West Mounted Police (later becoming the RCMP) to control the Indigenous population in 1873 and the subsequent implementation of the Indian Act of 1876 (Borrows 1997; Campbell 2000). The Indian Act granted the Canadian government authority over the management of Indigenous Peoples, their lands and other natural resources, monies, spiritual practices, education and enfranchisement. In the decades following the creation of the Indian Act, Canada carried out a series of systemic and structural policies to further its mandate: residential schools, the pass system, the denial of the right to vote until 1960 for First Nations Peoples, the Sixties Scoop, the Millennium Scoop, and the insufficient and ineffective inquiry into the epidemic of Missing and Murdered Indigenous Women, Girls and Two-Spirit (MMIG2S) people. There is no doubt that these approaches have had a detrimental effect on the health and well-being of Indigenous Peoples.

SOCIAL DETERMINANTS OF HEALTH

The enduring legacy of these colonial systems and structures has been far-reaching and long-lasting. In particular, their impacts can be seen in the inequities experienced by Indigenous Peoples in the social determinants of health. The social determinants of health are social factors, as opposed to medical factors, which influence a person's health and well-being. The WHO lists the following examples: income and social protection; education; unemployment and job insecurity; working life conditions; food insecurity; housing; basic amenities and the environment; early childhood development; social inclusion and non-discrimination; structural conflict; and access to affordable health services of decent quality (WHO 2025).

Indigenous Peoples also have their own determinants of health that contribute to their overall well-being. These may include

- continued kinship bonds;
- relationships with Elders;
- land-based teachings;
- traditional diet; and
- access to cultural and spiritual practices. (First Nations Health Authority 2025)

For Indigenous Peoples, both Western and Indigenous determinants of health have been disrupted by colonization. For example, consider food insecurity. Indigenous Peoples living in Northern communities have reached what some call a "crisis level" of food insecurity, which is driven by poverty and lack of availability, along with disruptions to land-based food sovereignty and Traditional Indigenous Knowledge. A Canadian study on childhood nutrition by Anna Banerji, Veronique Anne Pelletier, Rodney Haring et al. (2023) in remote Northern communities shows that inadequate access to appropriate food can follow children through to adulthood and impact their overall quality of life. Food insecurity "can lead to malnutrition and can have significant impacts on the physical, intellectual, emotional and social development of a child, often with lasting effects across the life course" (1). The impacts of food insecurity also show up in the Indigenous population in the above-average rates of type 2 diabetes, which reduces their life span. Food insecurity is a good example of how colonial disruptions to traditional lifeways engender inequity in the social determinants of health and impact mortality rates.

INDIGENOUS MORTALITY RATES AND THE SOCIAL DETERMINANTS OF HEALTH

Indigenous people have an average life expectancy that is 12–15 years lower than the national average (Park 2021), and they are more likely to die from violent and untimely deaths, such as suicide, homicide, accidents and avoidable health-related deaths. Further deepening the disparity is the fact that Indigenous people living on-reserve experience higher occurrences of violent death than Indigenous people living off-reserve. The disparity between Indigenous and non-Indigenous life expectancy has been known for decades. However, few studies have looked at the specific details that contribute to Indigenous mortality rates. Only recently have studies been aimed at understanding the underlying mechanisms that contribute to those higher mortality rates. The Canadian Public Health Association (2025) explains the disparities:

> Indigenous (First Nations, Inuit, and Métis) Peoples in Canada experience some of the most significant health inequities due to historical and systemic barriers to healthcare access, socio-economic challenges, and the effects of colonialism. Addressing these inequities is not only a matter of social justice but also a critical public health priority. The Canadian

federal government must take an active role in addressing these disparities, ensuring that Indigenous peoples have access to quality healthcare and the resources needed to achieve better health outcomes.

More recent studies aim to show "detailed information on mortality rates and causes of death for First Nations men and women on a national scope" (Park 2021: 4) by examining cause-specific mortality rates for on- and off-reserve Indigenous people via data from Canadian Census Health and Environment Cohort. Jungwee Park's study showed that two-thirds of mortality rates for Indigenous Peoples were caused by unintentional injuries, diabetes, suicide, assault, heart diseases, and chronic liver disease and cirrhosis, with on-reserve Indigenous people experiencing higher rates of each compared to off-reserve Indigenous people. The mortality rate difference between Indigenous and non-Indigenous people was greater for people under the age of 50 as well. Many people feel that these premature deaths were avoidable, and it is undeniable that the underlying social conditions are a result of colonization and that this long history has contributed to these preventable deaths. By applying a deeper understanding of the impact of colonization, death can be understood as systemic and structurally based, versus rooted in individual choices and behaviours.

Rates of Homicide, Suicide and Other Violent Deaths

The following statistics on Indigenous mortality rates illustrate exactly how disparities in social inequities impact the lives of Indigenous people:

- Homicide rates for Indigenous people are six times higher than the rates for non-Indigenous people.
- Suicide rates are three times higher for Indigenous people than non-Indigenous people, and Indigenous men have a higher rate of suicide than Indigenous women.
- Indigenous people have a rate of accidental death that is 2.6 times higher than non-Indigenous people.
- Indigenous people account for 10 percent of overdose deaths, despite being only 4.6 percent of the overall population. (David and Jaffray 2022; Kumar and Tjepkema 2019; Lavalley, Kastor, Valleriani and McNeil 2018)

Infant Mortality Rates

Indigenous people have higher infant mortality rates across all cultural groups when compared to non-Indigenous people.

- Inuit have a 3.9 times higher infant mortality rate.
- First Nations have a 2.3 times higher infant mortality rate.
- Métis have a 1.9 times higher infant mortality rate (Public Health Agency Canada 2018).

MEDICAL RACISM

Because of the insidious nature of systemic and structural racism, it is difficult to pinpoint precisely how many Indigenous people die from medical racism. However, we do know that medical racism disproportionately affects all members of the Black, Indigenous and People of Colour (BIPOC) community. A 2023 survey showed that up to 30 percent of Indigenous people living off-reserve reported experiencing some form of racism from a medical professional in the preceding twelve months (Statistics Canada 2024). Medical racism contributes to higher mortality rates for Indigenous people because it causes distrust towards the medical system and medical professionals, preventing people from seeking out much-needed treatment, which lowers their lifespan. Worst-case scenarios of medical racism result in death when health-care professionals dismiss the valid concerns of Indigenous people, chalking their symptoms up to racist tropes.

One of the most notorious cases of death by medical racism is the case of Joyce Echaquan, a 37-year-old Atikamekw mother who used her remaining moments to record hospital staff making racist remarks about her and dismissing her pain as symptoms of withdrawal from addiction despite Joyce having a pre-existing heart condition. Joyce died in her hospital bed of a pulmonary embolism while the staff told her she was "stupid as hell" and "only good for sex" (BBC 2021). Joyce's death was ruled by coroners to have been caused by racism. This incident occurred in 2020, and a group of concerned community members continue their fight to get Joyce's Principle legally recognized:

> Joyce's Principle aims to guarantee to all Indigenous people the right of equitable access, without any discrimination, to all social and health services, as well as the right to enjoy the best

possible physical, mental, emotional and spiritual health. Joyce's Principle requires the recognition and respect of Indigenous people's traditional and living knowledge in all aspects of health.
(Principe de Joyce 2024)

The above case studies and statistics show that higher-than-average mortality rates for Indigenous people are connected to colonization and social inequities. As Park indicated in his study, many deaths among Indigenous people are preventable. Indigenous health and wellness need to be addressed at the foundational level by increasing access to both Western and Indigenous social determinants of health, ensuring positive health outcomes for the entire Indigenous population.

CONTEMPORARY INDIGENOUS APPROACHES TO DEATH CARE

A presentation of Indigenous mortality rates in Canada can leave you with a feeling of hopelessness, particularly if you are Indigenous. However, it is important to note that Indigenous Peoples have long supported their own practices of care and well-being and continue to do so, despite colonization. Indigenous people take care of their living and dead by, for example, building and operating their own funeral homes and training and serving as death doulas. Death-care practices and institutions are ways that Indigenous people are supporting their own end-of-life processes in culturally meaningful ways. The Aboriginal Funeral Chapel in Winnipeg, Manitoba, is one such example. The chapel, which has been operating since 1991, serves over sixty nations in the province. Its website describes their organization, simultaneously highlighting the need for Indigenous-led funeral services: "Aboriginal customs surrounding death are distinct from the funeral practices of most others in our society so we focus on supporting the traditions and cultural rituals that provide those we serve with comfort and a sense of dignity at a time of loss." The chapel is open twenty-four hours, which accommodates cultural practices like wakes, and has a kitchen for use by their patrons, enabling grieving families to hold feasts, as is customary for many Indigenous groups.

Indigenous Funeral Homes

While a funeral chapel in an urban centre is good for servicing the wide range of people belonging to diverse Indigenous groups, some prefer to build a funeral home on their own nation. The Peepeekisis Cree Nation in Saskatchewan began construction of their nation-run funeral home in

June 2025, which will make it one of the only Indigenous nations in Canada to have their own funeral home (Favel 2024). The creation of institutions like these supports Indigenous sovereignty around culturally appropriate approaches to death care.

Death Doulas and End-of-Life Care

In recent years, there has been an increase in Indigenous death doulas. Typically, a doula is associated with bringing babies into this world and supporting the family through the birthing process. A death doula is much like a birth doula — they are someone who provides support to individuals and family members during a major life transition. In the case of death doulas, however, that life transition is end of life. Death doulas can provide respite for tired family members who need a break from the constant demands of care for their dying loved one. They can provide bedside companionship for the dying person or help cook meals and tidy the house to give the caregiver a break. Death doulas are also familiar with the laws regarding death in their province and able to advise the grieving family on what their rights and the rights of the deceased are. An Indigenous death doula performs all the typical services while also providing culturally appropriate support, and they are aware of and trained to deal with any systemic racism that Indigenous families and individuals experience in the medical system.

Many non-Indigenous end-of-life care professionals have also been working on being better prepared to support Indigenous people during periods of death and grief. The website Canadian Virtual Hospice offers free culturally specific training units on death and grief to support professionals who may be working with people from different cultures, including First Nations, Métis and Inuit Peoples. There are multiple videos one can watch, which share stories and experiences from Indigenous people on death, grief and the spiritual practices associated with both. According to the site, the resources on death and grief across different cultures are designed for the following:

- Healthcare providers can easily access evidence-informed, leading tools to better care for and communicate with people living with illness and their families.
- Educators can access content to supplement lectures and develop assignments for students.
- Researchers can share their latest findings, enabling healthcare providers to stay on top of important developments. (Canadian Virtual Hospice 2025)

From Indigenous-run and -owned funeral homes to Indigenous death doulas and the efforts of non-Indigenous medical professionals, culturally specific training and services provide meaningful pathways to navigating the challenging and complex experience of death and grief. Death and mortality rates look different today than they did prior to colonization, and it is important to note how these ways have shifted and what has remained through cultural adaptation.

INDIGENOUS MORTALITY PRE- AND POST-CONTACT

It is difficult to know precise pre-colonial population numbers in North America (an important geographical distinction since Indigenous groups were nomadic and colonial borders did not yet exist). With many points of entry for settlers across Turtle Island and its neighbouring land masses, historical accounts of local demographic information vary, and historians have yet to agree on a number for the pre-contact Indigenous population. Estimates suggest that the Indigenous population was anywhere from eight million to a hundred million (Dunbar-Ortiz 2014). What is known is that contact with Europeans resulted in the spread of foreign diseases to which Indigenous populations had little to no immunity. Indigenous populations everywhere were overwhelmed by influenza, smallpox, measles, mumps, whooping cough, tuberculosis, typhoid and diphtheria. The rapid spread of disease was coupled with intentional biological warfare on behalf of settlers and disruptions to traditional diet and cultural and spiritual practices, all aimed at eradication of Indigenous populations.

As colonial powers attempted to claim the land for themselves, they enforced restrictions on Indigenous hunting and gathering practices, going so far as to decimate entire populations of primary food sources, as was the case with the bison population both north and south of the Medicine Line (Duke 2006). Increased demand for sustenance for the growing settler population and increased commerce through the fur trade were combined with concerted efforts to actively annihilate the population because "every buffalo gone [was] an Indian dead" (Phillips 2018: 25). Colonial attempts at disrupting Indigenous lifeways were comprehensive in their efforts, and Indigenous populations, whatever their numbers, were markedly impacted, and their decline is indisputable.

According to Indigenous Oral Stories and paleo-archaeological records, Indigenous Peoples in Canada experienced comparably good health and mortality rates prior to colonial contact (Liebmann 2021). While lifestyles and diets varied from culture to culture on Turtle Island, Indigenous groups would have enjoyed active lifestyles, spiritual practices and healthy, traditional diets appropriate to their local climates and geographies, all of which contributed to their overall well-being.

Disease was present, of course, as it was across all societies. Records indicate that Indigenous Peoples would have experienced some infectious diseases such as streptococcus and staphylococcus and other physiological impairments like osteoarthritis, likely from overuse and repetitive motions from their hunter-gatherer lifestyles (Johnston 1979). People may have died from war and accidents at an average rate as well. However, there is no evidence in the paleo-archaeological record to suggest that diabetes was present or that cancer rates were as high as they are today (Walker 2019). The increase in these health issues, like many other health issues affecting Indigenous Peoples today, can be directly linked to colonial contact. Disease and mortality rates drastically increased upon contact with European explorers and settlers. The effects of colonial contact on mortality rates are evident in the decline in population numbers across Turtle Island.

GRIEVING PRACTICES PRIOR TO COLONIZATION

What we know today of end-of-life and grieving practices prior to colonial contact comes from knowledge passed down through Indigenous Oral Traditions and ethnographic accounts from early anthropologists, which are not always reliable due to their Eurocentric perspectives. Indigenous mortuary customs on Turtle Island varied from culture to culture and region to region. Indigenous Peoples cremated their dead, buried them in mounds and pits, placed *jiibegamig* (spirit houses) atop burial mounds, mummified their dead, performed tree burials by placing their dead in boxes on platforms in trees, and created and maintained group ossuaries. An ossuary is a chest, box, clay pot or site of the final resting place for the bones of the deceased. The method of disposal of remains depended on the unique culture and geographical location.

Traditionally, when an Anishinaabe person died, their family would comb their hair, paint their face, dress them in ceremonial clothing and jewellery and wrap them in blankets. Anishinaabeg buried their dead in the ground, often placing spirit houses on top of the grave. Inside the grave, they would place the personal items of the deceased, such as tobacco, pipes, bowls, kettles and medicines to help them in their journey to the Land of Souls (Johnston 1995).

Indigenous death customs did not end after the disposal of the deceased. After the death of a community member or loved one, Indigenous groups had different approaches to mourning. Although not comprehensive, the following list contains some common rites and rituals performed after the death of a community member:

- burning a sacred fire for four days;
- hair cutting;
- mortuary poles;
- not marrying for one year after death of a spouse;
- not speaking the name of the deceased for one year;
- never whistling at the northern lights because they are dancing spirits;
- donating the deceased's belongings to family or friends;
- rearranging the furniture in the house of the deceased so that if their spirit returns they are confused and continue their journey on the spirit path; and
- feasting after one year has passed.

Many death rituals are informed by an Indigenous understanding of time, which often sees time as cyclical rather than linear. "In order to understand death, one must first embrace the circle of life. Birth, life, death and afterlife are four stages of the journey of the human spirit" (Longboat 2002: 5). Anishinaabe tradition explains that as a people we come from the stars and that is where we return when our physical bodies cease to exist in this world. When we die, a person leaves their physical body on earth to become an ancestor, and their loved ones will do what they can to help them along that journey by not calling them back to Earth, which is what many of the above rituals ensure.

Traditional Anishinaabe Funerals

I (Audrey) am an Anishinaabe and an Indigenous death doula, and I am eternally grateful for the efforts to preserve our culture that cultural knowledge holders have undertaken. One such example is Lee Obizaan Staples and Chato Ombishkebines Gonzalez's detailed guide on how to conduct a traditional Anishinaabe funeral, entitled *Aanjikiing/Changing Worlds: Anishinaabe Traditional Funeral* (2023). The 170-page manual describes each step of the funeral process and explains why each step is taken. Lee Obizaan Staples states that he was compelled to share by a spiritual calling:

> The reason I am having this written down is that in the future there are going to be fewer people who know how to send the Anishinaabe spirit to that other world. This is my thinking: Why should I be stingy with what I have been taught? I do not own it. This teaching belongs to and was gifted to the Anishinaabe people. There will be no merit if I try to hold on to all this for selfish reasons and take it all with me when I pass on. It is meant to be shared so there are others in the future who can carry on these teachings. (2023: 5)

Obizaan's words illustrate the generous and reciprocal nature integral to Indigenous cultures. At the same time, non-Indigenous people should be cautioned against freely appropriating and recreating these cultural practices for their own purposes, particularly in a monetary capacity.

The guide is written in both Anishinaabemowin and English, with Anishinaabemowin on the left page and the English translation on the right, an effort which works towards preservation of traditional death language. Over seven chapters, Obizaan and Gonzalez teach the reader how to conduct the pre-funeral feast, the wake, conversations with close relatives, the funeral itself, the post-funeral feast and the one-year memorial feast. At each stage, the authors detail when to offer tobacco and when to pray, smudge, smoke, sing and offer food to their recently departed ancestor. They also describe the path that the deceased, whom they refer to as Waasigwan (Shining Feather), will take when journeying from the physical world into the spirit world, the Land of Everlasting Happiness. The guide is one of the best descriptions of Indigenous funeral rites written by and for Indigenous people, which is an important distinction from early ethnographic accounts written by settlers, who romanticized and exoticized Indigenous Peoples for a European audience.

CONTEMPORARY INDIGENOUS END-OF-LIFE RITUALS

Contemporary Indigenous approaches to grieving are as varied as the number of Indigenous cultures on Turtle Island. As we learn in the previous pages of this chapter, Indigenous Peoples have experienced disruptions to their traditional ways of life because of colonization, and the impacts of colonization on grieving practices are no exception. The current Indigenous population in Canada is dispersed across urban areas as well as more rural and remote locations. Each of these locations is traditional Indigenous territory, but due to colonial disruption, personal agency and the human desire for migration,

Indigenous people today may or may not be living on their own traditional territory or have the cultural connection they would have had in the past.

Grieving practices today are often referred to as "syncretic," a term used by anthropologists to refer to a combination of Indigenous and Christian traditions (Stewart 1999). Cultural evolution and adaptation are natural processes in human societies; no culture stays the same forever, and cultures do not evolve linearly, meaning that not all cultures will arrive at the same destination. Indigenous Peoples worked hard to retain their cultural practices despite attempts at genocide and assimilation. It makes sense that while adapting to colonization and simultaneously working to retain traditional knowledge that there would be a melding of traditions and beliefs between Indigenous and settler customs and values.

Contemporary Anishinaabe Funerals

Chippewas of Nawash citizen and law professor Lindsay Borrows (2015) describes her experience with on-reserve funerals as so varied that no two are the same. Her description below is an example of how many different approaches can be taken during an Anishinaabe funeral:

> Days before the actual funeral, people gather and talk about the deceased. This is a time to honour the individual's life, shed tears with relatives and laugh! There is always humour as people get together and discuss memories. The older people speak Anishinaabemowin (our language), and we sing. The songs may include drumming, hymns in Anishinaabemowin or in English, or a special song that reminds people of the deceased. Sometimes the funeral is held at the community centre, other times at either the Catholic or United church on reserve. Both of these buildings are over three generations old. Sometimes a three-day wake is held at the home of the deceased. This protocol varies depending on the family and their needs.

Funerals may take place in English or Anishinaabemowin, in a church, community centre or at home, with drumming and singing, hymns or traditional songs; the needs of individuals and their families are unique. Personally, I have been at large gatherings and memorial services where the event is opened with smudging and prayer, and the prayer is the Lord's Prayer recited in Nêhiyawêwin (Cree), which is a good example of religious syncretism.

INTANGIBLE, SYMBOLIC AND AMBIGUOUS LOSSES

Grief in Indigenous experiences may be triggered by many kinds of losses. While Indigenous people certainly experience the more commonly understood forms of grief, like grief from death, divorce or moving, that are ubiquitous in much of the literature on grief, many Indigenous populations around the world face unique grieving experiences that are created by conditions of colonization and span several generations. When I was conducting the research for my master's thesis, which looked at urban Indigenous experiences of grief and bereavement, many of my collaborators shared stories of loss of language, land, tradition and land-based teachings, as well as relating to climate change and other colonial interventions such as a family history of residential school attendance, surviving the Sixties Scoop or Millennium Scoop, the MMIG2S epidemic and more. These types of losses can be understood as intangible, symbolic or even ambiguous losses.

Intangible loss refers to losses like the loss of cultural practice, loss of social cohesion and loss of dignity. Many people I spoke to shared that the primary source of grief in their lives came not from death but from the loss of cultural connection, and not having that cultural connection to rely on during times of grief made their grieving processes more challenging and healing less complete. Conducting community-based traditional healing ceremonies, such as a Sundance or a Sweat Lodge, was deemed illegal by the Canadian government until the laws changed in the 1950s, which was coupled with the government's child removal policies, seen through residential schools and the still disproportionately high number of Indigenous children in the child welfare system. As a result, many families have not had the opportunity to pass down their traditional knowledge and people today face challenges in engaging in their cultural traditions.

Symbolic loss comes from the loss of relationships, such as when an interpersonal relationship ends, but those in the relationship remain living. For example, survivors of the Sixties Scoop, a process that resulted in Indigenous children being forcibly removed from their homes and families and placed in non-Indigenous foster homes, may experience symbolic loss because of the severed relationship between themselves and their parents and communities. I know several Sixties Scoop survivors, and each one has a story of loss that resonates with the others, where they long for their relatives who they know are alive but have no contact with, and they grieve for the connection with their parents that was severed.

Ambiguous loss refers to a loss that has no closure, such as soldiers who have gone missing during war. In an Indigenous context, people may be living far from home for a number of reasons, such as access to education or health care that is not provided in their home community. When someone dies back home, people often find that they are unable to return because it is too costly to travel back to their community. Thus, they are unable to grieve the loss of their loved one with others in the community. People who experience this report that they have been unable to gain closure because they couldn't grieve alongside other community members.

Disenfranchised Grief

Many of the grieving experiences of Indigenous people today can be understood using Kenneth Doka's (1989) concept of "disenfranchised grief." Disenfranchised grief is grief that is not, "or cannot be, openly acknowledged, publicly mourned, or socially supported" (37). For example, grief from pet loss may be classified as disenfranchised if the individual feels that their grief is not valid because people do not take the loss of a pet's life as seriously as they do a close relative or loved one.

The discussion about intangible, symbolic and ambiguous losses illustrates how, for Indigenous people, grief may be caused by occurrences unrelated to death that may have been occurring over generations, making it difficult to readily pinpoint the inciting event. As a result of lengthy processes of loss and grief, spanning hundreds of years and affecting many generations, it can be challenging to understand where and when Indigenous grief comes from and how actions in the past can continue to adversely affect Indigenous people today. Physical and mental health professionals, social workers and the public can easily overlook the complex dynamics that influence Indigenous grief if they lack education on the matter and are without the substantial lived experience that is often necessary for a fulsome understanding of an issue.

Why Should We Care?

Understanding disenfranchised grief and the role it plays in the lives of Indigenous people is important for several reasons. First, Canada is a nation that has only recently begun to acknowledge the impacts of colonialism on Indigenous Peoples, meaning that their instrumental role in causing different forms of loss and grief is only now being understood and accepted in wider society. I grew up in the 1990s, and at that time, the narrative from settlers that I consistently heard about Indigenous people, including myself, was that we were inherently flawed, uneducated and dirty drunks. When we shift that narrative to see the role colonization has played in that so-called deficit, we can better support a change in the narrative. There can be no reconciliation without truth first.

Second, when Indigenous people see themselves adequately represented in literature on grief, intergenerational grief and trauma, coupled with efforts to shift the narrative and speak truth to Canada's genocidal foundations and ongoing part in the inequities many Indigenous people still face, we can take a step towards collective healing and thriving alongside one another. Finally, when health-care professionals are fully aware of the underlying mechanisms that lead to disparities in Indigenous mortality rates, they are better equipped to use their positions of power to help, both immediately and at a policy level. Just like we saw in the section on contemporary Indigenous death care and funerals, Indigenous people have been working to ensure their well-being through their own means.

CULTURE AS HEALING

Since time immemorial, Indigenous Peoples have had strong spiritual connections through ceremony, song, dance, art and land-based teachings and language. All these practices have been disrupted by colonization, and as we have seen here, Indigenous health suffers for it. In recent years, studies, programs and lived experiences all indicate that cultural connection and cultural practice are significant when it comes to healing. Indigenous and non-Indigenous health-care professionals and researchers and Indigenous community members have been exploring the ways that culture can provide meaningful pathways to healing across a whole range of specializations, from physical and mental health care and treatment for addictions to suicide prevention and healing from loss and grief, all of which are interconnected. We cannot look at one of these issues without looking at all of them.

Culture for Addiction Treatment

Indigenous cultural practices are being successfully used for treatment of addictions for Indigenous people alongside more conventional Western approaches (Auger, Howell and Gomes, 2016; Rowan, Poole, Shea et al. 2014). Indigenous people in Canada face higher rates of drug addiction and death from overdoses. A culturally competent approach to addiction treatment may involve cultural (re)connection, such as attending Sweat

Lodge ceremonies while staying in a residential treatment centre or when transitioning back into society in a halfway house. Incorporating cultural practice into addiction treatment provides an additional level of healing from colonialism, which can intervene with the pain of colonial-imposed loss, resulting in a decrease in the need for pain-numbing behaviour like substance abuse. One of my favourite quotes on addiction comes from Dr. Gabor Maté (2015), who reminds us to ask, "Why the pain?" when looking at addiction, and not "Why the addiction?". Incorporating culture into addiction treatment has been proven to increase the success of these programs. The findings from my thesis research also indicate that culture is used as a form of support when healing from grief and as a form of building resiliency against suicide (see also Barker, Goodman and DeBeck 2017). It stands to reason that continued access and reconnection to cultural practice, at any and all levels, is an important path to Indigenous well-being.

> **The Text Within:**
> **Love and Humour Through the Darkness (Audrey)**
>
> My father is Anishinaabe from the Wasauksing Nation, in Parry Sound, Ontario, and we are both citizens of the nation. My mother is the daughter of a first-generation immigrant couple from the Netherlands and Germany, respectively. My grandparents on my father's side were institutionalized at different residential schools and sanatoriums, and their children were taken away from them during the Sixties Scoop. On my mother's side of the family, my Oma was born in Berlin in 1940, and her formative years were spent in the midst of the atrocities of World War II. What these histories mean for me is that intergenerational grief and trauma have had a considerable influence on my life and the lives of my family members. While it can be easy, at first glance, to assume that one's life is overly determined by grief and trauma when it has been such a present theme, I urge readers to remember that humans contain multitudes and that love and humour always find a way to make themselves known through the darkness. Art, poetry, dance, drumming, singing, beadwork, Storytelling and laughter are always present in the lives of Indigenous people. They are a powerful coping mechanism born from darkness and exist beautifully alongside our trauma. We are capable of so much, and I look forward to seeing what the future brings for the growing body of Indigenous grief and death workers on Turtle Island.

CONCLUSION

Indigenous approaches to end-of-life and mortuary customs are as varied as the numerous Indigenous cultural groups and nations across Turtle Island. While traditional ways of death care and body disposal have been interfered with through processes and systems of colonization, and mortality rates are disproportionately high for First Nations, Inuit and Métis Peoples, each group continues to work to address the conditions that led to those disparities in the first place. The interconnected web of colonization, high mortality rates, complex experiences of grief and nuanced understandings of loss are being addressed through community initiatives like suicide awareness and prevention training, Indigenous death doulaship, and the allyship of medical professionals adequately trained in cultural competency. Further, the more the average person is educated in these topics and understands how the underlying mechanism of settler colonialism works to perpetuate its goal of domination, the more that harmful narratives devaluing Indigenous lives will shift (Razack 2015). Therefore, it is with hope that I look to the future for Indigenous Peoples, knowing all the ways we stand here today as survivors of colonization and with the ability to support a thriving future.

IN-CLASS ASSIGNMENTS

1. Go to the Living My Culture website (livingmyculture.ca), select one of the thumbnails on First Nations, Métis or Inuit people, and watch one of the videos. Many of the videos are under two minutes long, so you may be able to watch more than one in the time allotted for this exercise. What did you learn? What was surprising?
2. Make a list of your own cultural practices, paying particular attention to the ones that are important to death and grief. Swap with your neighbour and discuss which cultural processes are most important to you when you experience the death of someone close and also for you when you die.
3. Discuss what you do to care for yourself during times of grief or loss. Is there a cultural component to your practice?

SELF-REFLECTION AND THOUGHTFUL CONVERSATIONS

1. Discuss with your group a time you experienced loss that was not related to death. What kind of loss was it (perhaps intangible, ambiguous or symbolic) and discuss the impact it had on you.
2. Are you aware of some instances of death by medical racism for Indigenous people in Canada? Google the topic with your group. Discuss what you think can be done to address this issue.
3. Discuss some of the underlying mechanisms that contribute to higher mortality rates for Indigenous people. Were there any that surprised you in this chapter?
4. How important is it to you that you experience a good death? What would be some necessary requirements for you to have a good death (example: dying at home, dying with loved ones around, food or drink preferences, music playing, culturally appropriate practices available and honoured, etc.)? What do you think your experience would be like if you were denied what you needed to have a good death?
5. What can non-Indigenous people do to support Indigenous people during loss, grief and death?

CHAPTER 11 REFERENCES

Due to the dearth of literature in this area, we have kept the specific references for this chapter as a stand-alone item as your resource.

Auger, M., Howell, T., and Gomes, T. 2016. "Moving Toward Holistic Wellness, Empowerment and Self-Determination for Indigenous Peoples in Canada: Can Traditional Indigenous Health Care Practices Increase Ownership Over Health and Health Care Decisions?" *Canadian Journal of Public Health* 107, 4-5: e393-e398, <doi: 10.17269/cjph.107.5366>.

Banerji, A., Pelletier, V.A., Haring, R., Irvine, J., Bresnahan, A., and Lavallee, B. 2023. "Food Insecurity and Its Consequences in Indigenous Children and Youth in Canada." *PLOS Global Public Health* 3, 9. <doi: 10.1371/journal.pgph.0002406>.

Barker, B., Goodman, A., and DeBeck, K. 2017. "Reclaiming Indigenous Identities: Culture as Strength Against Suicide Among Indigenous Youth in Canada." *Canadian Journal of Public Health* 108, 2 <doi: 10.17269/CJPH.108.5754>.

BBC News Online. 2021. "Joyce Echaquan: Racism Played Role in Death, Coroner Finds." October 6. <bbc.com/news/world-us-canada-58819203>.

Borrows, J. (1997). The Royal Proclamation, Canadian Legal History, and Self-Government. *Aboriginal and Treaty Rights in Canada: Essays on Law, Equity and Respect for Difference*, 155–172.

Campbell, D. 2000. "A Search for Justice in First Nations Communities: The Role of the RCMP and Community Policing." Doctoral dissertation, Carleton University.

Canadian Virtual Hospice. 2025. "About Us." <virtualhospice.ca/en_US/Main+Site+Navigation/Home+Navigation/About+Us.aspx>.

CTV News Online. 2024. "Sask. First Nation Will Be One of Few in Canada to Have Its Own Funeral Home." August 7. <www.ctvnews.ca/regina/article/this-sask-first-nation-will-be-one-of-few-in-canada-to-have-its-own-funeral-home/>.

David, J., and Jaffray, B. 2022. "Homicide in Canada, 2021." *Juristat: Canadian Centre for Justice Statistics*. <www150.statcan.gc.ca/n1/pub/85-002-x/2022001/article/00015-eng.htm>.

Doka, K.J. (1999). "Disenfranchised Grief." *Bereavement Care* 18, 3: 37–39.

Duke, D.F. (ed.). 2006. *Canadian Environmental History: Essential Readings*. Canadian Scholars' Press.

Dunbar-Ortiz, R. 2014. *An Indigenous Peoples History of the United States*. Boston: Beacon Press.

First Nations Health Authority. 2025. "Our History, Our Health." <fnha.ca/wellness/wellness-for-first-nations/our-history-our-health>.

Indigenous Services Canada. 2023a. *An Update on the Socio-Economic Gaps Between Indigenous Peoples and the Non-Indigenous Population in Canada: Highlights from the 2021 Census. A Compendium Report to the Department's 2023 Annual Report to Parliament*. <sac-isc.gc.ca/eng/1690909773300/1690909797208>.

Isenberg, A.C. 2020. "The Destruction of the Bison: An Environmental History, 1750–1920." Cambridge University Press.

Johnston, R.B. 1979. "Notes on Ossuary Burial Among the Ontario Iroquois." *Canadian Journal of Archaeology/Journal Canadien d'Archéologie* 3: 91–104.

Johnston, Basil. *The Manitous: The Spiritual World of the Ojibway*. New York: Harper Collins Publisher, 1995.

Kumar, M.B., and Tjepkema, M. 2019. "Suicide Among First Nations People, Métis and Inuit (2011–2016): Findings from the 2011 Canadian Census Health and Environment Cohort." June. (CanCHEC) <www150.statcan.gc.ca/n1/en/catalogue/99-011-X2019001>.

Lavalley, J., Kastor, S., Valleriani, J., and McNeil, R. 2018. Reconciliation and Canada's Overdose Crisis: Responding to the Needs of Indigenous Peoples. *Canadian Medical Association Journal* 190, 50. e1466-e1467, <doi: 0.1503/cmaj.181093>.

Liebmann, M. 2021. "Colonialism and Indigenous Population Decline in the Americas." *Routledge Handbook of the Archaeology of Indigenous-Colonial Interaction in the Americas*. Routledge.

Longboat, D.M. 2002. "Ian Anderson Continuing Education Program: Indigenous Perspectives on Death and Dying." University of Toronto. <cpd.utoronto.ca/endoflife/Modules/Indigenous%20Perspectives%20on%20Death%20and%20Dying.pdf>

Maté, G. 2015. "Gabor Maté: How to Build a Culture of Good Health." *Yes! Journalism for People Building a Better World*. <www.yesmagazine.org/issue/good-health/2015/11/16/gabor-mate-how-to-build-a-culture-of-good-health>.

Murray, K. 2015. "Reflecting on Death: First Nations People." *Life and Death Matters*. <lifeanddeathmatters.ca/reflecting-on-death-first-nations-people>.

Native Women's Association of Canada. 2022. *Misconduct, Missing and Murdered: The Experiences of Anti-Indigenous Racism in Reproductive Healthcare among Indigenous Women, Girls, Two-Spirit, Transgender, and Gender Diverse People, and the MMIWG2S+ Genocide*. https://nwac.ca/assets-knowledge-centre/9-Dec-Racism-in-Healthcare.pdf.

Park, J. 2021. "Mortality Among First Nations People, 2006 to 2016." *Health Reports* 32, 10. <doi.org/10.25318/82-003-x202101000001-eng>.

Phillips, N. 2018. "Skin and Bones: The Decimation of the Plains Buffalo." *Mount Royal Undergraduate Humanities Review* 5. <doi.10.29173/mruhr463>.

Principe de Joyce. n.d. "Joyce's Principle." <principedejoyce.com/en/index>.

Public Health Agency of Canada. 2018. *Key Health Inequalities in Canada: A National Portrait*. Ottawa: Public Health Agency of Canada. <www.canada.ca/en/public-health/services/publications/science-research-data/key-health-inequalities-canada-national-portrait-executive-summary.html>.

Reidpath, D.D., and Allotey, P. 2003. "Infant Mortality Rate as an Indicator of Population Health." *Journal of Epidemiology and Community Health* 57, 5: 344-6. <doi: 10.1136/jech.57.5.344>.

Rowan, M., Poole, N., Shea, B., Gone,. J.P., Mykota, D., Farag, M., Hall, L., Mushquash, C., and Dell, C.. 2014. "Cultural interventions to treat addictions in Indigenous populations: findings from a scoping study." *Substance Abuse Treatment, Prevention, and Policy* 9.

Roy, J., and Marcellus, S. 2019. *Homicide in Canada 2018*. Statistics Canada. <www150.statcan.gc.ca/n1/pub/85-002-x/2019001/article/00016-eng.pdf>.

Statistics Canada. 2024. "Health Care Access and Experiences Among Indigenous People." *The Daily*. <www150.statcan.gc.ca/n1/daily-quotidien/241104/dq241104a-eng.htm>.

Razack, S., 2015. *Dying from Improvement: Inquests and Inquiries into Indigenous Deaths in Custody*. University of Toronto Press.

Stewart, C. 1999. "Syncretism and Its Synonyms: Reflections on Cultural Mixture." *Diacritics*, 29, 3.

Walker, S. 2019. "The Persistence of Place: Hunter-Gatherer Mortuary Practices and Land-Use in the Trent Valley, Ontario." *Journal of Anthropological Archaeology*, 54. <doi.10.1016/j.jaa.2019.03.002>.

Chapter Twelve

THE CHANGING FACE OF CREMATION, FUNERAL AND BURIAL PRACTICES

IN THE LAST TWENTY YEARS, the funeral and burial industry has changed in dramatic ways. There has been an increase in cremation rates compared to traditional burials, a large number of women are entering the funeral and embalming profession, and there is a plethora of new products and services aimed at dealing with the final disposition of deceased persons. This has included green, ecological and "natural" funerals, celebrations of life, living wakes and funerals, burials at sea, drive-thru funerals, burials in space and in egg-shaped burial pods, and coffins made from mushrooms, among others! As well, there are many new ways to make use of cremated remains (often called ashes), for example, placing them in jewellery, infusing them into glass ornaments, garden statues and stones, adding them to paint to create an image of the deceased on canvas or another medium, mixing them with soil to plant trees and shrubs, adding them to stuffed toys, mixing them with ink for tattoos and other uses too numerous to mention.

Cremation has been practised in Europe since 1400 BCE, although the advent of Christianity brought cremation to a virtual halt at about 100 to 200 CE, "Eventually, neglect and the unsanitary conditions of European cemeteries brought about a surge in the popularity of cremation during the early 1800s" (Tipper 1989: 10). Canada's first crematorium was built in Montreal in 1901.

Around 75 percent of Canadians now chose cremation rather than traditional burials, in part due to financial concerns (Canadian Funerals Online 2025). The costs of cremations differ widely across Canada and among funeral homes, as well as depending on the types of services available. The cremation process involves reducing the body to bone ashes and bone fragments using intense heat. The water content of the body evaporates, and the carbon content is incinerated, leaving inorganic bone ash. The cremation chamber may reach temperatures of 2,000–2,500°F, thereby reducing the human body to five to seven pounds of ashes and bone fragments within an hour and a half.

As the costs of so-called traditional funerals with caskets and earth burials increase, a social movement known as the Fair Funerals Campaign started in the UK to make visible the challenges faced by individuals who are facing "funeral poverty," which they defined as follows:

> Funeral poverty is where the price of a funeral is beyond a person's ability to pay. This problem is getting a lot worse because funerals are getting much more expensive at the same time as support from the government is drying up. Funeral poverty has increased by 50% in just three years.

This campaign ended in 2018, but its work has been taken over by Quaker Social Action, which focuses on tackling funeral poverty through its Down to Earth project.

Funeral poverty became topical in Canada in 2024, when newspaper articles appeared about unclaimed remains being left at funeral homes because families could not afford to collect them and have them taken to a place of final rest. Authors Kyawsoe Oo and Anna Mehler Paperny (2024) write in *Reuters*, "In Canada, bodies go unclaimed as costs put funerals out of reach." They report that some Canadian provinces have logged a jump in unclaimed dead bodies in recent years, with next of kin citing funeral costs as a growing reason for not collecting loved ones' remains. The phenomenon has prompted at least one province to build a new storage facility, and the incidence of memorial fundraisers has surged. The overall cost of a funeral in Canada at the top end has increased to about $8,800 from about $6,000 in 1998, according to industry trade group estimates. In Ontario, Canada's most populous province, the number of unclaimed dead bodies rose to 1,183 in 2023 from 242 in 2013, says Dirk Huyer, the province's chief coroner. In most of those cases, the next of kin were identified but unable to claim the body for a variety of reasons, the most common being lack of money (Roberts 2025). In a *CBC News* article, Anthony Germaine and Mike Moore (2024) point out that in the province of Newfoundland and Labrador, unclaimed bodies are being stored in large freezers outside the Health Sciences Centre at Memorial University in St. John's, because there is nowhere else to put them.

While the financial costs to individuals are clearly an impediment to a traditional burial, this practice also represent a negative impact on ecosystems. They require vast amounts of land for cemeteries, contributing to urban sprawl and the loss of natural habitats. As urban areas expand, precious ecosystems, flora and fauna are displaced, disrupting the delicate balance of the environment. Embalming, a common practice before burial, involves the use of chemicals such as formaldehyde, a carcinogen that's been proven to pose health risks to people who have regular exposure to the it and which can leach into the ground, contaminating soil and nearby water sources, posing a threat to the environment and wildlife.

On a CBC Radio news broadcast journalist Darren Bernhardt (2016) talks to a funeral director in Ontario who uses only natural materials and in-earth decomposition of the deceased: "[Rather] than taking approximately three to five years to disintegrate you in the ground it just does it in a quicker process." Protection of the environment and preferring not to use materials that harm it are increasingly becoming key issues for many. As the earth's resources continue to decrease, there will undoubtedly be more who choose these options. Some, like those in the Urban Death Project, view it as a recycling endeavour: "Recomposition is a process that gently converts human remains into soil, to nourish new life after we die. Our goal is to offer recomposition as an alternative choice to cremation and conventional burial" (Spade 2016).

Another important area of social change in the past twenty years in Canada is the dramatic increase in the number of women entering the funeral business. In a *Globe and Mail* article, author Allison Dunfield (2024) suggested that "women are changing the face of the death care industry, with increasing numbers owning funeral homes and making up the majority of graduates from college programs focused on funeral directing. At Ontario's Humber College, which offers one of two such programs in the province, 70 percent of students enrolled are women." One reason why women are entering this profession, previously thought unsuitable, is that they are daughters of the retiring funeral directors who want to carry on the family business. As well, funeral directing is one of many professions encouraging more women to become involved.

THE IMPACT OF COVID-19 ON THE FUNERAL INDUSTRY

While the COVID-19 pandemic affected every aspect of life, it was especially difficult for those working in the funeral services because families could not see their deceased loved ones or participate in for funerals and celebration-of-life services in person. Funeral directors were not able to support those who were grieving with hugs and other face-to-face comfort measures. Because masks were required in most facilities, communication was restricted to the eyes. Bans on gatherings meant that mourners could not be together religious events, where, for some, comfort could be found amongst the clergy and other parishioners. Travel restrictions around the world also impeded family and friends from attending services and in-person sharing of stories and memories of the deceased. Many funeral directors saw a fall in revenues, while for others, these challenges had an impact on what types of services they offered. For example, some funeral directors replaced on-site funerals with virtual ones.

In a scoping review of the literature on the impact of COVID-19 on funeral services, Andie MacNeil, Blythe Findlay, Rennie Bimman et al. (2021) examined databases of fifteen medical, social sciences and other journals. The authors identified two main themes: grief responses and meaning making. About the first category, the authors state:

> The literature frequently reported that the use of virtual funeral practices during the COVID-19 pandemic has fundamentally changed how people grieve. The inability to gather in person and collectively mourn creates challenges for people to process their grief in traditional ways. The absence of familiar rituals may lead to complicated grief responses, such as prolonged grief and disenfranchised grief. Furthermore, because COVID-19 fatalities often exemplify characteristics that are indicative of a "bad death," such as physical discomfort and social isolation, bereaved loved ones may experience heightened feelings of guilt and anger throughout the grieving process.
>
> In addition to complicated grieving experiences, bereaved families have also been deprived of the simple practices that would traditionally bring comfort during a time of mourning, such as physical touch with loved ones. These challenges are compounded by the broader social isolation and psychological distress that characterize the COVID-19 pandemic. For many bereaved individuals, the grieving process has been disrupted by external stressors related to COVID-19, such as financial stress, precarious employment, and concerns over their health and the health of their loved ones.

This scoping review provides an excellent overview of the ways in which the funeral industry changed traditional ways of conducting funeral services, which fundamentally changed the ways in which people were able to deal with grief and bereavement in challenging times. The authors note in their conclusions:

> In the absence of traditional funeral practices, many bereaved individuals and families have been forced to reconcile uncomfortable and unfamiliar changes in grief responses. However, the adoption of virtual funeral practices has also highlighted the resilience of families and communities during the grieving process, and the ability to find new avenues of meaning despite the inability to gather in-person.

Another aspect of the funeral industry impacted by COVID-19 is the increase in drive-thru funerals, especially in the US, UK and the province of British Columbia. As most funeral homes in Canada are increasingly being owned by American funeral organizations, especially in larger provinces such as Ontario, Quebec, Alberta and British Columbia, it is likely that we will see more of these services in Canada. According to the Titan Casket company in the US, one of the largest in North America, a drive-thru funeral is

> also known as a drive-thru visitation or drive-thru viewing, it is a unique way to pay respects to a deceased person. It is quite different from a traditional funeral, where mourners gather at a funeral home, a community centre or a place of worship to view the casket or urn, offer condolences and attend a service. In a drive-thru funeral, however, there is a designated drive-thru area where the casket or urn of the deceased person is placed. Mourners can drive past this area and remain in their vehicles even as they complete the viewing. This effectively allows people to pay their respects without the need to park their vehicles or physically interact with other mourners. (Prout 2024)

The Titan website considers the following to be some of the benefits of drive-thru funerals:

- They are quicker than traditional funerals and save time.
- It is easier for many people to drive through and pay their respects.

- They ensure safety and social distancing, especially during critical periods like the pandemic.
- It helps people who are estranged from other mourners bid goodbye to the deceased person in private.

Drive-thru funerals are less expensive than traditional ones because there is no reception afterwards. As well, the drive-thru funeral allows the funeral home to display its expertise in the presentation of the deceased, therefore increasing potential sales. Most studies on the impact of COVID-19 have been conducted in North America, but there are doubtless significant impacts on the grief and mourning rituals in other countries that experienced high death tolls from the pandemic.

FINAL DISPOSITION SERVICES

Whereas it would have been common for our grandparents and possibly parents to be buried in a cemetery attached to a local church or cremated and the ashes placed in an urn, today the choices for the final disposition of the deceased are vast. I discuss some below, but many others exist (see, for example, FuneralResources.org 2023).

Rather than be placed in a coffin and then put into the ground, we can now be wrapped in a woven shroud, basket or biodegradable cardboard box and be buried or placed directly in a woodland area or some other green space. Alternatively, our ashes, or even our entire body, if folded into a fetal position, can be placed in an egg-shaped pod and then buried with a tree on top of us. This product of Italian design is called a Capsula Mundi, and according to an article by Emanuela Campanella (2016), people who choose this option would become part of a natural forest.

Another alternative for the final disposition of the deceased is an Eternal Reef:

> An Eternal Reef combines a cremation urn, ash scattering, and burial at sea into one meaningful, permanent environmental tribute to life.
>
> An Eternal Reef is part of a designed reef system created from individual reef balls made of environmentally safe, marine grade concrete that quickly assimilate into the natural ocean environment. These permanent memorials placed on the ocean floor create new marine habitats for fish and other forms of sea life.

> Eternal Reefs takes the cremated remains or "cremains" of an individual and incorporates them into a proprietary, environmentally safe cement mixture designed to create artificial reef formations. The Eternal Reefs are then placed in one of our permitted ocean locations selected by the individual, friend or family member.

According to the Eternal Reefs website, the reefs are predominantly sold in the US, and the cost varies from $2,500 to almost $8,000.

Also available predominantly in the US are memorial space burials, where there is a choice between four different space cremated ash burials available from Celestis Memorial Spaceflights, costing $3,495 to $12,995 in 2024. Another method for the final disposition of human remains is that of Resomation or Aquamation, brand names for alkaline hydrolysis, a process whereby an alkaline solution is used to dissolve human remains and then drain the effluents into a municipal sewer system; it is a system of cremation by water rather than fire (Cremation Association of North America n.d.).

After cremation, by whichever method an individual chooses, there are many options for the disposition of the cremains or ashes other than scattering, burying or placing them in a columbarium. As mentioned earlier, this can include infusing them into jewellery, glass or stone ornaments for the home or garden, using them in paint to create a picture of a subject the deceased may have enjoyed, having them placed in an hourglass, having them turned into diamonds, placed into a teddy bear or some other soft toy and so on. A recent addition to the eco-friendly burial option is to be buried in a mushroom-based coffin. According to In the Light Urns (n.d.), a mushroom coffin is

> a new innovation that uses a mixture of fungus as a means to decompose human remains in a way that improves the environmental aspects of burial and gives people another option over cremation. Not only is this an eco-friendly way to deal with end of life, it is a way in which a human body can give back to the natural world.

A popular item available on several websites is a living urn tree kit, which can be made of recycled paper, wood, metal, stone and other materials and be used outside or in the home. The kit includes the urn and a tree of your choice to plant in the urn.

A huge number of companies provide products and services related to this topic. Most are in the US and Europe, but all can be purchased and delivered to Canada. Although most of these procedures for the final disposition are yet to be available freely in Canada, either due to costs or laws regarding what can occur with human remains, it is undoubtedly just a matter of time before they come to our shores in greater numbers.

Because of the increased costs involved in traditional funeral services, two new social movements have emerged in Canada and elsewhere. One is the funeral cooperative or memorial society, which is a community-based initiative aimed at providing its members with compassionate, high-quality funeral arrangements on a not-for-profit basis. They are owned and operated by their members and do not exist to make profits, but rather to meet the needs of bereaved families, whatever their funeral budget may be. The cooperative/memorial society models guarantee the quality of services and commitment to people who make use of their services. One of the oldest funeral cooperatives in Canada was founded in Sudbury, Ontario, in 1952, and this movement has grown across the country since then.

The first memorial society in Canada was founded in British Columbia in 1956. Unlike some funeral cooperatives, it requires a $40 lifetime membership fee and notes that selecting the a funeral cooperative or memorial society is a benefit to family members who do not have to worry about how to finance this event (Memorial Society of BC). Its website notes that while there are financial consequences to individuals and families not being able to afford funerals, there are also emotional and distressful elements because the bereaved may feel shame, guilt and stigma about not being able to provide a decent "send-off" to people they love.

In Canada, the death benefit has also been lowered; presently it provides up to $2,500 for a family member if they have paid into the Canada Pension Plan for at least ten years. This amount was established in 2019 and has not increased since then despite increases in the cost of living. A *CBC News* item pointed out that the Canadian Pension Plan Death Benefit, which assists low-income individuals to pay for funerals, fall short of what is needed:

> A change to the Canada Pension Plan to provide a flat-rate death benefit to help low-income families cover funeral costs falls short of what funeral homes say is needed to cover the cost of a final farewell. After meetings this week, federal and provincial finance

ministers set the death benefit at a flat $2,500, regardless of how long or how much someone had paid into CPP. Leading up to the meeting, the Funeral Services Association of Canada lobbied governments to raise the value to $3,580 — back to what it was in 1997 before finance ministers of the day imposed a sliding scale benefit based on an individual's contributions to the CPP, capped at a maximum benefit of $2,500. (Canadian Broadcasting Corporation 2017)

The challenge of funeral poverty will presumably continue as long as individuals wish to have traditional funerals for their deceased loved ones, as the costs of these services continue to rise. One can now purchase a funeral insurance policy which enables the surviving family member to use the benefit to cover funeral expenses, final bills or however they see fit. An internet perusal of insurance companies in Canada revealed that the costs of these plans range from $30 per month and up.

Funeral directors are involved in a series of public and private events that assist in the final disposition and disposal of the dead. This work fits within the dramaturgical schema presented by Erving Goffman (1959) in his analysis of occupations and their settings. The "frontstage" arena, as invoked by Goffman, is the setting where the public has access to the work of the funeral director. It is in the funeral home or parlour that audiences visit the main foyer, viewing rooms, reception area, chapel and family rooms, where mourners can grieve in private. The frontstage is usually located on the first floor of the funeral home, whereas "backstage" work is conducted in the basement. Embalming may be carried out backstage, as well as other procedures for the dead, such as cosmetically preparing and dressing the body for viewing. The business offices and casket display areas are private in terms of being accessible primarily only to those who work in the funeral home. Not only are physical settings in the funeral home designed to facilitate specific tasks, but so too are those who work within them. It is the role of the funeral director to "stage" a presentation of the dead, to ensure that those attending the funeral service are orchestrated in such a way as to perceive a sense of solemnity, calm and peace and to escort the deceased and mourners to the final resting place of the "dearly departed."

The following three interrelated issues need to be addressed when discussing the disposal industry:

1. the role that funerals, or increasingly in Canada and elsewhere, cremation services, play in the death process;
2. the non-public behaviour in the funeral home: "presenting the dead";
3. the industry as part of consumer capitalism.

All cultures hold ceremonies for marking deaths. These ceremonies, regardless of where they are performed, seem to have the following two major functions: 1) to separate the body of the deceased from the community of the living, and 2) to assist mourners in adjusting to their loss and restructure their life without the presence of the person who has died. In this sense, the funeral enables the mourner to structure their relationship with the deceased from one of presence (i.e., living, interactive and responsible) to a relationship of memory.

Types of burial sites differ across cultures because each type was originally dictated by the local availability of materials or by climatic conditions. Among some Indigenous Peoples of the Arctic, surface burial was common. Because one cannot dig through frozen ground and there are no trees for a funeral pyre, the bodies were covered with stones to form a rock vault (Fulton and Metress 1995). In hot, desert-type countries, bodies are buried deep in the sand and covered with roots and stems to keep the sand from blowing away. Because of the heat and the flesh-eating insects living in the sand, decomposition of the body is rapid.

In less technologically developed communities, death has a profoundly disruptive effect on everyday life and is therefore accorded prominence in cultural behaviour. In close-knit rural areas, the death of a community member is noticed more than in a large city. As a society becomes more industrialized and therefore highly structured, death has less impact on the community, as individuals perform a variety of social roles. In these circumstances, institutions and agencies evolve to handle death work and thereby reduce the amount of time and commitment that individuals devote to the loss of a family or community member. Funeral directors are professionals who direct all this organization.

There are four functions to most funeral and cremation services. First, they provide supportive relationships for the bereaved. The bereaved receive the support of concerned family, friends and communities, and may also receive the support of religious or philosophical meanings for the death. People can be supportive symbolically but also physically by their presence and by "acceptance," such as the physical touching of the bereaved.

Second, such services do the work of reinforcing the reality of death. When an open casket is used, the dead body is a physical object visible to all. The third function is to make possible the acknowledgment and open expression of the mourners' feelings of loss and grief and to share these experiences with others. Fourth, services mark a fitting conclusion to the life of the person who has died. Like birthdays celebrate the day of birth, funeral and cremation services celebrate the day of death, including the achievements and relationships that occurred in the deceased's life. The funeral or cremation service, then, is a symbolic ritual in every culture that displays change and transformation in human life and death. The funeral is a social event in which mourners are surrounded by a group that shares some of their loss and that joins them in marking the end of a relationship with dignity and support and allows the opportunity for visible expression of grief.

BEHIND THE SCENES IN THE FUNERAL PARLOUR

The undertaker or funeral director's work consists of the following four main tasks:

1. removal of the body;
2. embalming of the body;
3. presenting the dead;
4. arranging funerals or cremation services, selling caskets, urns, flowers, cards, graves and plots, headstones, music and total services on either a pre-arranged or fee-for-service basis (Howarth 1996; Pine 1975; Leming and Dickinson 1988).

A funeral director normally removes the dead body from the place where death occurs, usually taking it to a funeral home. Most "removals" are from institutions (hospitals, hospices and nursing homes). "Removals" also occur from private homes and accidents or other emergency sites. Removals from institutions are usually straightforward. Death certificates are completed by the funeral director, and all necessary identification forms are usually available at the funeral home.

Removals from private homes may be more complicated. The funeral director's work is more visible in private homes, and they must appear professional, sympathetic and caring. Removals from private homes also enable the funeral director to contact family members and discreetly act as a salesperson for their firm. In the case of accidents or emergency "removals," the funeral director is usually instructed by police, physicians or others to get the "body out of here," and less reverence may be shown to the deceased.

Embalming is the process whereby body fluids, including blood, are drained from the dead and replaced with preserving fluids, which are said to sanitize and remove odours from the decaying corpse, so it may be viewed by family and friends, if necessary, prior to burial. Embalming is clearly relegated to the non-public arena of the funeral home. As Michael Leming and George Dickinson observe:

> Embalming, by definition, is the replacement of normal body fluids with preserving chemicals. This process is accomplished by using the vascular system of the body to both remove the body fluids and to suffuse the body with preserving chemicals. The arterial system is used to introduce the chemicals into the body, and the venous system is used to remove the body fluids. The intravascular exchange is accomplished by using an embalming machine. (1988: 444)

It is during the embalming process, whether by using chemicals or essential oils, that the issue of "presenting the dead" becomes paramount. It is now that efforts are made to "restore" the face of the deceased to a "natural likeness." The act of restoration involves creating a "memory picture" of the deceased person that enables family and friends to recognize and remember their loss. There is much cosmetic work involved in restoring the dead to a lifelike appearance. When we die, our blood drains to the lowest parts of our body, our eyes involuntarily stay open, and our mouths gape. Much emphasis is on the face and hands because they are the body parts most visible to viewers.

It is the surface appearance, the cosmetic effect, rather than the tissue preservation itself, that makes embalming an important part of the modern North American way of life. Embalming came to North America in the 1800s. Prior to that time, corpses were kept on ice to allow travel time for distant friends and family to attend the viewing and funeral. During the mid-nineteenth century, two undertakers in the UK introduced a coffin known as a corpse cooler, which had a special compartment for holding ice and was fitted with a tap for draining water as the ice melted. During the US Civil War, between 1861 and 1865, the federal government made available research funds for the creation of new techniques for preserving bodies. Funeral directors could apply for grants to research techniques that would enable them to preserve the war dead longer, to bring them home for burial. The first school of embalming in North America was opened in Cincinnati in 1882. Earlier, in the UK, another war, the Crimean War of 1854–1856, caused governments to fund research for embalming techniques (Mayer 1996).

In some smaller communities across the country, there is only one funeral director, who may also run the ambulance service, so they have easy access to referrals. In such places, there is usually not much competition for services. The consumer can be in a difficult position if they are not satisfied with the services they receive from the funeral director. Unlike many products, which can be returned due to faulty manufacture or lack of consumer satisfaction, it is highly unlikely that a body would be removed from a funeral parlour due to a lack of appropriate service. The lack of competition and choice hinders access to services if a person is not satisfied with the local director.

Other items and services that the undertaker "sells" besides caskets, urns, funeral services and burials or cremations are limousines, plots, receptions, clothing, jewellery and travel cars. The funeral director may complete the obituary and place it in the paper or on their website, and arrange and sell flowers, music, candles and church rentals or other services (sometimes on a commission basis if not directly supplied by the funeral home). Memorial cards and registers may be sold as well as vaults, vault liners and urns. They may also sell a video recording of the funeral to send to family members or others not able to attend the service and/or provide a livestream of the service.

It is no longer necessary to have a funeral arranged by an undertaker or funeral director. It is possible to handle all the details of the disposal of a loved one in an informal manner if the necessary forms and permissions are provided by the doctor or hospital, depending on the location of death. As well as informal disposal arrangements, celebrations of life are becoming more common than traditional funerals, with mourners remembering the deceased with stories, poetry, music, jokes and tributes, without a religious or spiritual facilitator or funeral director. Celebrations of life honour and respect the dead by celebrating them and their accomplishments, rather than dwelling on their absence from those who knew and loved them. Another area of social change regarding funerals, cremation services and burials is in music choices. An internet search in 2024 provided a plethora of sites which suggest the types of songs and music that could be played at end-of-life services, and many enable the reader to select genre, style and mood of the songs or music required to celebrate or recognize the end of a life.

LIVING FUNERALS AND WAKES

Since MAID was legalized in Canada, there have been more people interested in living funerals and wakes. These services, provided across the country by most funeral directors, involve holding events while an individual is alive. Recently, a friend of Jeanette's held such a service on the Saturday prior to her MAID appointment the following Monday. Lisa, who was sixty-three, was living with a heart condition for which there was no further cure or hope, so she was granted approval for MAID. With the help of family, friends and a few palliative care providers, a living funeral was planned. Even though Lisa had to wear an oxygen mask and be in a wheelchair, she still enjoyed a good time at the celebration of her life prior to her death. She was even able to "dance" to one of her favourite songs when a group of four friends encircled her wheelchair and held her while they moved her around the floor to "When We Were Young" by Adelle.

Journalist Heidi Petracek (2024) writes about a young Nova Scotian woman who is planning her own funeral after being granted access to MAID. The article speaks of "A Nova Scotia woman [who] has defied convention and societal norms by hosting her own living funeral, allowing people to celebrate her while she's still around. Once a performer herself, April Hubbard planned the event like a night at the theatre." The article quotes April:

> I always kind of thought that I would have to end my own life at some point in some way, even before MAID (medical assistance in dying) was legalized in Canada. But I don't think anybody expected it to be this soon for me and for me to have such a quick decline suddenly.

According to the article, when April was seventeen, she was diagnosed with tethered cord syndrome, a condition in which the spinal cord becomes attached to the tissue surrounding the spinal column. The article acknowledges that April "has been an outspoken advocate in the disability community and realizes her choice to seek MAID can be controversial." April held her living funeral in a local theatre. She concluded that her living funeral was "really a celebration of the way I lived my life."

Those who support the idea of living funerals and wakes suggest that they provide opportunities to address unresolved issues, apologize or make amends with friends and family members. They are seen as an opportunity to discuss topics often left unsaid, like death, legacies and afterlife beliefs. Adam Binstock's (2023) "Living Funerals Guide" notes:

> Facing our own mortality can be a scary and traumatic part of life. A dying person might find a pre funeral to be therapeutic in dealing with the prospect of death. Having control of the funeral allows them to share their stories, wisdom, and lessons, and be remembered as they wish to be.

CEMETERIES

Cemeteries can be places of great solitude and peace, where there is a lavish tradition of remembering the dead. Cemeteries were initially thought of (in the 1800s in Europe) as places for meeting with the dead, places for private meditation and prayer, and as settings to display symbols of love and respect for the dead. They also served the purpose of recording that people once lived and who they were related to. Europeans in the 1800s believed that stone or any hard "natural" surface had the power to preserve and retain memory. Furthermore, the hard, natural surface of marble, granite or stone can retain words by which loved ones can be acknowledged as well as remembered. These surfaces, being costly, help to remind viewers of the grave or marker that expenses were involved in the memorialization of this loved person. Such materials were also used to create art — sculptural denials of the ugliness of death. Poorer people, who could not afford such monuments to loved ones, brought flowers to beautify the final resting place of those they loved. Gravestones do not honour death, but life. It is our way of celebrating human relationships.

If we examine graveyards themselves or pictures of them, including those available on the internet, we can observe that there have been several motifs used throughout history to honour the dead. I am fortunate in growing up in England and visiting there frequently, because I have been able to visit some very old burial places, such as Westminster Abbey and Highgate Cemetery. However, even in our Canadian cemeteries, especially older ones, we can see many common symbols used to remember and honour the dead.

Graveyard Symbols

Graveyard art includes religious symbols such as praying hands, crosses and angels, as well as archways or gateways, which provide a sense of the deceased going through a gateway to another reality. Following are a few common graveyard symbols:

- Nature: Often cemeteries are in spacious open areas surrounded by trees and large expanses of green. These are places of quiet, peace and solitude — good settings to rest in. Often benches are situated throughout the cemetery to encourage private contemplation. Some of the symbols of nature in cemeteries include flowers, made of stone, marble and more recently plastic; the sun and moon; animals, especially lambs; and wishing wells. In nature symbols there is a sense of the cycle of life continuing without the deceased. The processes of birth, life and decay are also invoked in such symbols, presenting the reality that life goes on. These images may call to mind the Garden of Eden, the idea of "dust to dust" or the return to the land.
- Sleeping figures are often seen on memorial markers or gravestones, signifying that death is peaceful, a final resting; we go to sleep to awaken in heaven or wherever else we believe eternity to be. Angels are often presented on headstones, presumably to accompany us in eternity.
- Wreaths are present at funerals and gravesites. They represent never-ending circles joined together to invoke beginnings and endings. Wreaths also suggest life and are reminiscent of the cycle of nature. Flower wreaths provide colour to a sombre occasion and remind us that even in death there can be beauty. Snakes eating their tails present the idea of everlasting life.
- Praying hands suggest togetherness in eternity and the notion of meeting again in the afterlife.
- The hourglass with wings, often seen on gravestones, reminds us that we will all die, that time flies and time passes.

Cemeteries provide us with the hope of immortality, and some in Europe, like Highgate in London and Père Lachaise in Paris, provide guided tours. St. Paul's Cathedral and Westminster Abbey in London and many similar places throughout Europe provide the opportunity to view death and burial statutory as works of art. They are like museums of the famous. James Curl expresses his displeasure at the present-day lack of cemetery art:

> The neglected cemeteries, poorly designed crematoria, and abysmal tombstone designs of the present insult life itself, for death is an inevitable consequence of birth. By treating the disposal of the dead as though the problem was one of refuse-collection, society devalues life. We could learn much from the funerary

architecture of the past if we are to give new significance to a celebration of life in our own time. (1993: 367)

Grave Blankets

During the December holidays, there are many advertisements in local and national newspapers and magazines advertising "grave blankets" that have seasonal themes. A grave blanket is a "living" blanket of evergreens which are placed on the grave site to keep it "tidy" and as a way for the bereaved to remember their loved ones with a floral tribute. To find out more about this phenomenon, I went on the internet and found more than 842,000 websites dealing with this topic. Apparently, grave blankets can be purchased throughout the year, and they can include flowers as well as evergreens. They can be changed according to what is seasonally available so that the grave is always covered in fresh greenery or flowers. According to some of the websites, grave blankets are a way for the living to remember the dead, they create a pleasant and attractive ambience for visitors to cemeteries, and they help keep graves tidy.

CARDS OF CONDOLENCE

The greeting card industry creates memorial and remembrance cards to either commemorate a life or to raise philosophical notions of the afterlife and nature of death. These contain touching stories and poems, such as the following example:

> *I Am Not There*
> Do not stand at my grave and weep.
> I am not there. I do not sleep.
> I am a thousand winds that blow.
> I am the diamond glints on snow.
> I am the sunlight on ripened grain.
> I am the gentle autumn rain.
> When you awaken in the morning's hush
> I am the swift uplifting rush
> Of quiet birds in circled flight.
> I am the soft stars that shine at night.
> Do not stand at my grave and cry.
> I am not there; I did not die. (Tim Tiley Prints, Bristol, England)

CONCLUSION

In this chapter we highlighted some of the key changes that have occurred in the funeral industries and other organizations dealing with the final disposition of human remains. In this ever-burgeoning industry there is no doubt that many other forms of remembrance of the deceased will be created, at least in Western parts of the world and in capitalist countries, where individuals are willing and sometimes able to afford such resources.

SELF-REFLECTION AND THOUGHTFUL CONVERSATIONS

1. What would be your idea of a perfect funeral or celebration of life?
2. Do you think alternative funerals will be a continuing trend in the future? Why or why not?
3. Would you consider a green or eco funeral for yourself or a loved one? Why or why not?
4. Write up your own obituary and discuss it with the class.

VISIT YOUR LOCAL CEMETERY

1. What do you take to be the plan by which this cemetery was developed? (Notice where the earlier burials are located, the way the roads are arranged, etc.)
2. Which memorial markers seem more durable: marble or granite? Are all the inscriptions still readable? What colours of granite can be found?
3. Examine the inscriptions, and look for some that contain more than a name, dates and a short saying (such as "Rest in Peace"). What religious symbols can you find? What artistic motifs are found, and what does each mean to you? Do the names show who lived there as a community or a faith group? Make sketches and record some interesting gravestone epitaphs.
4. Record the age at death of a dozen females taken at random. Do the same for a dozen males. What is the average age at death for each gender? What significant difference, if any, is there in these averages?
5. In areas where there is an option, why do you think hillsides rather than valleys are usually chosen for cemeteries?
6. What considerations do you think are important in selecting a cemetery or a family plot within it?

Chapter Thirteen

LEGAL AND ETHICAL ISSUES IN DEATH AND DYING

SEVERAL LEGAL ASPECTS TO DYING need to be attended to prior to death to ensure that individuals' wishes are met after they die. They include the following:
- making a legal will, a living will or health-care directive;
- registering for organ and other body product donations (if previously chosen by the deceased);
- financial planning for our important ones; and
- choosing a health advocate or power of attorney.

Legislative concerns affect us prior to death, at the time of death and after death. Prior to death, we all ought to prepare our will, living will or health-care directive and perhaps select someone to act as our power of attorney and/or health guardian, depending on the laws in each province. Many people put this aside and do not consider it necessary until it is too late. At death, a certificate is legally required prior to the removal of a body from an institution, a home or the scene of an accident or suicide. After death, the following legal issues must be taken care of: organ, tissue, and body donations; disposition of assets; and taxes.

LIVING WILLS AND ADVANCE HEALTH-CARE DIRECTIVES

There are two types of living wills or advance health-care directives. One is an instructional advance directive, which talks "about what decisions you would want made or you describe your values and beliefs to guide a decision maker about what you would have wanted in a given situation." Instructional advance directives are also known as living wills. A proxy directive allows an individual to specify "who you would want to make decisions for you" when you are no longer able to make the decisions yourself. This type of directive is also known as durable power of attorney for health care (Health Law Institute n.d.).

All provinces recognize advance health-care directives, even though they may have different names. For example, in Alberta, the Northwest Territories and Nova Scotia, the legislation is known as a Personal Care Directive, while in British Columbia and Ontario, the Advance Care Planning Act sets out the laws for this process. In Manitoba, Saskatchewan, New Brunswick and Prince Edward Island, the term used is health-care directive or living will; in the Yukon the term is advance directive, and in Quebec the legal term is "in case of incapacity." For more information on any of these pieces of legislation, their most current form and name, and the necessary forms which need to be completed to arrange such procedures, you can go directly to the Health Law Institute website or to your provincial department of health. In all cases the goal of these laws is to encourage Canadians to consider "what may lay ahead, what your care needs might be, what might be the choices for your care and the type of decisions that may be required in the future" (Canadian Virtual Hospice n.d.). The Canadian Virtual Hospice is an excellent online resource for any Canadians seeking articles, assistance, guidelines or help with end-of-life issues. The group called End of Life Planning Canada developed a set of guidelines in a document titled *Patient Rights Booklet: Your Rights and Options at the End of Life* (2016). This handbook is used to assist individuals and families who wish to make end-of-life decisions and is available online.

PREPARING A LEGAL WILL

Each province in Canada has regulations regarding the disposition of a person's estate after death, and there are also provincial guidelines as to what form of will is acceptable. The purpose of a will is straightforward; it states what an individual wants to have happen to their assets: who gets what, when and under what conditions. A will could also state wishes regarding funeral and burial arrangements or who would care for young children if parents or guardians predecease them, and it may include last words of comfort to specific family members and friends.

The issue of living wills and advance health-care directives is separate from but interconnected with the following issues: the right to die with dignity; the right to request or refuse treatment; the rights of the mentally challenged or incompetent adult patient; the criteria for the determination of death; MAID; and civil and criminal liabilities of health-care professionals. With so many interwoven threads of legal, personal and professional interests, living wills and medical directives represent an interesting legal challenge and have an impact on social, political, religious and medical practices and decisions about the end of life. Many people prefer selecting a proxy, which would be a person who knows you well and whom you trust, who would be able to make complex decisions based on knowledge about you, given situations that sometimes cannot be set out in advance on paper.

> **The Text Within:**
> **Completing a Health-Care Directive (Jeanette)**
>
> When I completed a health-care directive, at the suggestion of my family physician, it had the advantage of causing me to reflect on what sorts of medical intervention I would require if faced with specific medical situations. In our discussion, I also became more informed as to what types of medical procedures were required and available in my area. Completing a medical directive, then, has the additional advantage of enabling us to be better, more informed consumers of health care in Canada. As well, it can provide a relatively non-threatening opportunity for a frank and open discussion between patient and physician, as well as between the individual and their family and other important ones.

ETHICAL WILLS

An ethical will is a way for individuals to share their values and beliefs with family and friends who are left behind. Ethical wills are usually written as separate documents attached to a legal will. Two individuals Jeanette knows prepared ethical wills on videotapes for their grandchildren. Ethical wills were initially described in Hebrew scripture, so they are not a new concept. In an article in *My Jewish Learning*, Rabbi Jack Riemer talks about using an ethical will to pass on a written spiritual legacy to one's grandchildren:

> There is a lovely Jewish custom, one that is unfortunately not sufficiently known in our time, of writing what is called an ethical will. Parents would write a letter to their children in which they would try to sum up all that they had learned in life. ... They would leave these letters behind because they believed that the wisdom they had acquired was just as much part of the legacy they wanted to leave their children as were all of the material possessions. (Riemer n.d.)

Rabbi Riemer also raises interesting questions related to personal reflection when writing ethical wills:

> An ethical will is not an easy thing to write. In doing so, one confronts oneself. One must look inward to see what are the essential truths one has learned in a lifetime, face up to one's failures, and consider what are the things that really count. Thus, an individual learns a great deal about himself or herself when writing an ethical will. If you had time to write just one letter, to whom would it be addressed? What would it say? What would you leave out? Would you chastise and rebuke? Would you thank, forgive, or seek to instruct?

Riemer notes that an ethical will reflects the "voice of the heart" in that it is a "love letter to your family." Some common themes include "important personal values, important spiritual values, hopes and blessings for future generations, life's lessons and forgiving others and asking for forgiveness."

In Jeanette's experience of working with and for older persons, she has seen a great interest in ethical wills. When conferences and workshops are being planned, this topic is often popular. Older persons see the ethical will as a way of passing on their values and beliefs to their grandchildren in a legitimate, if not legal, manner. The writer of an ethical will has the opportunity to reflect upon and articulate their values and experiences, so it is a way to affirm the past and to be positive about the future. There will be an increasing interest in the ethical will, in our view, and we expect to see more people attaching this document to their legal wills.

ORGAN DONATIONS

Most Canadian provinces have their own version of the Anatomical Gift Act, which determines the procedures by which organs, tissue, blood products, other body parts and even entire cadavers may be donated by individuals. Most provinces require donors to sign a specific section of their driving licence, while others have a separate form to fill out.

According to Canadian Blood Services' website,

> Blood and blood products are a critical part of everyday medical care including major surgeries, medical procedures, cancer treatments and managing diseases and disorders. As a blood donor, you form a vital link in Canada's lifeline, helping many Canadians wake up healthy each day. (2025)

You can find more information about how to donate blood, your blood type, rare blood types and what is required. There is also information about plasma, stem cells, and organ and tissue donation.

Health Canada (2023) states,

> Every year, many Canadians receive life-saving organ transplants, while thousands still wait, and hundreds die because not enough organs are available. Despite significant progress in organ donation rates, Canada is still unable to meet the needs of all patients waiting for an organ. With 3,777 people in Canada waiting for a transplant as of December 2022, and only a fraction of Canadians registered as donors—the need for donors is critical.

According to Health Canada, "a total of 2,936 solid organ transplants — such as kidney, heart, lung, liver, etc. — were performed in Canada in 2022. This is an increase of 6.8 percent compared to 2021 and a 31.4 percent increase compared to ten years ago. As of December 31, 2022, 3,777 Canadians were on wait lists to receive a transplant."

As well as issues related to whether or not Canadians should be compensated for donating blood, tissue, cell products and organs, there is concern about the time factor in most organ transplants; therefore, hospital deaths are more suitable for all transplants except cornea and skin. The length of time within which organs may be used after the death of the donor are as follows: "Heart 4–6 hours, Lungs 4–6 hours, Liver 8–12 hours, Kidneys 24–36 hours" (DonorAlliance 2025). In 2022, journalist Kate Dubinsky reported that "human cadavers are a key teaching tool for future doctors and dentists, but in some medical schools, donations have dropped since the start of the COVID-19 pandemic."

The Government of Canada (2025c) website provides provincial rules and information as to how to donate blood products, tissues and organs. No doubt, as the need for a ready supply of these essential products continues to increase, not only in Canada but globally, more rules and regulations will be required to ensure that these supplies are forthcoming.

FINANCIAL PLANNING

Making financial plans for the disposition of an estate prior to death can help the executor or personal representative to administer an estate in accordance with the individual's wishes. There are a variety of tax and other legal considerations, which include identifying the location of important documents like the birth certificate, social insurance number, will, insurance policies, mortgages, deeds, tax bills, leases, debts and bank accounts. As well, the executor should know about any death benefits the deceased is eligible for, which include survivors' benefits, military pensions and the Canada Pension Plan death benefit. Along with financial planning, many Canadians also prefer to make prepaid arrangements for their funeral, again to save their bereaved loved ones this difficult task and to participate in discussions with loved ones while making these decisions. Most provinces have memorial societies, funeral cooperatives and other groups that provide lower-cost or prepaid services. As well, most banks in Canada have financial planners that clients can meet with, or tax accountants and funeral directors may be able to help with financial arrangements, normally for a fee.

CHARITABLE DONATIONS

Many organizations seek legacy donations from individual Canadians who are passionate about or have been touched by a specific cause. The Canadian Cancer Society, Doctors Without Borders, and many other health-related organizations benefit from financial donations that individuals choose to make as part of their will. Such a gift could also go to a local group related to the arts, literary pursuits or theatre; it could be for a shelter housing women experiencing violence or an animal rescue organization. Historically, "tithing" was giving a regular donation (often 10 percent of annual income) to support one's own community or place of faith. Some people become a regular monthly donor during their lifetime, and they may also leave money to those same causes after they die. These charitable donations have legal implications for estates, taxes and wills.

This gift-giving option is available to anyone but may be particularly relevant for individuals who do not have children or whose family has become estranged, those who have great wealth, people with a community-based sense of responsibility or those who have priorities not shared by their immediate loved ones. In a society in which we see increased geographical mobility and families separating through divorce, individuals do not always live in the same town or even country as their children and grandchildren. This can add to reasons why people may elect to create a section in their will related to local community-based and more global and conscientiously driven donations. Do you have a cause you deeply believe in that you would like to support?

Sometimes individuals die without doing any estate planning. Have you ever seen a sign at a house that says "Estate Sale — everything must go"? Sometimes there is no immediate family, and no plan or will has been made by the individual living there. At times such as this, the state (an appointed public trustee) will take on the responsibility of disbursing that person's estate. Valuable artifacts are sometimes found — paintings, precious gems or jewellery, or simply, many pairs of shoes and collectables the owner bought over a lifetime. What should we do with those items? Donating to a shelter or thrift store allows these once cherished items to have a second life — someone in need (e.g., refugees and newcomers) can benefit from the leftover furniture, clothing and dishware. Sometimes, an abandoned home can also reveal a treasure trove of history. Whose right is it to decide what to do with these items if the owner had no family and made no plans? How a family should decide can be a broad ethical terrain as well, depending on siblings and loved ones to agree. In a day and age when we all collect many items of personal value, and sometimes monetary value, the disbursement of our things after death can be a legal and ethical quandary, not easy for loved ones to solve.

PREPARING YOUR OWN DEATH PLAN

It is common for parents in Canada to produce a detailed birth plan, which contains their wishes for the process of the birth of their baby. For the past twenty years, while teaching sociology courses about death and dying, both in the classroom and online, we have required students to complete a similar kind of plan — a death plan. The objective of this assignment is to take full responsibility for how, given the choice, we would like to spend our final days. The plan may include directions as to our funeral or memorial service and the final disposition of our body. As well as we may describe those behaviours, values and traits that we want others to remember about us. Included in the death plan might be the following if one is choosing MAID: the place of death, with whom (or alone), if the individual wants medication or pain control, what happens after death, and all the elements of a funeral or memorial service (from types of music and flowers to food and drink). The death plan may also respond to your death if it is unplanned (e.g., what should happen in the event of a car accident or plane crash?) or the ways in which you choose palliative care over MAID. The plan includes who, if anyone, would be pallbearers or speakers at the memorial service, who would preside at the interment and so on. It may include making decisions about a tombstone and the font used for your name! Or would you rather have your ashes strewn by airplane over some beloved spot?

In this plan, you may also make decisions about charitable donations, who should get your things of value. In some cases, we find that older adults who passed away had pets who are themselves older and need loving care. Animals are an important part of the equation — who will care for them? Your death plan may also indicate who should care for the beloved cactus you nurtured for years, or the quilt your grandmother sewed for you (which probably holds no monetary value but was made with love for you). A death plan may also state more esoteric wishes for the loved ones who will bury you — to buy a home with the inheritance for their own emotional stability, for two warring factions to sort out their differences, for spiritual guidance for a young person in trouble or well wishes for loved members of your community. A death plan may express a prayer or a desire for the future well-being of your loved ones, or it may state what you want your own legacy to be (e.g., a plaque or memorial located somewhere special).

Most students find this a fascinating and rewarding exercise. Many include letters to important ones saying final goodbyes, write poems or select songs they want presented at their wake. This assignment brings death closer to home, helping us to realize how much work is involved in making final decisions and how we can take some responsibility for tying up loose ends.

CONCLUSION

As you can see in this chapter, there are many financial and legal aspects to deal with prior to and after death, for the individual and their important ones. Some of these challenges can be dealt with through various community-based organizations, banks, financial institutions, lawyers, accountants and funeral homes.

SELF-REFLECTION AND THOUGHTFUL CONVERSATIONS

1. Is it important to make a will and a living will? Why or why not?
2. If you were to produce a medical directive, what features would you include?
3. What might be some of the personal and social consequences of organ donation?

IN-CLASS ASSIGNMENTS

1. Find out what legal requirements for living wills or medical directives are necessary in your province. Do the same for organ donations and your provincial equivalent of a medical proxy or health guardianship.
2. Write an ethical will.
3. Write up your own death plan.

Chapter Fourteen

CAUSES AND PREVENTION OF SUICIDE IN CANADA

Catherine White

(This chapter was written by Dr. Catherine White, a recently retired occupational therapist working in mental health and related fields. Her recent experience includes six years as an assistant professor in the School of Occupational Therapy, Dalhousie University, five years in New Brunswick with Horizon Health Network as prevention coordinator (Suicide Prevention and Mental Health Promotion), part-time teaching (Gerontology) at St. Thomas University and one year as an assistant professor (Family Studies and Gerontology), Mount Saint Vincent University).

> **The Text Within: Encounters with Suicide (Catherine)**
>
> I answered the phone one Sunday morning, only to hear my mother say, "She is gone ... your sister is gone." Gone? Where had she gone? My sister's life had taken a path quite different from my own. As a family, we had feared her untimely death might result "by accident" from the risky behaviour she often chose, but we were unprepared to learn she had intentionally taken her own life. At the age of forty-eight, she was gone. Not coming back. Many questions and no opportunity to have them answered. That is what suicide is like — the unfathomable. This was not my first brush with suicide. My professional role placed me right in its path. As I reflect on my twenty-five-year career as an occupational therapist practising in the field of mental health, I can visualize many of the distressed clients I encountered. I recall chasing one girl out the back door of the hospital, my heart pounding as I realized she might outrun me, and I would never see her again. "Cathy, why won't you let me die?" she shouted back at me. I later realized she wasn't running from me; she was running from her atrocious past. Thoughts she could no longer cope with. I recall thinking, "I don't know what to do here. I can't make it go away." All I could think of was "Be yourself, be here for her. Show her you care."

IN A WORLD WHERE PEOPLE GO TO GREAT LENGTHS to preserve or extend their lives, it can be challenging to understand why others would take steps that intentionally lead to death, yet each year in Canada, an estimated 4,500 people die by suicide (Public Health Agency of Canada 2024b). Many others live in despair with suicidal ideation (taunted by thoughts of suicide that vary in intensity), in the aftermath of an attempt or in mourning for someone lost to suicide. Even though suicide can be traced long into history, it remains an enigma. The legalization of medical assistance in dying (MAID) in Canada in 2016 adds a new perspective, socially sanctioning the choice to end your life, although it is not accessible to those solely with a mental health concern (Government of Canada 2024c). While there are cultural differences, death by suicide is generally considered a tragic outcome for people across the lifespan and around the world.

Accurate and timely statistics regarding suicide are difficult to obtain as investigations are often lengthy and complex, and Canadian provinces document suicides differently, making national compilations challenging. Age and gender are commonly referenced when discussing suicide. For example, according to the most recent Government of Canada reports, three times more males as compared to females die by suicide each year, but females are more likely to experience suicidal ideation. Males from sexual minorities, as well as Indigenous, middle-aged, and military personnel are particularly vulnerable (Oliffe et al. 2021). Men experiencing loneliness and isolation, feeling like a failure and experiencing stress and emotional pain as they relate to suicide risk have been discussed as research priorities (Bennett et al. 2024). Females are generally more likely to seek help, but John Oliffe, Mary Kelley, Gabriella Montaner and colleagues (2021) discuss the need for employers in male-dominated professions, such as the military and first responders, to make help-seeking in the face of mental health challenges more acceptable.

With regard to age, suicide deaths in preteens are extremely rare, but for youth and young adults up to age 34, it was the second leading cause of death (second only to accidental deaths), accounting for almost 40 percent of all suicide deaths, in Canada in 2021. Stressors old and new are to blame. Being victimized by bullying (including cyberbullying) has been identified as a major risk factor for youth suicide (Li et al. 2024). In fact, cyberbullying has been called "a gateway to suicidal thinking" (Steffens 2019: 41). Amanda Todd, Jenna Bowers-Bryanton and Rehtaeh Parsons are just a few examples of youth in Canada who exemplify this tragic outcome. Their suicide deaths in the aftermath of bullying/cyberbullying and similar events have led to increased focus on laws meant to prohibit such actions, but the stated outcomes to perpetrators (they might "have their devices taken away, have to pay their victims and may even face jail time") remain inadequate, and bullying/cyberbullying remain a devastating concern.

Sexual and gender diverse youth are among those with a higher prevalence of suicidality (Richardson, Connell et al. 2024). The risk of suicidal thoughts, plans and attempts for Canadian youth aged 15 to 17 with sexually diverse identities as compared to their heterosexual peers was three times higher.

Other contributing factors, such as lower life satisfaction and reduced emotional well-being, have been implicated (Huertes-Del Arco et al. 2024), but given their variable precursors, specific causes are unclear. Ana Huertes-Del Arco, Eva Izquierdo-Sotorrío, Miguel Carrasco and colleagues discuss humiliation, feeling like a failure and being unable to escape from a painful situation as possible contributors. Substance abuse, being a victim of violence (physical or sexual), conflict with family or friends, knowing someone who recently died by suicide and other stressful life events have also been linked to suicide risk in youth (Steffens 2019). Newer stressors such as concern for the environment, climate change (known as ecoanxiety) and response to catastrophic events are being explored, and preliminary results show linkages to depression and risk for suicide in youth (Cianconi et al. 2020).

As the Statista (2024) report indicates, over 40 percent of the suicide deaths in 2021 were attributed to those over age 50. Older adults may face losses related to physical and mental health, resulting in a declining quality of life and increased dependence on others, which may become too great (Erlangsen et al. 2021). Attempts made by older adults are more likely to be lethal (especially for men), with one in four attempts resulting in a suicide, as compared to ten to twenty attempts for every one suicide in the general population (Van Orden and Conwell 2016). Research suggests a focus on protective factors — such as finding reasons to live, enhancing social supports and relationships and engaging in meaningful community activities, perhaps outside of their comfort zone — as a positive step in suicide prevention (Deuter et al. 2020). Furthermore, as Gordon Flett and Marnin Heisel point out, mattering, or having a sense of purpose in life, is critical. They state, "The feeling of mattering provides a sense of connection and comfort and a source of resilience that is a strong buffer of life problems and feelings of stress and distress" (2021: 2452).

Overall, the age group from 25 to 64 reflected the highest number of suicide deaths in the Statista report. Thus, middle age, especially for men, presents the highest risk for suicide. While age and gender offer interesting vantage points to examine suicide, a variety of other viewpoints, including those of higher-risk groups, need to be considered. This chapter explores theoretical perspectives, high-risk groups, risk and protective factors and prevention.

THEORETICAL PERSPECTIVES

Historically, sociologist Émile Durkheim (1951 [1897]) is credited as the first person to advance a theory of suicide. Durkheim's work identified both inter- and intra-personal contributing factors, including altruistic (over-integration to a group; suicide for the benefit of a group), egoistic (limited social integration), anomic (inadequate moral regulation, inattention to social norms) and fatalistic (excessive moral regulation; not meeting self-imposed standards) perspectives that may explain suicide, confirming a range of causes (Auger 2019; Zhang 2019). His theory also identified protective factors, including social integration (presence of social ties) and moral regulation (alignment with social norms).

Many of the newer theoretical understandings draw on this early work but integrate a focus on the transitions that occur in the ideation-to-action framework (Klonsky and May 2015). For example, Thomas Joiner's interpersonal theory of suicide posits that suicide is the result of thwarted belonging and perceived burdensomeness, accompanied by hopelessness and the acquired capability to act (Van Orden et al. 2010). Other theories add a focus on unbearable pain (often psychological pain, or psychache) (Klonsky and May 2015; Shneidman 1993), response to a negative life event (Conejero et al. 2018) or the interplay between risk factors and protective factors (Brown and Schuman 2021).

Fluid vulnerability theory adds the perspective that suicidality is both individualized (given the variability of baseline and acute risks one might face) and dynamic (given the fluctuations in mood and intent that may occur) (Rudd 2006; Rugo-Cook et al. 2021). In this theory, each person has baseline risk factors, or an array of predisposing factors that have accumulated throughout life. Examples might include adverse childhood events or genetic vulnerability. Acute risks or stressors can then interact with baseline risks and trigger the activation of "suicidal mode," defined as "an active suicidal episode that is triggered by an environmental stressor" (1081). This may occur more readily in those with greater baseline risk factors, thus explaining why two or more people can experience the same acute stressor (such as a devastating diagnosis or a military deployment to a war-torn area), but not all experience the same outcome.

While these theories consider predisposing factors and the accumulation of adverse events across the lifespan alongside acute or emerging stressors, they offer little attention to the varying contexts in which we live. From a critical suicidology perspective, Jennifer White observes that suicide prevention often focuses on solutions that "target individuals for change, but leave the specific social, political and cultural context of people's lives — including the corrosive effects of structural inequalities — unaccounted for" (2017: 472). Individual approaches are not enough.

The critical-ecological framework acknowledges the need to broaden the view beyond the individual — to examine the situation and be prepared to act — by combining Bronfenbrenner's focus on context, including the interdependent levels of the environment (macrosystem, exosystem, mesosystem and microsystem), with action-oriented critical theory (Norris et al. 2013). In this theory, the individual is nested at the centre of interdependent levels. The microsystem includes direct contact with family, work/school and neighbours. The mesosystem focuses on the interaction between microsystem influences. The exosystem includes government agencies and community resources, and the macrosystem includes culture and ideologies. The critical component of this theory incorporates the process of becoming critically conscious, examining power imbalances and oppression, and envisioning a different future. The social-ecological suicide prevention model adds to this understanding specifically with regard to suicide prevention, focusing attention on the need for integrated multi-level approaches across the ecological levels that do not solely situate the problem in the individual and do not wait for the individual to become suicidal before acting (Cramer and Kapusta 2017). To gain a better understanding of the ways in which suicidal ideation emerges, and how it evolves toward action, as well as what can be done to support prevention, one theory is not enough. Given the personal and contextual variability between individuals and the fluctuations within each person, each of the theories discussed can play a role.

Risk Factors and Protective Factors

Although a wide variety of assessment tools are used to assess the risk of suicide, trying to predict if and when a suicide might occur is generally considered a fruitless effort. There is far too much variability between and within individuals. As Jeanette A. Auger concludes, "Suicide involves a highly complex set of interconnected interactions that involve psychological, societal, cultural, genetic, biochemical and social factors" (2019: 249). The constellation of risk factors and protective factors is ever-changing and differs for each person. Some people live with chronic suicidality, sometimes making their imminent risk or cries for help fall on deaf ears. For others, the notion of suicide seems to "come out of nowhere" as they may keep it to themselves. As AnnaBelle Bryan, Jacqueline Theriault and Craig Bryan discuss (2020), thoughts of suicide may be *discontinuous*, fluctuating in the days and hours immediately preceding a suicide attempt. They found that 75–90 percent of individuals who attempt suicide did so without advance planning and only made the final decision to act within the preceding hour.

Although suicide is impossible to predict, the most common approach to assessing risk and choosing targets for change is to examine risk factors and protective factors. Warning signs include increased talk about death, hinting that they won't be around, calling people to say goodbye and giving away valuables. The *National Suicide Prevention Action Plan 2024–2027* (Public Health Agency of Canada 2024c) clarifies that risk factors include anything that increases the likelihood of serious thoughts of suicide, suicide attempts and/or death by suicide, while protective factors decrease the risk and may support mental health and well-being overall. The action plan points out that risk and protective factors can be seen at the individual level, the interpersonal level and the community level, aligning well with the ecological perspectives. Individual risk factors discussed in the action plan include physical or mental health challenges, including chronic pain, substance use, life stressors such as job loss or loss of a relationship, homelessness, low income, low education level and disability. Having a previous suicide attempt, a family history of suicide or experiencing a suicide loss also increases the risk of suicide. At the interpersonal level, adverse childhood experiences, loneliness and bullying (either in-person and online) are identified as risk factors. Finally, at the community level, discrimination, exposure to violence (physical, sexual or emotional), living in a socially or economically deprived area, living in a rural or remote area, and historical and intergenerational losses are discussed as risks.

Other authors have discussed risk factors relevant to specific populations. For example, newcomers to Canada may experience culture shock, loneliness and isolation as they adjust to a new country (Aran et al. 2022). Among older adults, negative impacts on independence, sense of usefulness, value, dignity and pleasure in life have been identified as risks for suicide (Fässberg et al. 2016; Kjølseth et al. 2010; Obuobi-Donkor et al. 2021). Impacts on independent functioning, such as loss of mobility, impaired ability to complete self-care tasks and loss of driving, can impact autonomy regarding social and community activities, resulting in increased sense of burden and impacts on quality of life (Mournet et al. 2020; Westefeld et al. 2015). The diagnosis of dementia can be a risk factor, especially in the first year following the diagnosis, when the person may have insight into the likely trajectory and still be able to plan and carry out suicide. As Timothy Schmutte, Mark Olfson, Donovan Maust and colleagues (2022) point out, given the concerns of the first year, suicide risk assessment is an important accompaniment to confirming a diagnosis of dementia. Social isolation and loneliness have also been implicated in the suicide of older adults (see, for example, Heuser and Howe 2019; Niu et al. 2020; Obuobi-Donkor et al. 2021). This may include losing social supports due to the death of intimate partners and friends, retirement (which removes one from an important social network) and health changes (Bonnewyn et al. 2014; Westefeld et al. 2015). A further concern relates to the macrosystem issue of ageism, where older adults no longer see their role in life and may feel expendable or disposable (Flett and Heisel, 2021).

Rebecca Richardson, Tanya Connell, Mandie Foster et al. (2024) discuss risk factors for youth at the individual, relational, community or societal level. They found that individuals in gender and sexual minorities and those with mental health disorders, problem behaviours, previous suicidality, self-harm or who were female experienced the greatest vulnerability, and bullying victimization presented the highest risk factor for suicide. They also highlighted research discussing how exposure to childhood maltreatment, community violence, parental separation and hopelessness could increase risk factors for suicidal behaviour. In another study, Black youth who were experiencing bullying/cyberbullying as well as perceiving themselves to be over or underweight placed them at increased risk for suicide (Richardson and Gunn 2024). As this study discussed, the intersectionality of race and identifying within a sexual minority increased the likelihood of bullying/cyberbullying, thus increasing suicide risk.

Protective factors, to mitigate risk, are often considered the opposite of risk factors, or the absence of risk factors, but specific protective factors are also identified. The national action plan lists effective coping and problem-solving skills, a sense of cultural identity, religious and spiritual beliefs, an optimistic outlook, self-esteem, a sense of meaning and reasons for living as protective factors in the face of individual risk factors. To mitigate interpersonal risk factors, the plan discusses having strong personal relationships and social support networks with peers, friends, partners and family. Regarding community risk factors, feeling connected to the community and having a safe and stable environment, timely access to appropriate health care and restricted access to lethal means (weapons, medications) are key protective factors.

For older adults, a variety of protective factors have been identified. The presence of strong social supports, social connectedness and the opportunity for social interactions are among the strongest protective factors. Other factors include overall health condition, receiving timely and appropriate care for mental and physical health problems, having a sense of purpose in life, effective coping skills and being adaptable to change (Aviad and Cohen-Louck 2021; Cabello et al. 2020; Obuobi-Donkor et al. 2021). Opportunities for helping others, such as offering informal support, can decrease perceived burdensomeness and help with social connection (Smith et al. 2020).

Among youth, as Richardson, Connell et al. (2024) note, anti-bullying campaigns, efforts to enhance inclusivity and connectedness and timely access to health care are essential. They also suggest a shift in classroom culture from competitiveness to collaboration to enhance the sense of belonging and safety.

High-Risk Groups

While the risk of suicide crosses all socioeconomic groups, all ethnicities, all sexualities, all genders, all ages (except for the very young) and all ability levels, some clusters of the population face increased vulnerability. The rest of the chapter discusses some examples.

SUICIDE AMONG INDIGENOUS PEOPLES

Rates of suicide are disproportionately high among Indigenous Peoples, at three to five times the national average (Dunn et al. 2024). It is especially concerning that in some communities, Indigenous children up to age 15 have suicide rates fifty times higher than their non-Indigenous peers (Kumar and Tjepkema 2019). Suicides in Indigenous communities are known to reflect socioeconomic inequality and are notably influenced by disparities in the social determinants of health, especially in remote areas (Dunn et al. 2024). The Government of Canada's (2024d) report *Suicide Prevention in Indigenous Communities* suggests that a focus on the disparities in the social determinants of health and promoting a sense of hope, purpose, meaning and belonging may be effective in promoting life and preventing suicide for Indigenous Peoples. In the report, Indigenous Services Canada identified suicide prevention and life promotion as a priority for Indigenous communities, clarifying the need to address the many contributing factors, including the consequences of colonialism, discrimination, community disruption and the loss of culture and language. One initiative in alignment with the recommendations of the Truth and Reconciliation Commission (2015), specifically regarding the social determinants of health, relates to education. Education institutions have been encouraged to increase the number of Indigenous students pursuing postsecondary education, especially in health-care professions. As Nolan Hop Wo, Kelly Anderson, Lloy Wylie and Arlene MacDougall (2020) point out, many First Nations communities with more autonomy and control over their health-care services report no incidents of youth suicide. Experiencing cultural continuity and native language use are associated with lower suicide rates. While some steps have been taken to increase the number of health professionals with Indigenous roots, Hop Wo and colleagues discuss how pursuing a postsecondary education is increasingly stressful for all students, with an increased number reporting hopelessness and depression and seeking help with complex mental health needs. Their study draws attention to the fact that although there is increasing focus on mental health in general in postsecondary institutions, little attention is directed to the specific needs of Indigenous students who are distanced from their home and culture and are more likely to experience mental health issues, such as depression, anxiety, increased self-harm, suicidal ideation and suicide attempts as compared to their non-Indigenous peers.

If institutions continue to offer "training to Indigenous peoples without a deeper understanding of the Indigenous connections to ceremony, protocols, language, spiritual teachings, community, stories, and the impact of history, they will repeat the cycle of colonization and assimilation" (Steinhauer and Lamouche 2015: 152). Like all initiatives to address the prevention of suicide, culturally relevant practices are essential but "there remains a paucity of safety planning practices that are tailored to Indigenous peoples" (Dunn et al. 2024: 223). Canada's suicide prevention action plan acknowledges the importance of self-determination and Indigenous-led strategies to ensure they are informed by the culturally specific needs of First Nations, Inuit and Métis communities. The action plan observes, "Some Indigenous approaches … shift from an exclusive focus on individual problems to one that centres on community strength and capacity in the face of oppressive policies and condition" (5), thus reflecting an ecological perspective to the prevention of suicide.

SUICIDE AMONG THE 2SLGBTQ+ COMMUNITY

As many as 82 percent of individuals in gender and sexual minorities reported having experienced suicidal ideation, and 39 percent had attempted suicide at some point in their lives, compared to 13 percent of the general population who experienced suicidal ideation and 4.6 percent who had attempted suicide, reflecting an increased risk (Coleman et al. 2024). Multiple contributing factors, such as interpersonal conflict/relationship issues, being victims of violence, emotional issues/mental illness, stress related to life circumstances and minority stress related to sexuality and gender identity have been found (Ferlatte et al. 2024). The risk has been further discussed in relation to minority stress across age groups, whereby acceptance, choices around concealing one's identity and fear of social exclusion have been implicated as contributors to suicidal ideation (Canen and Brausch 2024).

A better understanding of the contributing factors is important to inform relevant approaches to suicide prevention within this community. Ecological models that take context into consideration are particularly poignant (Pharr and Batra 2024). For example, some people may be battling intra- or interpersonal conflicts or family exclusion, while others are dealing with policy decisions, stigma or discrimination at a broader level that impact their everyday lives. A scoping review regarding youth in this population identified a wide range of factors across the levels of the social-ecological model (Wallace et al. 2024). Examples of risk factors included a religious upbringing with unresolved shame (intrapersonal); interpersonal violence, referred to as "enacted stigma" (903), family rejection (interpersonal); minority stress at school/work, lack of identity-appropriate health care (organizational/community level); and societal stigmatization, victimization and discrimination (policy and societal level).

Jennifer Pharr and Kavita Batra (2024) adapted the social-ecological model, defining individual, family, community and societal influences specific to suicidal ideation among sexual and gender minorities. They highlighted that being "out" (where one's identity was known by others) was a risk factor for some and a protective factor for others. Those who were guarded and vigilant (not wanting others to know in anticipation of potential discrimination or stigma) were at higher risk for suicidal ideation (individual level). Families could be either protective or detrimental depending on their response — acceptance or rejection (family level). Bearing the brunt of discrimination in social, institutional or workplace settings could negatively impact mental health (community level). Living in a location where laws and policies contributed to marginalization and vulnerability (societal level) was an additional risk factor.

As with other populations, multiple risk factors are identified, but there is insufficient evidence to confirm a "cause and effect" relationship, thus making the prediction of suicide impossible. Individuals in sexual and gender minorities face many barriers to inclusion across multiple ecological levels but can draw on personal resilience and additional protective factors as they navigate challenges and move toward a positive future. These may include self-esteem, self-efficacy, positive academic self-concept and reframing social rejection (intrapersonal); familial connectedness, cohesion, acceptance, social support, positive coming out experiences and 2SLGBTQ+ friendships (interpersonal); community 2SLGBTQ+ services and resources, access to inclusive health care and chosen name used at school and within the community (organizational/community level); and inclusive 2SLGBTQ+ policies and legislation, funding for mental health services, anti-bullying policies and engagement with activism (policy/societal level) (Wallace et al. 2024). Emma Wallace, Siobhan O'Neill and Susan Lagdon (2024) conclude that addressing minority stress and combating bullying, victimization, interpersonal violence, marginalization and discrimination through policies and legislation are essential to mitigate suicide risk in the 2SLGBTQ+ population. Critical perspectives, whereby a critically conscious stance is taken, provide a lens through which to perceive and contest oppression to make way for a different future and may lend well in this situation (Brookfield 2005).

SUICIDE AMONG THE ARMED FORCES AND VETERANS

The risk of suicide is a concerning issue for the armed forces, both for serving members and for veterans. A wide range of risk factors is relevant to military populations. Stressors commonly faced by military members include frequent relocations and adjustment to new environments, impacting social connections and sense of belonging, prolonged separation from family and friends during deployments and facing the risk of personal harm on a regular basis (physical and psychological) in both training and active duty. Although rates of suicide are generally higher for veterans, both veterans and active members may experience mental or physical health problems, exposure to cumulative trauma (including sexual trauma) and medical or involuntary discharge from the military (Sadler et al. 2024).

The 2023 *Report on Suicide Mortality in the Canadian Armed Forces* compared male and female suicide deaths. At the time of their suicide death, among males, 25 percent had depressive disorders, 16.7 percent had anxiety disorders, 8.3 percent had post-traumatic stress disorder (PTSD), and 25 percent had other trauma and stress-related disorders. Addiction or substance use disorder was reported in 8.3 percent of male suicide deaths, and 16.7 percent had a traumatic brain injury. In comparison, at the time of their suicide death, 33.3 percent of females had depressive disorders, 33.3 percent had anxiety disorders, 16.7 percent had PTSD, 16.7 percent had other trauma and stress-related disorders. Addiction or substance use disorder was reported in 33.3 percent of female suicide deaths, and 33.3 percent had been identified with a personality disorder (Boulos 2023). As the report noted, 100 percent of males and 83.3 percent of females who died in the reporting period experienced at least one additional work/life stressor, including a failing relationship, friend/family suicide, family/friend death, family and/or personal illness, excessive debt, work problems and legal problems. Post-traumatic stress, depression and substance use disorders have also been linked to suicide risk for both veterans and current military members (Bryan et al. 2015).

Veterans and military members may have also been exposed to moral injuries, the "invisible injuries of war ... deeper rooted injuries to the soul," including actively engaging in unacceptable behaviour or passively witnessing another doing so, being unable to prevent suffering or death, assaulting or inflicting harm on the innocent and being exposed to human remains (Richardson and Lamson 2022: 145), resulting in profound shame, guilt and anger, as well as "immense moral dissonance" (152). Engaging in such activities that "severely shake a combatant's moral code and challenge basic expectations of right and wrong" can result in suicidal ideation and suicide (Levi-Belz et al. 2023: 625). Military members experiencing moral injury may be reluctant to seek help due to stigma, denial or mistrust of the military health system (Houle et al. 2022). A strong research base regarding moral injury is lacking, but similar to PTSD and traumatic brain injury, it can be linked to suicidality (Parry et al. 2023).

While the military is paying increased attention to the mental health and well-being of its members, the culture that values physical strength, endurance and emotional fortitude may unwittingly convey that self-identifying and asking for help could be a career-limiting move. Military members (particularly females) have not always received support when reporting unwanted sexual advances. As Andrea Brown, Heather Millman, Linna Tam-Seto and colleagues (2024) report, in the study period, 57 percent of military sexual trauma incidents among Canadian Armed Forces members went unreported, and many victims did not seek mental health treatment. Reasons given included safety concerns or fear of further violence or repercussions, potential negative impacts on their career, fear of being blamed or treated differently, belief that reporting would be futile and concern that confidentiality would not be respected. This is a concerning situation given the correlation between military sexual trauma and adverse mental health outcomes, including risk for suicide.

SUICIDE AMONG PRISON INMATES

Risk of suicide is a significant concern among prison inmates, particularly for those with lengthy sentences and little hope of release. Incarcerated individuals are nine times more likely to die by suicide than the general population (Marks et al. 2024). One in five prisoners who attempt suicide have done so before; half of all who die by suicide in prison have previously attempted; and one in ten prisoners will attempt suicide during their incarceration (Favril et al. 2022). The culture of punishment within prisons perpetuates emotions such as fear, anger, anxiety, mistrust and lack of safety, which can lead to aggression, trauma, depression and suicide (Bloom and Bradshaw 2022). Prisoners are separated from family, friends and supports, and meaningful activity, while often being treated in a dehumanizing manner. The seemingly endless loop of punishment for violation of rules that are virtually impossible to follow can lead to hopelessness. As Tina Bloom and G. Bradshaw observe, "The current prison staff culture inflames conflict between prisoners and staff, exacerbates prisoners' distrust of authority, increases a sense of alienation, and undermines any prosocial behavior" (142). Attempting suicide is indicative of a high level of distress that can build up in these circumstances. Louis Favril, Jenny Shaw and Seena Fazel found a variety of additional prison-related factors that related to suicide risk. Examples include bullying, problems with staff, being less likely to be engaged in purposeful activities and concerns regarding the living conditions. Having a mental disorder, previous attempts and those with low levels of self-directedness, cooperativeness and affective stability were more at risk. Inmates who fared better were those who perceived autonomy, safety and good relationships with staff.

In secure settings such as prisons, it is challenging to engage in suicide prevention strategies that might work in other settings because of the environmental limitations and governing policies that dictate what prisoners can do, when and where. While making changes in prison environments is challenging, some factors are modifiable. Bloom and Bradshaw (2022) discuss the need for a culture shift to provide nature-based settings, trauma-informed approaches, empathy and compassion to support healing while maintaining the integrity of the prison setting. Better access to appropriate health care for both physical and mental health issues, increasing opportunities for purposeful activity, meaningful social support and enhancing safety for those who are victimized are factors that could be considered to mitigate suicide risk (Favril et al. 2022). Supporting staff to increase suicide awareness and enhance suicide prevention skills has been suggested, but more innovative approaches that overcome the constraints of the environment are needed (Freese et al. 2023).

SUICIDE PREVENTION SPECTRUM

As we shift our focus to prevention, we often think of actions that can be taken once we have detected that a person is suicidal. What to do — phone 911? Walk away and don't get involved? So much to think about. As much as this critical moment demands attention, the prevention of suicide can happen long before, along what is known as the suicide prevention spectrum.

Given that suicide attempts are often correlated with declining mental health, treatments are often biomedical in nature. Medications to address diagnoses such as major depression disorder, bipolar disorder, anxiety disorders, post-traumatic stress disorder and schizophrenia are commonly prescribed. Counselling or psychotherapy are often useful adjuncts, but although these treatments may mitigate symptoms, they are individual in nature and often not sufficient to fully reverse thoughts of suicide. For example, as the interpersonal theory of suicide suggests, thwarted belonging and perceived burdensomeness are key contributors to suicidal ideation (Van Orden et al. 2010). Feeling that one belongs and is not a burden are not the expected outcomes of biomedical treatments. A broader ecological approach is required.

The social-ecological suicide prevention model focuses attention on the need for integrated multi-level approaches across the prevention spectrum (prevention, intervention, postvention), using universal, selective and indicated approaches (Cramer and Kapusta, 2017). While indicated approaches are important interventions when encountering someone who is in suicidal mode, selective and universal strategies can cast a wider net, "catching" people before they become acutely suicidal. Indicated approaches often involve the use of a safety plan, a collaboratively developed plan that can be implemented in the face of imminent risk for suicide (Knapp 2023). Such plans can include specific coping strategies, contact numbers for supports and useful activities that will help a person navigate a crisis. Of note, the previous mental health professional practice of "contracting for safety" is no longer an acceptable practice as it did not provide useful guidance on how to navigate a crisis and had limited impact on reducing suicide attempts (Knapp 2023). Selective initiatives (focused on high-risk groups) may address issues such as social isolation at a community level (such as increased intergenerational activities to ensure inclusivity for older adults). Universal approaches are targeted at the overall population. They can target ideologies such as ageism and can offer widespread awareness or broader policy changes to address social determinants of health, such as social supports, employment opportunities and battling discrimination (de Mendonça Lima et al. 2021; Sakashita and Oyama 2019).

This model describes prevention as an upstream approach with a focus on environmental factors, which may be reflected primarily in the macro and exosystems. At this level, universal approaches to prevention are called for. This might include awareness campaigns or anti-stigma initiatives, such as addressing racism in the community or cyberbullying in schools. These universal-level approaches are directed at the general public or to broad populations where the prevention of suicide may be a general concern.

In a recent example, researchers developed a universal prevention program and piloted it in school classrooms comprising a range of students. The focus of the intervention, known as the PositivaMente program, was to improve students' knowledge and attitudes regarding mental health, help them develop socio-emotional competencies, promote timely help-seeking, reduce the overall stigma surrounding mental health and support them to better manage crisis situations (Díez-Gómez et al. 2024). While results were limited in actual reduction of suicide, the process was effective in creating a forum where positive mental health could be discussed, warning signs to watch for in themselves and others were identified, support for help-seeking was provided and students were exposed to relaxation techniques to promote coping with crisis situations. Like most universal approaches, there are challenges in measuring outcomes, but nonetheless, creating an environment that encourages open discussion of mental wellness and support for timely help-seeking is generally viewed as positive.

Returning to the prevention spectrum, intervention is the next consideration. Intervention is typically focused on those who have given an indication that they may be suicidal or who have overtly stated their intentions. Thus, the approaches are either selective or indicated. Some people in this situation will self-identify to health-care services or be noticed by family or other close contacts and supported to seek help, but it is here that those with "gatekeeper training" can also come into play. Gatekeeper training embraces the notion that we are all gatekeepers. We can all be the "eyes and ears" in our various environments and become increasingly comfortable in doing something when we perceive an issue. This intervention is commonly implemented to increase alertness to those who are struggling, facilitate help-seeking behaviour and increase overall suicide awareness. Such training focuses on increasing knowledge about suicide (what to look for) and gatekeeper comfort level when asking individuals if they are considering suicide. An affirmative (or ambiguous) answer can result in referrals or connections with appropriate mental health services (Spafford, McWhirter Boisen et al. 2024). An immediate call to Canada's 988 Suicide Crisis Helpline can be made by a person considering suicide or by someone worried about the safety of another. A wide range of other community-based services and supports may also be contacted.

Gatekeeper and other trainings include the range of programs offered by LivingWorks, a company best known for in-person, two-day Applied Suicide Intervention Skills Training. This approach helps gatekeepers to intervene when they have identified someone with current thoughts of suicide, help them develop a safety plan and support them to access help. The half-day, in-person SafeTALK training prepares gatekeepers to be more alert to someone thinking of suicide and connect them with help. The Mental Health Commission of Canada, HealthCareCAN and the Canadian Association for Suicide Prevention have developed a series of modules geared more toward health-care providers entitled *Suicide: Facing the Difficult Topic Together*. The Centre for Suicide Prevention offers a variety of other programs, many of which are focused on Indigenous populations (Little Cub, River of Life, Walk with Me) and youth (Looking Forward, Skills for Safer Living). Another program, QPR (question, persuade and refer) Online Gatekeeper Training, is a two-hour online crisis response program that focuses on how to question, persuade and refer someone who may be suicidal. Sources of Strength is a youth-oriented program focused on upstream approaches that increase well-being, help-seeking, resiliency, healthy coping and sense of belonging. While these programs and others are widely used as interventions, more research is needed to provide clarity on whether and how they work to prevent suicide (Spafford, Silverman et al. 2024).

Finally, the suicide prevention spectrum focuses on postvention. Postvention, commonly directed toward those who have experienced a suicide loss but sometimes directed at those who have survived a suicide attempt, is also an approach offered at the selective or indicated level. People bereaved by suicide are known as "survivors of suicide" (Honeycutt and Praetorius, 2016). A survivor is "a person who has lost a significant other (or a loved one) by suicide, and whose life is changed because of the loss" (Andriessen 2009: 43). Some people are *exposed* to suicide (such as losing a classmate or acquaintance), while others are *affected* by suicide (such as the suicide of a family member or close friend) (Cerel et al. 2014). Those who are affected by suicide are most likely to experience emotional distress and increased risk of suicide themselves, with parents who have lost a child being at greatest risk due to the intensity and duration of symptoms, including depression and prolonged grief (Hamdan et al. 2020).

Survivors of suicide face challenges as they reflect on the days and weeks leading up to the suicide. Should they have noticed something? Should they have done more? They may play over their last encounter with the loved one and question if something they said or did or did not say or do may have pushed the person to act, thus taking on blame. Trauma is often associated with learning of the suicide itself, including in some cases being the person who is present or discovers the remains of the deceased individual (Harrington-LaMorie et al. 2018; McGill et al. 2023). The death itself demarcates a dramatic life change. One person reported, "Emotions surge, bodies shake, legs buckle. Call it a grenade, an earthquake, or an avalanche. Plans evaporate" (Walker 2017: 635). In addition to emotional upheaval, the routines of daily life are disrupted and must be gradually reconstructed over time, incorporating the loss (Dransart 2016). People bereaved by suicide may be up to nine times more in need of professional help than those mourning those lost to other causes of death, but, for various reasons, many neither seek nor receive the help needed (Froese et al. 2020). Appropriate services may be non-existent, inconsistently available (timewise and geographically) or perceived as not suitable or helpful, often leaving families to handle the situation on their own.

Individuals and families respond differently to suicide loss, often dependent on the relationship the deceased individual had with each individual and the family as a whole, making it difficult to address their needs. Some of the main challenges they may face in the postvention stage include: 1) navigating the intense grief, often considered different from grief typically experienced following a death due to the trauma, shock and guilt that may arise; 2) managing interpersonal impacts, such as the reactions of others to the death, and dealing with stigma and shame which may limit their willingness to seek help; 3) dealing with practical challenges, starting on the first day with legal interrogations about the death, and resuming daily activities such as eating and sleeping and responsibilities such as parenting, work, school and household tasks; 4) seeking support, including emotional and practical support (noting that needs change over time); and 5) undertaking post-traumatic growth, whereby survivors appreciated being listened to and took action to honour the person by establishing a legacy of some sort in remembrance (McGill et al. 2023).

While addressing most of these challenges would be considered an "indicated" approach handled for the most part on the individual or family level, the context in which the survivors reside plays an important role. For example, even in a close-knit family, not all family members will feel the same about a suicide. Some may be angry, some relieved, some devastated. Some family members may experience "conflicted grief," especially if they experience relief that their loved one had ended their suffering, for example, in the case of a severe and chronic mental illness (such as PTSD), addiction or other painful circumstances (Dransart 2016; Harrington-LaMorie et al. 2018). Extended family members may rally around or, conversely, pull away. As Ann Nguyen, Robert Taylor, Linda Chatters and colleagues (2017) found, those who had frequent contact with close family and friends had lower rates of suicide ideation and attempts themselves, reflecting a support network that would be a valuable resource in the face of a suicide loss. Such frequent contacts aligned with a sense of belonging, while limited or negative interactions reflected thwarted belonging, a risk factor discussed in the interpersonal theory of suicide risk.

In some cases, the context can play an even greater role. For example, in the case of a suicide loss of a military member, dependent spouses and children not only have to experience the tragedy of the immediate loss, but also navigate the future, often separate from the well-established military lifestyle. In addition, military suicides are often seen as dishonourable, "a disgrace to the victim and the profession," regardless if PTSD or other mental health disorders were incurred directly from duty, creating an additional challenge for families to face (Harrington-LaMorie et al. 2018: 145).

CONCLUSION

As we work toward the prevention of suicide, it is important to remember that suicide is not only an individual problem. A continued focus on medicalizing suicide and placing blame on the individual "risks losing the means to understand and engage with the complex and changing contexts in which suicidal individuals are formed and suicides occur" (Marsh 2016: 26). A wide variety of interventions, initiatives and approaches within and outside of traditional health care that could lend well to changing the discourse on mental health and address individual needs with environmental responses long before suicide enters the picture are needed. As Karen Whalley Hammell points out, "The need for both the ability and opportunity to experience and express pleasure, purpose, accomplishment, and meaning in life through engagement in roles and occupations ... is of central importance to human wellbeing" (2020: 106).

White (2017) introduces perspectives of critical suicidology where we might shift away from pathology toward life-activating questions. What really matters to people? As Flett and Heisel point out in their research about mattering, "It is about whether the individual feels seen and heard and valued versus invisible and unheard and someone who does not count to the people in their lives and perhaps society as a whole" (2021: 2450). That says it all!

SELF-REFLECTION AND THOUGHTFUL CONVERSATIONS

1. Medical assistance in dying (MAID) is now legal in Canada, but those with solely a mental health diagnosis are not eligible. Discuss the pros and cons of limiting access to this population.
2. White (2017) supports the idea that our suicide prevention practices could become more life-activating, hopeful, justice-seeking, community-building and creative. Do you agree, and if so, how might you make this happen?
3. There is a lot of talk about using the proper language when discussing suicide. For example, the term "commit suicide" has been replaced with "died by suicide." Do you think language matters as a means of reducing stigma? (See these references for more information: <suicideinfo.ca/local_resource/suicideandlanguage, camh.ca/-/media/files/words-matter-suicide-language-guide.pdf> and <canada.ca/en/public-health/services/publications/healthy-living/language-matters-safe-communication-suicide-prevention.html>)

IN-CLASS ASSIGNMENTS

1. With partners, create an initiative that could address suicide prevention in your community at the "universal" level.
2. Older adults benefit greatly from "intergenerational" interactions (rather than always attending activities with those of similar age). If you were a recreation planner in your community, how might you implement this?
3. Review the Mental Health Commission's roots of hope model and the five pillars <mentalhealthcommission.ca/roots-hope>. For each pillar, think of an action or activity you or a small group could undertake.

Chapter Fifteen

DEALING WITH GRIEF AND BEREAVEMENT

Give sorrow words, the grief that does not speak knits the overwrought heart and bids it break. (William Shakespeare, *Macbeth*, Act IV, Scene III)

GRIEF REPRESENTS THE EMOTIONAL, PHYSICAL, PSYCHOLOGICAL AND SOCIOCULTURAL reactions that we experience due to loss. Bereavement is the process of learning to deal with sustained losses throughout our lives. The two terms are often used interchangeably and may refer to our reactions to losses of all types, not just those as a result of death. The loss inventory in Chapter 2 lists some of the losses we might experience throughout our lives, and we encourage you to reflect on this at the end of this chapter in a fresh way.

Grief is usually experienced as deep or intense sorrow; it encompasses our total emotional response to loss. To ignore grief or to postpone the process of bereavement may only intensify pain later. It does not go away by itself, and when we grieve, we engage our total selves in the process. Physically, grief can be measured by stress levels on the body and mind. In assisting those who are grieving or when reflecting on our own losses, it is useful to examine the modalities of grief. Being able to talk about where the feelings of grief are located in our bodies or in external physical sites — what it smells, tastes and looks like, as well as identifying the colours of grief — can add a concreteness to the experience that helps individuals articulate their awareness more fully.

Psychologically, grief is a highly personal experience influenced by who we are and how we deal with challenges throughout our lives. Therese Rando (1984) identified the factors that influence individual reactions to grieving over a death. These factors depend on the roles the deceased occupied in the family or social system and are as follows: personal coping behaviours; personality characteristics and mental health; level of maturity and intelligence; past experience with loss and death; social, cultural, ethnic, religious and philosophical background; amount of unfinished business with the deceased; sudden versus unexpected death and length of illness prior to death; age of both the deceased and the grieving; and the number and type of resources available within the local community.

Individuals do not often have different coping strategies for different kinds of losses, but we might employ them to varying degrees and in a variety of ways. Culturally, we tend to view death as the most profound of losses, and because of this, we are not as supportive or responsive to "smaller" losses. However, learning to recognize and work through all losses may result in a greater set of resources to assist us with losses that occur because of death. The death of a pet or moving away from a neighbourhood can be very painful and may remind us of other larger and more human-oriented losses in our lives.

However, it is important not to create a hierarchy of loss, with death as the major one, or to diminishing how someone else may experience a loss differently than you do. All people experience different types of losses in different ways, and all loss should be recognized for what it is — a deeply distressful event that challenges our ability to deal with everyday life and causes us to question who we are without the missing person, a certain location (because of relocation due to immigration, the loss of a home, change of schools, employment and so on), a beloved object (a gold necklace your mother gave you), a dear pet or an annual event.

Mourning may include aspects of grief and bereavement. In particular, different communities, cultures and social groups have long-standing ways to mourn: a religious funeral, a wake or a length of time for grieving and rituals associated with clothing, prayer and food. Immediately following a death, there is a sense of shock, numbness and disbelief that can last minutes or weeks. The person may feel panicked and overwhelmed and may experience strong physical reactions. This period enables the person to take in information at a slower pace and prepare for the adjustments that lie ahead.

Grief Objective: to move from denial to acceptance that the loss really has occurred; to regain a sense of our self and balance, without the physical presence of the deceased. It is important not to medicalize grief at this time — there are many healthy ways to grieve that do not look the same from one person to another.

SOCIAL RESPONSES

After the death of a loved one, it is common for some to withdraw from usual activities. Sometimes others remove themselves from the bereaved. In classes and community workshops led by both Jeanette and Kerstin, many participants state that once the funeral, cremation or celebration of life is over, no one brings meals, telephones, writes, emails or checks in to see if the person is okay. Some of this behaviour may be because of embarrassment, not wanting to witness others' sadness, not knowing what to say, not wanting to encourage dependency or other such fears. People also move on with their lives and simply forget that the grieving person may still need them in specific and concrete ways.

Many people who are grieving say that the best thing to do is just "be there" for them. Being there may involve sitting in silence together, eating a meal, going for a walk or talking about the deceased. It is important to feel able to be there, and, if you can't, it is important to be honest and open about your inability to do so. A grieving person can also find many online and community-based resources to create a broader set of options for their healing.

PHYSICAL RESPONSES

Physical responses to grief can vary according to the individual. Some people experience headaches, sleeplessness, nausea and dizziness. Others have no physical reactions at first but may develop them after some time has passed. It is crucial to remember that everyone experiences grief in their own unique way. Some say that having to notify family and friends, arrange the funeral, deal with the final disposition of the deceased and keep themselves busy delays physical responses to grief, which materialize some weeks or even months after the death. Unless medical concern is warranted, it is important to know that grief can show itself in real physical symptoms; this can be confusing and may even result in deep grief being medicalized as an illness.

EMOTIONAL RESPONSES

Many conflicting emotions occur in grief. Individuals may feel relief that the deceased is no longer suffering, yet guilt because they feel this way. A person may feel anger or resentment for being left by their loved one, or joy because they have a sense of freedom from an abusive or hurtful relationship. It is important not to judge feelings, others or our own, but to accept them for what they are, reactions to events.

SPIRITUAL RESPONSES

For some, grief involves strong spiritual responses — either relying on religious faith or questioning the beliefs and rituals of faith. In our work in classes and the community, participants sometimes ask, "How could God allow this to happen?" or "Why did God do this to me?." In these cases, individuals question their faith in a higher power. On the other hand, when people of faith experience the death of a loved one, especially unexpectedly, their faith may help them through the extremely difficult time. Others examine the meaning of their own lives in terms of questioning karma, whether there is life after death, if they believe that God or some other deity has a plan for them which has yet to manifest itself or the possibility of having missed their path in life. Some people feel "called" to do something new, stepping away from their chosen lived path, and others abandon their faith altogether.

When an important one dies, we experience both physical and emotional pain. The former is usually easier to deal with because we can seek assistance from outside sources, such as physicians, health centres and complementary therapies like massage, aromatherapy, grief counselling and so on. Emotional pain may be more difficult to articulate and understand, especially if conflicting feelings are experienced. In such cases, it is useful to keep a journal of thoughts and emotions to keep track of how we are reacting to the death. It is often useful to write a letter to your loved one telling them all the things you wished you had said, positive and negative, to let your feelings out and to come to some sort of workable resolution of your pain.

As the first strong responses wear off, the person grieving may begin to feel the emotional pain of daily living even more. The intensity of grief may surprise and frighten them, but the pain is healthy and can soften over time. The time required for this work will be affected by the quality of the person's support network, other losses, the preparation they may have had for the death and the nature of the relationship with the person who died.

Grief Objective: To acknowledge, experience and work through feelings of hopelessness, yearning and despair.

RECONNECTING

As an individual's grief becomes more resolved, the person may have the energy and desire to reconnect with the world once again. They may begin to see their loss in perspective and as part of the past.

Grief Objective: To adjust to a life without the person who died; to invest in new or old activities and new or old relationships. Although most of the literature on grief assumes that there are five main phases, it is important to reiterate again that everyone grieves in their own unique way. If we want to be able to assist others and ourselves in dealing appropriately with grief, we need to ask what works for them, what they need and how we can help. Responses will be as varied as the individuals who respond, so attentive listening is crucial. Setting a timeline for the end of grief is not helpful, since we know that grief can last a year or more, or simply transform into a new way of being, as we discuss later.

TYPES OF GRIEF AND BEREAVEMENT

A great deal of literature has been written on grief and bereavement over the past thirty years and more (see, for example, Sigmund Freud 1957; Bowlby 1980; Doka 2002; Kübler-Ross 1973; 1993; Rando 1984, 1986b, 1988, 1993; Whipple 2006; Tamor 2005 and many others). Out of this vast body of work, which includes material dealing with children as well as adults, a grief classification system has emerged. We have selected but a few examples below, with the understanding that many types of grief have been recorded in the literature.

- Open: Open grief refers to the process whereby the griever feels comfortable with expressing their feelings about the loss of a loved one. Open public expressions of grief are healthy and real; think of the rituals of some cultures where public wailing and mourning are appropriate and necessary.
- Anticipatory: This type of grief is experienced by patients as well as by the loved ones of patients. When grief is anticipated, individuals may live in constant grief, sadness or fear of their loved one's (or their own) death. This is especially true for those with terminal diagnoses that have a long trajectory; families of Alzheimer's patients feel anticipatory grief, as do parents of children with long-term chronic diseases.
- Disenfranchised: This is also referred to as hidden. This is grief that cannot be publicly expressed, e.g., experienced by 2SLGBTQ+ individuals, someone in an unrequited love situation or in the case of an abortion, miscarriage or stillbirth.
- Unresolved: As it sounds, the grief is always there. Grief will wait for us until we are ready, but it does not go away! People experience unresolved grief for a variety of reasons, sometimes because it is easier to hold on to grief and all that it represents in terms of one's attachment to the deceased, especially if it sustains a sense of belonging to

that relationship. This may be related to a conflict or negative relationship prior to the person dying. It can be associated with someone who lived far away, and we did not have a chance to say goodbye. For others, the loss may be connected to people or material possessions, and the complexity of connections is difficult to unravel.

It is also crucial to recognize that the way death occurs can influence the grief process. In general, it seems to be the case that sudden or accidental death, including suicide, causes more complicated grief reactions than expected death (Rando 1986b, 1993). Even when death is anticipated, if there is unfinished business between the dying person and the bereaved, this non-closure can prolong the grief process.

How we deal with losses in our lives affects how we grieve after the death of a loved one. It has been said that grieving teaches you how to live! Our strategies and tools for daily life are heightened and come to the fore during our grief. As well, we learn how to grieve from our familiar surroundings and our cultural and spiritual heritage. Those with religious beliefs who believe in Heaven may not fear death because they see it as everlasting life. For those who believe in reincarnation, death is a sad event but also a pathway into the next life. We learn from our parents initially the most appropriate ways to show our sadness at the loss of important people, pets and events in our lives. It is important to reflect on how such deaths were dealt with when we were young, so that we can learn how we developed our later reactions to loss.

There are many newer ways to deal with and express grief, including grief walking groups, cyber-grieving, grief cafés, grief doulas, online grief support services and groups, and traditional grief counsellors.

GRIEF WALKING GROUPS

Across most provinces in Canada, where hospices and palliative care programs exist, grief walking groups have been established to assist mourners to speak about and share their grief while walking with others with comparable experiences. Most groups last about eight or nine weeks and all are facilitated by hospice palliative care volunteers. There are no costs to participants of these programs. An example is the Hospice Palliative Care bereavement group in Vancouver, which states on its website: "The Bereavement Walking Program combines fresh air, exercise and companionship for those who have suffered the loss of someone in their life.

The group is facilitated by trained hospice volunteers. Participants walk at a casual pace for about an hour, followed by the option of coffee and continued conversation."

Author Adriana Barton (2011) states that while such groups are

> unfamiliar to many academics who study grief, walking groups for the bereaved have been formed in recent years in cities including Winnipeg, Hamilton, Edmonton and Waterloo, Ont. Some are modelled after one of the first Canadian groups, organized by the Victoria Hospice Society in 1986, after a woman in the community suggested there must be a better way to reach out to others than sitting around in a circle talking about loss.

CYBER-GRIEVING

Social media has become a forum for people of all ages to express their grief over the loss of friends, family and acquaintances. Whether it is Facebook, Instagram or another platform, social media has become a therapeutic place for people who are more likely to express themselves online than in person. This is an example of how technology has the potential to allow some people to express themselves more openly. People are attracted to dealing with loss through this means because they can communicate with others without having to have face-to-face contact, avoid being embarrassed by disclosing personal feelings and feel that they are heard (read) more sympathetically by others with similar experiences, and they can choose to be anonymous.

GRIEF DOULAS

The website of the End of Life Doula Association of Canada states:

> An End of Life Doula is someone who supports a person faced with an illness or terminal diagnosis. The End of Life Doula can educate, advocate for, and empower clients by starting the conversation about death and embracing the dying process early. By aligning the client's needs with their expectations and wishes, the End of Life Doula can significantly improve the quality and dignity of the end of life journey. Some of their tasks and skills may include:

- advocate for the best possible experience for the client
- understand the physiology of death and the complexity of emotions that go along with the diagnosis of a terminal illness
- assist clients in creating and carrying out their health-care treatment decisions
- are knowledgeable about legalities, options, and tools in Canada.

Shelley Steeves (2023) reported on the increase of death doulas in Canada. She interviewed Ashley Brzezicki, a death doula in New Brunswick, who confirms that she assists people to find some comfort as they face their worst fears about dying: "We really only get exposed to death in our culture when we are butting up right against it." After facing her own fears about mortality, Brzezicki studied to become a death doula during the pandemic.

MUSIC THANATOLOGY DOULAS

There are also those who are trained in music therapy as music thanatology doulas, which, according to Music-Thanatology Association International is

> a professional field within the broader sub-specialty of palliative care. It is a musical/clinical modality that unites music and medicine in end-of-life care. The music-thanatologist utilizes harp and voice at the bedside to lovingly serve the physical, emotional and spiritual needs of the dying and their loved ones with prescriptive music.

Further, the website suggests that this music can

> help to ease physical symptoms such as pain, restlessness, agitation, sleeplessness and laboured breathing. It offers an atmosphere of serenity and comfort that can be profoundly soothing for those present. Difficult emotions such as anger, fear, sadness and grief can be relieved as listeners rest into a musical presence of beauty, intimacy and compassion.

DEATH DINNERS AND GRIEF CAFÉS

Our modern age is characterized by a strong reluctance to discuss our mortality. Death's detachment from everyday life — handled instead by hospitals and funeral services — makes it necessary to schedule specific times to discuss and exchange our personal views about death (Testoni et al. 2020). Now, imagine you have been invited to attend a dinner — no formal wear is needed, no gifts for the host, only a willingness to discuss your end-of-life wishes. A group of health-care and wellness leaders, led by Michael Hebb, are working to break the taboo around conversations about death and dying. Hebb, the founder of DeathOverDinner.org, created a free public website to initiate discussions about death and dying with family and friends while sharing a meal — a "death dinner." Hebb's book *Let's Talk about Death (Over Dinner)* (2018) recounts his personal realization that end-of-life conversations are needed prior to the onset of fatal illnesses. The book offers insights into twenty-two prompts that can help facilitate a death dinner. Having dinner is familiar and comfortable. Therefore, transforming the daunting conversation about death and dying to a safe space, such as the kitchen table, allows for anxieties and fears toward death to subside.

Andrea South and Jessica Elton (2017) used qualitative research methods to examine the importance of discussing one's death wishes. In the study, 240 volunteers aged 18 to 76 were engaged in end-of-life conversations using Death Over Dinner, an online platform that facilitates discussions of death and dying. The majority agreed that more conversations about death and dying with family and friends are necessary to eliminate anxiety. South and Elton conclude by acknowledging Death Over Dinner as an advantageous platform to use to stimulate conversation about death and dying. South and Elton, alongside Alison Lietzenmayer (2020), conducted another study using Death Over Dinner to analyze how humour is used when discussing death and dying. They examined eighty-three death dinners with 424 participants. Their study revealed six types of humour: entertainment humour, gallows humour, tension-relieving humour, confused/awkward laughter, group humour/narrative chaining and self-deprecating humour. Humour was used by participants to help them face their anxieties and fears concerning mortality — to share honest viewpoints without sounding morbid — and provided a "moment of release" for the participants (857). Again, the authors support the use of death dinners as a useful tool to promote death education.

Likewise, Emily Mroz, Susan Bluck and Krista Smith (2020) had 109 participants between the ages of 18 and 28 fill out a pretest or engage in a death dinner about advance care planning. The results conclude that the intimate setting of the kitchen table is a better suited medium to use to begin the end-of-life dialogue — during the death dinner the participants decreased their reservations toward advance care planning. To date, the above three papers are the only empirical studies that used Death Over Dinner to analyze conversations about death and dying. While death dinners may seem morbid, South, Elton, Lietzenmayer, Mroz, Bluck and Smith proved that they are effective for gathering data on people's views on mortality and end of life.

In a similar vein to grief walking groups, death and grief cafés are locations where individuals can gather to talk about grief and loss because of death. According to the Death Café website, death cafés are intended to provide people, often strangers, a place to gather to eat cake, drink tea and discuss death in all its aspects. Their objective is "to increase awareness of death with a view to helping people make the most of their (finite) lives." Death cafés exist in many locations around the world, including within death art galleries. There are also blogs on which people can post their concerns and feelings about many aspects of death, including grief. A student in one of our online classes attended a grief café in her neighbourhood. She mentioned in an email, "I feel like this is the only place I can go to talk about my Mom's death. The people here are so caring and supportive, and even though I didn't know any of them before I had the guts to come here, now I feel like they are true friends" (received in May 2018). Regardless of where people find support and encouragement to speak openly about their feelings of grief and bereavement, it is important that they can do so.

LIVING WITH LOSS

No one is immune to loss; we all experience it throughout our lives. Some losses affect us more deeply than others, and no matter the causes, how it is defined or how it is experienced, all types of grief require what is known as "grief work." The Canadian Virtual Hospice defines grief work as

> a multi-faceted human response to loss. Grief work emphasizes that grief is a process that we engage in as active participants. Grief demands attention, refusing to go away automatically with the passage of time. (Nelson 2017)

Grief work is as unique as each individual who experiences it — it has stages, it has tasks, and it must be worked through. Grief never ends fully, but it can get easier to manage. Grief work teaches us to acknowledge loss and thereby how to live our lives more fully, as we tend to grieve in similar ways to how we live our everyday lives. An excellent resource for finding information and resources dealing with grief can be found at the website of Grief Matters.

ASSISTING THE DYING PERSON

In terms of assisting others in the grief process, there are two main groups who are targeted as needing support: the bereaved and the dying person. Gere Fulton and Eileen Metress (1995: 372) suggest that the following guidelines may be useful in assisting those who are grieving:

1. *Don't rush someone through grief.* The grieving period is variable. Impatience with grief is a prevailing characteristic of our society.
2. *Don't trivialize someone's grief.* We may say hurtful things unknowingly, such as, "Be strong," or "She lived a long life," or "This was meant to be." We might also discount certain losses, such as that of a beloved pet.
3. *Make your support available, especially beyond the funeral period.* The bereaved are often "on their own" after the funeral. They need support and concern after this period, long after the funeral is over.
4. *Allow the deceased to be important during the grieving process.* We can do this by encouraging memories of the deceased.
5. *Give permission to grieve.* We can do this by talking about our own reaction to the death. By engaging in open talk about the deceased and our feelings, we can give the bereaved permission to do the same.
6. *Help the bereaved deal with any guilt or anger.* These are common components of grief and may be rational or irrational. Talking about them can be helpful.
7. *Realize the importance of obsessive review.* The bereaved may be preoccupied with memories of the deceased and how the death took place. Provide an environment that allows them to talk about the death.
8. *Remember that grief is highly individual.* Don't expect the bereaved to follow an established set of rules. Allow for individual differences.
9. *Help the bereaved to get on with living, to form new relationships.* Be there for them, but don't rush them into a premature "resolution" of grief.

Most books and websites that deal with grief recommend similar guidelines. However, it is important to establish your own grief goals, no matter how difficult, rather than to follow someone else's interpretation, whether for yourself or another.

CHILDREN AND GRIEF

Barbara Sourkes (1996) notes that a child's anticipatory grief manifests itself in symbolic terms, in questions about others, in projections onto a significant adult and in references to the possibility of their own dying. Even though Sourkes' research and work were conducted in North America, many of her experiences echo those Jeanette had in England when visiting children's hospices; she was struck by the level of maturity and openness that many children exhibited when speaking about feelings of their impending death and the deaths of those they loved. For example, Trevor (not his real name) was a 13-year-old boy suffering from leukaemia and a degenerative motor neuron disease. Although confined to a wheelchair, he gave Jeanette a tour of the hospice where he was living. He explained that he knew his mother was more frightened for him than he was for himself, because in the hospice, all the children talked about how they felt about dying. He thought that his mother would be "scarred for life" by his death, and that made him sad.

Trevor had been keeping a diary of his thoughts and feelings about his experiences during his life and his illness. He had included photographs of himself and friends at the hospice as well as pictures he had drawn during his art therapy sessions. He had asked the hospice to give his mom the diary after he died so that she would "always remember that he could be a little terror and a fun boy." Trevor knew that although he had come to terms with his illness and approaching death, his mother had not.

Kevin (not his real name), a 13-year-old cancer patient, told me, "We are all going to die, I'm just going to do it sooner than you, and adults can't cope with that." In children's hospices, a variety of techniques are used to encourage and assist children to discuss, draw, role-play, act out and generally communicate their feelings about death and grief. Jeanette feels that these therapeutic techniques would be useful in assisting all age groups to deal with grief. Many individuals are not comfortable talking through their feelings, as art and music therapists have long known (Bright 1996).

Children express universal realities about grief towards not only their own deaths but the deaths of those they love. Sourkes reminds those who counsel grieving children that the therapist

> must be capable of witnessing and tolerating the anguish of threatened separation and loss. ... In working with a child facing death, the therapist must be able to enter the threat with the child,

accompany him or her through the steps, while knowing that this may be a journey that they cannot complete together. (1996: 59)

THE LOSS OF A CHILD

There are many ways that parents, siblings, family and friends grieve the loss of a child, either through abortion, miscarriage, stillbirth, accident or illness. Parents who lose a child through miscarriage or fetal death often feel that their loss goes unacknowledged by others, and such deaths are not always recognized or supported by care providers who deal with grief. For the mother who was pregnant, such grief may also involve hormonal changes that further impact the way they feel physically, emotionally and mentally. For their partner, the experience may feel isolating if they think others don't understand their loss. Sometimes, older parents lose an adult child who may have their own family and life. This can be very difficult, whether it is due to illness or a tragic accident. Older parents never expect to lose an adult child before they themselves die, and this has its own kind of grief and bereavement.

Women who have chosen abortion for whatever personal reasons may feel relief or an overwhelming sense of guilt and loss or both. They might feel impacted right away, or perhaps the realization of the loss does not occur until much later. No matter what or when these feelings arise, these emotions are valid. Similar to miscarriage and prenatal death, for women who choose to end an unwanted pregnancy, grief is often not acknowledged or recognized.

LOSING A PET

When we invite a companion animal into our home and hearts, we recognize, as we do with our human loved ones, that at some time in our relationship they will die. For many people, a pet is one of their primary relationships — a best friend, the one who gives unconditional love, the one we count on when we are down or even happy and celebrating — and often an animal is the one who welcomes us when we come through the door, no matter what our day was like. The loss of a pet can be a devastating experience. It's important to grieve this loss and work through the emotions, and sometimes in society, other people do not relate or understand this kind of healthy and nurturing attachment. The loss of a pet can be as real as any other kind of loss.

For many younger people, their first loss is that of a pet. For many older persons, pet loss is one of many that we experience throughout our lives, and for those who live alone, pets are our constant companions who have often shared so many other losses in our lives. It is imperative that we recognize pet loss as an important source of grief for so many.

GRIEF IN OLD AGE

Although one would expect to find a great deal of material dealing with older persons' grief, this is not the case, either in Canada or globally. We might assume that older people, especially the very old (80 and over), would have a great deal of experience dealing with the loss of partners, friends, family members, pets, work as the result retirement, declining health, possible relocation because of institutionalization, giving up possessions to move into a nursing home and so on. These continued experiences of loss were termed "bereavement overload" by Robert Kastenbaum. However, in our work with older adults, we have found that with advanced old age, most people experience a sense of resilience and the ability to move on. Past and anticipated losses are acknowledged, and the coping skills acquired from dealing with them provide some resources for those to come. This is not to say, of course, that all older people deal effectively with grief, or that they welcome it. Rather, with age, for many, comes the ability to cope with life's challenging and inevitable changes.

Another related issue is the death of older people in our lives, within our families and communities. Sometimes, these deaths may be minimized; they are seen to be expected due to advanced age, or normalized in some way, yet the grieving person may experience the loss of a parent, aunt or grandparent as the loss of a whole set of childhood stories, valuable memories, cultural narratives or personal connection. Linking higher age falsely with an easier death or simple grieving for the bereaved, or somehow stigmatizing those who are grieving the loss of an older person, does not respect and address the many unique and individual ways that we may hold dear those older loved ones. History has shown us that when matriarchs die, for example, the whole structure of communication in families can change. We may see the loss of history in survivors of world events (e.g., the Depression, the Holocaust, the COVID-19 pandemic) as they are dying now through old age, and many other historical events, if not recorded, are then lost to new generations. In an era in which our Canadian (and global) population is aging, it seems highly relevant to find new ways to honour and celebrate the lives of those who have paved the path ahead of us.

GRIEF AS AN OPPORTUNITY FOR GROWTH

The best outcome for grief is to understand, no matter how challenging or difficult it may be at the time, that this is an opportunity for growth. It can be invisible, and this makes it harder to see and be a witness to. Grief and loss are shared experiences by each one of us on this globe, and while it can be terrifyingly lonely, we all experience grief and loss in our lifetimes. How might it change how we continue to live and be alive? What changes might we make for our own lives? How do we imagine coming out of grief and loss in the future? Some people say that they want to make those who have passed on proud and to carry parts of them with us in our goals and dreams. One day, someone will look to you as a role model and ask, "How can they carry on your legacy?" This is one of the richest and most powerful realities about being alive.

CONCLUSION

Grief is one of the topics in death and dying work that we most want and need to talk about. Historically and culturally, there are many variations to the rituals which are socially approved and sanctioned for the expression of grief and its healing processes. These can truly help communities come together, whether it is a personal loss or a communal one. These deeply ingrained rituals and rites may also create barriers for some and prevent much needed healing. We need room for long-standing traditions, room for growth around grief processing into the future and room for individuals to come forward and discover what they need to heal on a personal level. This can be a fragile and complicated process but one ripe with potential and possibility. We hope this chapter has made apparent some of the areas which need focus, growth and more research.

SELF-REFLECTION AND THOUGHTFUL CONVERSATIONS

1. Why is it so difficult to express grief openly, among colleagues and strangers? Are we ashamed to grieve publicly? Why or why not?
2. Do women and men grieve differently? Do we grieve differently about people at stages across the lifespan? Please describe. In what communities or cultural settings do you observe these differences taking place?
3. How might you describe the opportunities for growth that you yourself have experienced as a grieving person in the past?

IN-CLASS ASSIGNMENTS

1. Think for a moment of the losses you have sustained. Name one significant loss you have experienced. Describe what happened. What emotional and/or physical reactions did you have?
2. Complete the list of questions below below and be prepared to discuss your responses.

    Dealing With Our Own Grief: Questions
    a. Why does it matter if we deal with grief?
    b. How does grief affect our daily living?
    c. What happens when we let the feelings of grief/loss in/out?
    d. What is the worst part of grief?
    e. What is the best part of grief?

Chapter Sixteen

REVIVING INTEREST IN DEATH AND DYING AND IMMORTALITY

Sometimes we lie still and do not move. If air is still going in and out of our breathing holes, this is called sleep. If not, it is called death. When a person has achieved death, a kind of picnic is held, with music, flowers and food. The person so honoured, if in one piece, and not, for instance, in shreds or falling apart, as they do if exploded or a long time drowned, is dressed in becoming clothes and lowered into a hole in the ground, or else burnt up.

These customs are among the most difficult to explain to strangers. Some of our visitors, especially the young ones, have never heard of death and are bewildered. They think that death is simply one more of our illusions, our mirror tricks; they cannot understand why, with so much food and music, the people are sad.

But you will understand. You too must have death among you. I can see it in your eyes. (Atwood 1992: 126)

WE HAVE MUCH MORE INFORMATION about the physical, psychological, spiritual and social consequences of death in our many global cultures than ever before in our history. Yet despite all this information, we have relatively less knowledge, understanding or case about our own mortality, or what it is like to die, than we ever had. It is as if the more we know about who dies, the causes of death, where and how people die, the less likely we are to think about our own death. We remain a death-denying and a death-defying culture. Over the past thirty years, predominantly because of the hospice palliative care movement, there seems to be a revival of interest in matters related to death and dying. As well, a variety of goods and services are now available to help us deal with death, some of which we discuss throughout this book.

Our awareness of death and dying has been revived in great measure by the work of two important women, who both died in 2006: Elizabeth Kübler-Ross and Cicely Saunders. Kübler-Ross, a Swiss psychiatrist working in the US, began in the late 1960s to call for a more humane approach to care for the dying. She and her colleagues interviewed thousands of dying people, and her work has been published in many books. Initially, however, her findings were not well received by the medical profession, which was threatened by her ideas. Kübler-Ross did not just produce academic work from her research with the dying; she also appeared on television and radio talk shows, taking her message to ordinary people.

While Kübler-Ross was reviving an interest and awareness of the needs of dying persons on this continent, Cicely Saunders, a nurse who later became a physician, opened St. Christopher's Hospice just outside of London, England. This hospice was the first of its kind in modern times, and, as a model of "care not cure," has influenced every other hospice or palliative care unit since. Today, there are thousands of palliative care programs throughout the world. In Canada, according to the Canadian Hospice Palliative Care Association, there are currently 480 programs across the country. Palliative care and hospices have helped to spark the revival of interest in death and dying. People's stories about living and dying with diseases like cancer and AIDS are made visible in movies, music, books and TV shows, and this has also created a revival of interest in the subject. Given the many programs across Canada that train people on related topics, we also see an increased commitment to research and education.

Presently, in our daily lives, we seem to be experiencing a type of "pornography of death" (Gorer 1965), with a whole slew of violent, popular movies showing people being killed for "fun." Thrillers and everyday entertainment make light of death at the hands of deranged villains. Because of the increase in population and our awareness through social media, violent deaths on the street, in wars and at "home" have increased in our view and in a manner unparalleled in human history. Individuals like Sue Rodriguez, Nancy B., Dr. Jack Kevorkian and others involved in the right to die movement also raised awareness of death and dying. These factors, plus others, have increased medical, legal, religious, political and social discussion and debate about who should or will die, where, when, how and why.

Implicit in some of these discussions is the notion that there are "right" ways to die — at home, or at least in a hospice, surrounded by loving family and friends. Like the midwifery movement, which assured women it was better to have babies at home, hospice and palliative care philosophies tell the dying and their important ones that it is better to die at home. At the same time we note that some health-care providers in Canada, the US and the UK argue that such care is "Cadillac service" for a few. This argument suggests that all dying persons should receive quality holistic care, with high nurse-patient ratios and adequate pain and symptom relief. Palliative care should not be accessible only to a minority in Canada. The principles of palliative care include an ideology that suggests it is better for patients and their important ones to be open about death, to communicate their fears and feelings fully and to attend to their unfinished business. This ideology underpins the effectiveness of palliative care and may create a set of value judgments to which some patients and their loved ones may not adhere.

Michael Traber notes that death, "as part of a spectacle of violence, is the staple face of the mass media" (1992: 3). Death or mourning of ordinary persons, unless the death occurred in a tragic, newsworthy circumstance, is totally excluded from public view. As Traber notes, the invisibility of "real deaths" and the proliferation of newsworthy ones obscures some of the real human tragedies in our lives and allows us to confuse movie, soap opera, cartoon and other contrived deaths with the real thing. Trabor states,

> This is the century of the Holocaust, the century of mass starvation and infants' death, and a century of seemingly never-ending genocides and wars. It all fits into the general framework of the Western value system, expressed and reinforced by the mass media, that life on earth is cheap, that it can be disposed of easily, and that life is annihilated according to specific patterns related to status and power. (5)

DEMOGRAPHICS

Because of our aging population, with Canadians in general dying much later in life, there is a revival of interest in death and dying issues among older persons. How cultures deal with an ever-increasing number of elders and the diseases that affect them is also a contemporary topic.

As the world population continues to grow, concern is heightened regarding the use of land for burial rather than shelter or food production, as well as the pollution caused by funeral pyres, placing remains in rivers and crematoria waste. There is a renewed interest in what happens to the physical and material world because of people dying.

POLITICS

Politics is involved in all levels of decision making, and we see this clearly regarding MAID, the death penalty, and funding and training for those who want to work in palliative care or provide home care and other forms of chronic health treatment. Despite the notion that health care is accessible to all Canadians, with cutbacks to health-care programs across the country, the smaller provinces, i.e., those in Atlantic Canada, already geographically marginalized, are hit hardest when it comes to hospital closures. As well, there appear to be greater hardships for those in rural and Northern communities than those in larger population centres with greater tax revenues and political clout. This scenario applies to the Prairie Provinces as well, with their vast geographies, harsh winters, and many small towns and rural and Northern communities.

Those who provide services to the dying and their important ones at home normally utilize programs offered by palliative and hospice care programs run by volunteers, the Victorian Order of Nurses, the Red Cross and other provincial home care agencies. These organizations, usually funded through provincial ministries of social and community services, are also experiencing funding cutbacks. Although governments pay lip service to the care of the dying, few provinces in this country provide adequate resources to assist this group of citizens. Providing adequate care to the dying and their important ones is not politically a high priority, possibly because the dead do not vote!

RELIGION

The role of denominational religious institutions, for example, the Canadian Council of Catholic Bishops, in the MAID and abortion debates has also increased awareness of death and dying issues. Cases exist in all denominations in which individual religious leaders speak out in favour of openness, discussion and choice in these matters — but their congregations may not be in agreement, believing perhaps that even the discussion is morally suspect and sinful. At the same time, decriminalizing medical assistance in dying, for example, does not mean that it is for everyone. The deep stigma associated with even having related discussions (not even decision making) can mean that no one feels free to talk about a complicated topic — those who disagree with MAID are sometimes not welcome to speak out, and those who firmly believe in its value may feel silenced in other contexts. This is a deeply personal and profound issue for most people! Decisions are made in private and out of the public eye, so a large pendulum swing continues to exist in many communities and religious contexts.

Peter Berger (1967) noted that religion has always been involved in matters relating to death, particularly the notions of leading a "good" life until death, what happens after death and the very meaning of life and death. As organized religions grapple with issues such as abortion, reproductive technology and MAID, this creates a revival of interest, debate and discussion of the topic of death and dying.

LAW

As well as in the political realm, the MAID and the opioid and drug addiction debates take place within the legal profession, as we have seen with prominent cases like those of Terri Schiavo, Robert Latimer, Sue Rodriguez and Dr. Nancy Morrison. It is important to understand the nuances of all sides of the discussions surrounding life and decisions about death. Some members of the disability community have spoken out valiantly about their view on what it means to receive medical support and life-sustaining resources and be able to choose life. Many sides of the law discuss the reasons why choice is a good option but also highlight the "slippery slope" legal argument — that just offering decriminalization does not mean the service is a resilient offering for all people and in all contexts. Living wills and medical directives are also funnelled through legal jurisprudence.

Charles Corr, Clyde Nabe and Donna Corr note that the law is involved in issues related to death and dying in the following three important ways: 1) prior to death in legal matters such as "advance directives for the treatment of the dying"; 2) those that arrive with death itself, the "definition, determination and certification of death"; and 3) "those which may have been initiated prior to death, but whose real force is exerted after death, such as organ, tissue or body donation, and broader questions concerning disposition of one's body and property" (1997: 436).

MEDICINE

The field of medicine clearly plays a pivotal role in public awareness and the revival of interest in death and dying. Pain control, definitions and diagnostic abilities, comfort measures and definitions of death all fall within the public discourse of the medicalization of death. There is more awareness in Canada today that dying is a natural process which need not be medicalized or legalized. Medical advances with the ability to create life through reproductive technology, prolong and maintain it through life-saving machines like dialysis or end it via lethal injection all have an impact on public perceptions of how, where, when and if people die. For example, if we allow heart surgeries and the removal of brain tumours to sustain life, an ethicist might ask: Are those life-sustaining medical decisions the same or different than decisions specifically focusing on ending a life? If we say no to heart surgery, are we choosing life or death?

We also die and live depending on what resources are made available to us. This has become clear in discussions about MAID, where young people with chronic conditions find they cannot support their daily life on their own and, lacking resources, move towards MAID. These decisions are embedded in social determinants of health — poverty, health, sex and gender, race and housing. If a health-care system is unable to provide, or we cannot afford, the resources required to live a reasonable and healthy daily life, many opponents argue that the choice towards MAID remains a false one.

THE QUEST FOR IMMORTALITY: LIFE EVERLASTING, COULD WE REALLY LIVE FOREVER?

How we deal with death and dying and life after death tells us much about how we deal with life. The COVID-19 pandemic has taught us many things about how we deal with the dying. It has also taught us about ageism, homophobia, discrimination and gender differences in disease recognition and treatment options, and how our culture deals with certain types of death. The debates surrounding MAID have made us question notions of freedom of choice and ethical considerations about heath care and religion. In the past ten to twenty years, those interested in life extension technologies, such as cryonics, elective prosthetics, body modification devices and producers of vitamins and supplements, among others, have suggested that humans could vastly extend our life expectancy by engaging with technological advances.

Cryonic Suspension

The relatively new field of cryonics, whereby heads or entire bodies can be frozen until a cure is found for what killed them and can then be (theoretically) resuscitated, raises interesting questions about who our ancestors might be in the future. Hypothetically, in the year 2130, I could die at age eighty-five and be cryonically suspended for resuscitation a hundred years later. In the meantime, my daughter could have had a child, who could have had a child, who could have also had a child (up to five generations could have been born while I was in suspension). By the year of my resuscitation in 2230, the youngest of these children would know a "grandmother" who lived almost two hundred years before the child was even born. Talk about a generation gap! With cryonics, our current chronological sense of lineage and family ties could be dramatically altered. Although right now this is a question that affects only those rich enough to afford the technology, who can predict how many of us will be cryonically preserved by the year 2130?

The American-based Cryonics Institute (n.d.) suggests the following nine reasons for choosing this option at the end-of-life: another chance at life, renewed youth and health, reunite with loved ones, witness the future, future cures for today's diseases, live longer, organ preservation, new life for a beloved pet and preserve endangered species. Journalist Sharon Kirkey shares the story of "Patient 74," a 79-year-old woman from Kingston, Ontario, whose son suggested that she be cryopreserved. The article explained what was involved:

> In the end, Patient 74 "deanimated" — was pronounced dead — on Mother's Day of 2006. Soon after death, her body was placed in a hospital refrigerator, then packed in ice in a casket three hours later for the drive across the border to Clinton Township, Michigan, where, at the Faulmann and Walsh funeral home, her blood was drained through her jugular veins, burr holes were drilled into each side of her skull and first her brain and then her body perfused with cryoprotectants, chemical solutions that help protect tissues and cells from ice formation at deep-freeze temperatures. Once suffused with biological antifreeze, her head stuck inside a plastic box filled with crushed dry ice to accelerate brain cooling, the body was transported to the Cryonics Institute, a warehouse squatting in an industrial park outside Detroit. There, Patient 74 was zipped into a sleeping bag, placed inside a cooling chamber, slowly cooled to -196 C over six days, then strapped to a backboard and lowered inside a cryostat." (Kirkey 2023)

The American-based Alcor Life Extension Foundation defines cryonics as the "technology for freezing a person after a terminal illness or a fatal accident, in the hope that medical science will be able to revive that person in the future, when life extension and anti-aging have become a reality."

Noting that cryonic suspension is extremely expensive, from $80,000 to $150,000 for a whole body, Alcor (n.d) counters this cost with the "good news" that this can be paid by taking out a life insurance policy that names Alcor as the beneficiary, so that when a patient is pronounced legally dead, Alcor receives the insurance money. On this website, the producers claim that they are redefining death, which they suggest "is only permanent when the structures encoding memory and personality (necessary for consciousness) have become so disrupted that it becomes theoretically impossible to recover the person. The is called 'information-theoretic-death.' Any other definition is arbitrary and subject to revision." Alcor also claims that death is a process that can be paused through the process of vitrification, which is "the transformation of a substance into a glassy solid. High concentrations of cryoprotectants permit biological tissue to be cooled to very low temperatures with little to no ice formation. It is now possible to physically vitrify organs as large as the human brain, achieving excellent structural preservation without freezing." For those interested in being cryonically preserved in their search for immortality, this is a very interesting site to explore, as it goes through the entire process and the costs for whole or parts of bodies, as well as for pets.

The Cryonics Society of Canada is a Canadian non-profit corporation "dedicated to informing Canadians about cryonics in Canada." Its Facebook page has a great deal of information about cryonics, including posts dealing with religious, psychological, philosophical and ethical issues, among others. Because it is not selling products involved in cryonic suspension, it is a useful site for additional information on the topic.

Bionic Limbs

While produced initially to assist amputees who lost limbs to disease or accidents or who were born without them, elective prosthetics are now available to those who wish to improve their performance by replacing healthy limbs with bionic or robotic ones. Prosthetic limbs can be operated through the existing muscle system; they can be attached to existing muscles in the arm or leg, and the muscle use generates an electrical impulse, which makes the arm or leg move. Scientists are currently testing a system that sends impulses directly from the brain to the limb.

Body modification devices have always been present in human society: consider body piercing and painting, breast and penis implants, plastic surgery, circumcision, cosmetic dental work, eyeglasses, hearing aids and tattoos. Recent developments include having implants inserted into various parts of the body to enhance performance. *Tapestry* host Mary Hines interviewed self-proclaimed cyborg Lindy Wilkins, a teacher and artist at Toronto Metropolitan University about the sub-dermal modification devices she has inserted into her body. According to Wilkins, a cyborg is a being with both organic and biomechatronic body parts. She pointed out that cyborg is not the same as bionic, biorobot or android; it applies to an organism that has restored function or enhanced abilities due to the integration of some artificial component or technology that relies on some sort of feedback. Wilkins inserted a magnetic implant into her hand so that she can pick up metal objects, and she inserted into her chest wall a device which acts as a compass, so that she always knows which direction she is facing. She sees body modification devices and elective prosthetics as the future, with artificial intelligence creating new types of humans (Canadian Broadcasting Corporation 2018).

The techniques used to enhance and change humans are also known as nanotechnology. Authors Jacob Heller and Christine Peterson (2017) note:

> The long-term goal of nanotechnology is to be able to fully manipulate molecular and atomic structures. Since humans are made of the same building blocks as the natural world, nanotechnology will probably enable the ability to change human tissue and cells at the molecular level. This will open doors to medicine, thought impossible, and enable us to extend the length and quality of human life. It will also open the door to enhancements of the body — better IQ, appearance and capabilities. In the long run, nanotechnology would enable us to repair and enhance any physical ailment in the body.

Another term for the desire to alter, enhance and prolong human life is "transhumanism," which is an international intellectual movement that aims to transform the human condition by developing and making widely available sophisticated technologies to greatly enhance human intellect and physiology. The American-based Transhumanist Party has established goals for life extension policies in all areas of life. Elon Musk, the US billionaire, is a key player in the field with his company Neuralink, whose goal is to use artificial intelligence (AI) to "create a generalized brain interface to restore autonomy to those with unmet medical needs today and unlock human potential tomorrow." Using brain/computer interfaces, the Transhumanist Party website claims that, using surgical robots, organs, tissues, and other body products can be replaced with AI.

These quests for life extensions and immortality further increase the notion that we are afraid to die, that we deny the death imperative, in that we all die, but also these attempts to extend life hinder our ability to come to terms with death and dying. Even if it were possible to live forever, would we want to do so? When I ask students this question, both in the classroom and in my online courses, the clear majority say "No." Those who say that they would indeed like to live forever say that they cannot imagine a life without them in it, and they wonder at what the world would look like over the centuries.

Deathbots

The introduction of AI in many aspects of life has created a new trend in grief management and immortality in the form of deathbots, which are chatbots that imitate the conversational behaviour — content, vocabulary and style — of a person who has died. Based on generative AI systems that depend on a large collection of human-generated information, deathbots draw on text messages, voice messages, photographs, video recordings, emails and social media posts to mimic the speech or writing of a deceased person. The most common form of deathbot is based on text. However, deathbots with audio outputs are becoming more common. They draw on "digital remains," generating responses to prompts entered by a human which can resemble the conversational responses the now deceased person would have given (Skelly 2024).

Based on photographs, videos and voice messages, deathbots can also predict what a deceased person may look and sound like in the future; this technology is being used especially in cases where infants and children die so they can be "recreated" later in life. The manufactures of deathbots claim that they can facilitate a new way to process grief, but questions of ethics, morality, consent and so on raise more concerns than benefits.

CULTURAL DIFFERENCES IN THE QUEST FOR IMMORTALITY

Across the world, many cultures believe in some sort of afterlife, where the dead become ancestors who guide the behaviour of the living when asked to do so. As Audrey Medwayosh, one of the contributors to this edition and a member of the Wasauksing Nation in Parry Sound, Ontario, told us,

"Some of our cultural teachings (depending on the nation) are that death is not the end, but a step towards another stage in life. When we die, we begin our journey to the spirit world, where we become ancestors" (email correspondence with Jeanette, October 27, 2024). The belief in the guidance of ancestors is also common in East Asian countries, such as China and Japan, as well as some in Europe and many in Africa. Often referred to as "ancestor worship," but now more understood as "ancestor respect," this belief is prevalent, and in some African countries, it is also linked to new births. Benson Ohihon Igboin (2022) notes,

> Belief in the existence of ancestors is universal, though different religious traditions place different significance on it. In African Indigenous Religion, belief in, and veneration of, ancestors have a pivotal place not only because of the nearness of the ancestors to the living in terms of communality and spirituality but also because they are believed to reincarnate in new babies.

The idea that our ancestors are always with us and available to guide when requested is a comforting one to many who wish to seek guidance and support from those who have gone before. This may especially be the case for those who go to DNA-testing sites to find more information about their ancestors.

In an interview with Nobel Prize-winning molecular biologist Venki Ramakrishnan, journalist Jessica DuLong (2024) asked the eminent scientist about his research into life extension, which suggests that humans live twice as long as we did 150 years ago due to increased knowledge about diseases and their spread. She asked, "Does that suggest interventions to triple or quadruple our lifespan lie just around the corner?" His reply is a good way to end this chapter:

> I think this quest for immortality is a mirage. One hundred and fifty years ago, you could expect to live until about 40. Today, life expectancy is about 80, which, as author Steven Johnson has said, is almost like adding a whole extra life. But we're still obsessed about dying. I think if we lived to be 150, we'd be fretting about why we're not living to 200 or 300. It's never-ending.

> **The Text Within: Nothing Stays the Same (Jeanette)**
>
> We have learned much from researching, writing and revising the fourth edition of this book. Some of the topics covered in this version did not even exist when I wrote the third edition almost seven years ago. This shows how much things change in such a short period of time, especially when it comes to health-care procedures and technologically driven AI options to extend life. Some years ago, one of the icons of my past died — Dusty Springfield, the famous and fabulous British pop singer of the sixties. When she died, I received phone calls, letters and newspaper clippings from friends I had not heard from in years. Collectively, we mourned the loss of not only Dusty but of all that she represented to us: our youth; a culture without computers, microwaves, email or faxes. Her death reminded us that we are growing older and that, although nothing stays the same, friendships and memories last a lifetime.

CONCLUSION

As this book ends, we want to thank you for reading it. We have covered as many aspects of the social, historical and cultural aspects of death and dying that we could in the number of pages allotted to us. We hope that it has been a journey of discovery for you, not only on a theoretical level but also in a personal and reflective way. After thinking about and working in the field of death and dying for most of her life, Jeanette would like to pass on the inspiring words of Norman Cousins from *The Healing Heart*: "Death is not the enemy: living in constant fear of it is" (1989:69). May you enjoy life until the very last moment.

SELF-REFLECTION AND THOUGHTFUL CONVERSATIONS

1. Where do you hear, see or observe a revival of interest in death and dying? How have views about death changed since your parents' and grandparents' times?
2. Why do you think we grieve publicly over the deaths of celebrities?
3. If you could live forever, would you want to? Why or why not? Is this a quest for immortality also anti-aging (ageism)? What would happen if we all lived forever?

IN-CLASS ASSIGNMENTS

1. Look up newspaper, magazine or internet accounts of the death of a celebrity of your choice. What themes emerge from these stories?
2. Make a list of celebrities who have died in your lifetime. Rank them based on age, gender and cause of death. What impact did these deaths have on your life?
3. Count the number of movies you have seen with death as a main theme. What sorts of images were portrayed? Have others in the class do the same for pop songs, television shows and videos and compare your responses.

SELECT BIBLIOGRAPHY

Aderibigbe, I.S., and Falola, T. (eds.). 2022. *The Palgrave Handbook of African Traditional Religion*. New York: Macmillan Press.

Aiken, L.R. 2001. "The Arts and Philosophy." *Dying, Death and Bereavement*, 165–190. Lawrence Erlbaum Assoc. <https://cipra.cl/biblioteca/duelo/Lewis%20R.%20Aiken%20-%20Dying,%20Death,%20and%20Bereavement-Psychology%20Press%20(2000).pdf>.

Al-Ibrahim, D. 2023. "How Television Affects Audience Behaviour in the New Era: A Review of Cultivation Theory." *China Media Research* 19, 1: 1–71.

Alcor. n.d. "What Is Cryonics?" <alcor.org/what-is-cryonics/>.

Allred, M. 2023. "Mortality, Mortuaries, and Movement-Implications of Dance/Movement Therapy and Death: A Literature Review." *American Journal of Dance Therapy* 45: 150–168. <https://doi.org/10.1007/s10465-023-09391-8>.

Andriessen, K. 2009. "Can Postvention Be Prevention?" *Crisis: The Journal of Crisis Intervention and Suicide Prevention* 30, 1: 43–47. <doi.org/10.1027/0227-5910.30.1.43>.

Angus Reid Institute. 2018. "Opioids in Canada: One-in-Eight Have Family or Close Friend Who Faced Addiction." <angusreid.org/opioid-crisis>.

_____ 2022. "Canada Across the Religious Spectrum: A Portrait of the Nation's Interfaith Perspectives During Holy Week." Angus Reid Institute. <angusreid.org/canada-religion-interfaith-holy-week>.

Aran, N., Card, K.G., Lee, K., and Hogg, R.S. 2022. "Patterns of Suicide and Suicidal Ideation in Relation to Social Isolation and Loneliness in Newcomer Populations: A Review." *Journal of Immigrant and Minority Health* 25, 2: 415–426. <doi.org/10.1007/s10903-022-01422-9>.

Archer, D. MD. 2013. "Body Snatchers: Organ Harvesting for Profit Kidneys and Organs Are Selling to the Highest Bidder on the Black Market." *The Millenium Report* <themillenniumreport.com/2016/12/body-snatchers-organ-harvesting-for-profit/>.

Ariès, P. 1974. *Western Attitudes Towards Death*. Baltimore: Johns Hopkins University Press.

_____ 1975. "The Reversal of Death: Changes in Attitudes towards Death in Western Societies." In David E. Stannard (ed.), *Death in America*. Philadelphia: University of Pennsylvania Press.

_____ 1982. *The Hour of Our Death*. New York: Vintage.

_____ 1985. *Image of Man and Death*, translated by J. Lloyd. Cambridge, MA: Harvard University Press.

Arnup, K. 2013. *Death, Dying and Canadian Families*. Vanier Institute of the Family, 7. <caregiversns.org/images/uploads/all/DeathDyingAndCanadianFamiliesVanier.pdf>.

Atkey, M. 2006. *Broadway North: The Dream of a Canadian Musical Theatre*, First edition. Toronto: Dundurn Press.

Atwood, M. 1992. *The Good Bones*. Toronto: McClelland and Stewart.

Auger, J.A. 2019. *Social Perspectives on Death and Dying.* Third edition. Halifax: Fernwood Publishing.

Auger, J.A., Tedford-Litle, D., and Wallace-Allen, B. 2018. *From the Inside Looking Out: Competing Ideas about Growing Old.* Halifax, Fernwood Publishing.

Auger, J.A., and Alison Bursey. 1997. *Mind, Body and Soul: Exploring the Need for a Hospice in Kings County, Nova Scotia.* Kentville, NS: Victorian Order of Nurses, Kings County Branch.

Auger, M., Howell, T., and Gomes, T. 2016. "Moving Toward Holistic Wellness, Empowerment and Self-Determination for Indigenous Peoples in Canada: Can Traditional Indigenous Health Care Practices Increase Ownership Over Health and Health Care Decisions?" *Canadian Journal of Public Health* 107, e393-e398. <doi: 10.17269/cjph.107.5366>.

Aviad, Y., and Cohen-Louck, K. 2021. "Locus of Control and Purpose in Life as Protective Factors Against the Risk for Suicide in Older Adults." *Smith College Studies in Social Work* 91, 4: 295–308. <doi.org/10.1080/00377317.2021.1968323>.

Banerji, A, Pelletier, V.A., Haring, R., et al. 2023. "Food Insecurity and Its Consequences in Indigenous Children and Youth in Canada." *PLOS Global Public Health* 3, 9. <doi.org/10.1371/journal.pgph.0002406>.

Barker, B., Goodman, A., and DeBeck, K. 2017. "Reclaiming Indigenous Identities: Culture as Strength Against Suicide among Indigenous Youth in Canada." *Canadian Journal of Public Health* 108, 2. <https://summit.sfu.ca/item/18056>.

Barnes, J. 2010. "The Loss of Depth." *Levels of Life.* New York: Knopf.

Barnieh, L., and Manns, B. 2014. "We Should Compensate Living Donors for Their Kidney." <healthydebate.ca/opinions/we-should-compensate-living-donors-for-their-kidney>.

Barton, A. 2011. "Walking Groups Help You Through Loss One Step at a Time." <theglobeandmail.com/life/relationships/walking-groups-help-you-through-grief-step-by-step/article570272>.

Baum, D.J. 1977. *Warehouses for Death: The Nursing Home Industry.* Don Mills, ON: Burns and MacEachern.

BBC News. 2021. "Joyce Echaquan: Racism Played Role in Death, Coroner Finds." October 6. <bbc.com/news/world-us-canada-58819203>.

Bennett, S., Robb, K.A., Andoh-Arthur, J., et al. 2024. "Establishing Research Priorities for Investigating Male Suicide Risk and Recovery: A Modified Delphi Study with Lived-Experience Experts." *Psychology of Men and Masculinities* 25, 1: 85–98. <doi.org/10.1037/men0000448>.

Berger, P.L. 1967. *The Sacred Canopy.* Garden City, NY: Doubleday.

Bernhardt, D. 2016. "Bio-Cremation: Why Burn a Body When You Can Dissolve It?" *CBC News*, March 4. <cbc.ca/radio/the180/electric-cars-aren-t-green-pot-is-still-a-drug-and-we-need-to-rethink-the-canoe-1.3475291/bio-cremation-why-burn-a-body-when-you-can-dissolve-it-1.3475360>.

Bericat, E. 2016. The Sociology of Emotions: Four Decades of Progress. *Current Sociology* 64, 3: 491-513. <https://doi.org/10.1177/0011392115588355>.

Bertman, S.L. 1999. *Grief and the Healing Arts: Creativity as Therapy.* Routledge.

Binstock, A. 2023. "Living Funerals Guide: What Are They and How to Plan One." You Are Forever, October 24. <youareforever.com/en-ca/blogs/main/living-funerals>.

Blignault, I., Smith, S., Woodland, L., et al. 2010. "Fear and Shame: Using Theatre to Destigmatize Mental Illness Is an Australian Macedonian Community." *Health Promotion Journal of Australia* 21, 2: 120–126. <doi: 10.1071/he10120>.

Bloom, L.E. 2024. "Jewish Ghosts: Judit Hersko and Susan Hiller and the Feminist Intersectional Art of Post-Holocaust Memory." *Arts* 13, 2: 50. <doi.org/10.3390/arts13020050>

Bloom, T., and Bradshaw, G.A. 2022. "Inside of a Prison: How a Culture of Punishment Prevents Rehabilitation." *Peace and Conflict: Journal of Peace Psychology* 28, 1: 140–143. <doi.org/10.1037/pac0000572>.

Bogetz, J.F., Schroeder, A.R., Bergman D.A., et al. 2014. "Palliative Care Is Critical to the Changing Face of Child Mortality and Morbidity in the United States." *Clinical Pediatrics* 53, 11: 1030–1031. <doi: 10.1177/0009922814534767>.

Bolton, R. (ed.). 1989. *The Context of Culture: Constants and Constraints*. CT: Bergin and Harvey.

Bonnewyn, A., Shah, A., Bruffaerts, R., et al. 2014. "Reflections of Older Adults on the Process Preceding Their Suicide Attempt: A Qualitative Approach." *Death Studies* 38, 9: 612–618. <doi.org/10.1080/07481187.2013.835753>.

Bookey. n.d. "30 Best Uta Hagen Quotes with Image." <bookey.app/quote-author/uta-hagen>.

Borrows, J. 1997. "The Royal Proclamation, Canadian Legal History, and Self-Government." In M. Asch (ed.), *Aboriginal and Treaty Rights in Canada: Essays on Law, Equity and Respect for Difference*. Vancouver: UBC Press. <sfu.ca/~palys/Borrows-1997-Wampum_at_Niagara.pdf>.

Borrows, L. 2015. "Reflecting on Death: First Nations People." In Kath Murray *Life and Death Matters*. <lifeanddeathmatters.ca/reflecting-on-death-first-nations-people>.

Bosticco, C., and Thompson, T.L. 2005. "Narratives and Storytelling in Coping with Grief and Bereavement." *OMEGA-Journal of Death and Dying* 51, 1: 1–16. < https://doi.org/10.2190/8TNX-LEBY-5EJY-B0H6>.

Boulos, D. 2023. *2023 Report on Suicide Mortality in the Canadian Armed Forces (1995 to 2022)*. <canada.ca/en/department-national-defence/corporate/reports-publications/health/2023-report-on-suicide-mortality-in-the-caf-1995-to-2022.html>.

Bowlby, J. 1980. *Attachment and Loss: Vol. 3. Loss: Sadness and Depression*. New York: Basic Books.

Brabant, A. 1989–90. "Old Pain or New Pain: A Social Psychological Approach to Recurrent Grief." *Omega* 20, 4: 273-279, <doi.10.2190/YA0Q-45B2-JTJF-VH3H>.

Bracken, A. 2016. "How Canada Got Addicted to Fentanyl." *Toronto Globe and Mail*, April 8. <theglobeandmail.com/news/investigations/a-killer-high-how-canada-got-addicted-tofentanyl/article29570025>.

Brant, J.M., and Silbermann, M. 2021. "Global Perspectives on Palliative Care for Cancer Patients: Not All Countries Are the Same." *Current Oncology Report* 23, 5: 60. <doi:10.1007/s11912-021-01044-8>.

Brazil, K., and Thomas, D. 1995. "The Role of Volunteers in a Hospital-Based Palliative Care Service." *Journal of Palliative Care* 11, 3: 40–42.

Bright, R. 1996. *Grief and Powerlessness: Helping People Regain Control of Their Lives*. London: Jessica Kingsley Publishers.

Brookfield, S.D. 2005. *The Power of Critical Theory: Liberating Adult Learning and Teaching*. Jossey-Bass.

Brown, A., Millman, H., Tam-Seto, L., et al. 2024. "Increasing Understanding of the Barriers to Military Sexual Trauma-Related Reporting and Treatment Seeking in Canada." *Journal of Military, Veteran and Family Health* 10, 1: 101–106. <doi.org/10.3138/jmvfh-2023-0021>.

Brown, S., and Schuman, D.L. 2021. "Suicide in the Time of COVID-19: A Perfect Storm." *The Journal of Rural Health* 37, 1: 211–214. <doi.org/10.1111/jrh.12458>.

Browne, R. 2015. "The Rise of the Death Doula." *Maclean's*, March 15. <macleans.ca/society/death-doulas>.

Bryan, A.O., Theriault, J.L., and Bryan, C.J. 2015. "Self-Forgiveness, Posttraumatic Stress, and Suicide Attempts Among Military Personnel and Veterans." *Traumatolog* 21, 1: 40–46. <doi.org/10.1037/trm0000017>.

Bryan, C.J., Butner, J.E., May, A.M., et al. 2020. "Nonlinear Change Processes and the Emergence of Suicidal Behavior: A Conceptual Model Based on the Fluid Vulnerability Theory of Suicide." *New Ideas in Psychology* 57. <doi.org/10.1016/j.newideapsych.2019.100758>.

Buchanan, J. 2021. *Wellness, Wellplayed: The Power of a Playlist*. Calgary: JB Music Therapy.

Buchholz, K. 2022. "Where Most People Die by Assisted Suicide." <forbes.com/sites/katharinabuchholz/2022/08/12/where-most-people-die-by-assisted-suicide-infographic/?sh=530b708f49a3>.

Burgess, G.M. 2024. "Inviting Death In: Incorporating Death Education in Public School Music Classes." *The Canadian Music Educator* March 22, 65, 3: 8–13.

Cabello, M., Miret, M., Ayuso-Mateos, J.L., et al. 2020. "Cross-National Prevalence and Factors Associated with Suicide Ideation and Attempts in Older and Young-and-Middle Age People." *Aging and Mental Health* 24, 9: 1533–1542. <doi.org/10.1080/13607863.2019.1603284>.

Cait, C.A., and Lafreniere, G. 2024. "'Stop Imposing on Us': A Critical Examination of Ethnocultural Considerations in the Canadian Volunteer Hospice Palliative Care Landscape." *Journal of Social Work in End-of-Life and Palliative Care* 20, 2: 185–200. <doi.org/10.1080/15524256.2024.2321522>.

Callahan, A.B. 2011. "The Parent Should Go First: A Dance/Movement Therapy Exploration in Child Loss." *American Journal of Dance Therapy* 33, 2: 182–195. <doi.10.1007/s10465-011-9117-3>.

Callanan, M., and Kelley, P. 1992. *Final Gifts: Understanding the Special Awareness, Needs and Communication of the Dying*. New York: Barnes and Noble.

Calzo, J.P., and Ward, M. 2009. "Media Exposure and Viewers' Attitudes Toward Homosexuality: Evidence for Mainstreaming or Resonance?" *Journal of Broadcasting and Electronic Media* 53, 2: 280–299. <doi.10.1080/08838150902908049>.

Campanella, E. 2016. "Biodegradable Burial Pods Will Turn You Into a Tree When You Die." *Global News*, March 4. <globalnews.ca/news/2558634/biodegradable-burial-pods-will-turn-you-into-a-tree-when-you-die/>.

———. 2017. "Don't Want to Be Buried or Cremated? 5 Funeral and Burial Alternatives." *Global News*, July 15. <globalnews.ca/news/3595677/dont-want-to-be-buried-or-cremated-5-funeral-and-burial-alternatives>.

Campbell, D. 2000. "A Search for Justice in First Nations Communities; The Role of the RCMP and Community Policing." Doctoral dissertation, Carleton University. <collectionscanada.ca/obj/s4/f2/dsk2/ftp03/MQ52341.pdf>.

Campbell, I. 2024. "Members of Special Joint Committee on MAID Express Contrasting Views in Lead Up to Report." *Hill Times*, January 28. <hilltimes.com/story/2024/01/08/members-of-special-joint-committee-on-MAID-express-contrasting-views-in-lead-up-to-report/407460>.

Canadian Association of Retired Persons. 2017. "Opioid Poisoning on the Rise for Canadian Seniors." <carp.ca/2016/11/17/opioid-poisoning-rise-canadian-seniors/>.

Canadian Blood Services. 2016. *Organ Donation and Transplantation in Canada: Systems Progress Report 2006–2015*. <profedu.blood.ca/sites/default/files/odt_report.pdf>.

____ 2025. "Donating Blood with Canadian Blood Services." <blood.ca/en/blood/donating-blood>.
Canadian Blood Services and World Health Organization. 2012. *International Guidelines for the Determination of Death – Phase I*. <thaddeuspope.com/images/WHO_montreal-forum-report.pdf>.
Canadian Broadcasting Corporation. 2004. "Transplant Tourism." *The Passionate Eye*, October 14.
____ 2015. "Timeline: Assisted Suicide in Canada." February 5. <cbc.ca/news/health/timeline-assisted-suicide-in-canada-1.2946485>.
____ 2017. "Flat Rate CPP Death Benefits Panned as Sufficient to Cover Funeral Costs." December 16. <cbc.ca/news/politics/change-cpp-benefit-panned-funeral-costs-1.4452815>.
____ 2018. "The New Human." *Tapestry*, June 10. <cbc.ca/radio/tapestry/the-new-human-1.4696724>.
____ 2018. "Seniors in Long-Term Care Facilities Twice as Likely to Be on Opioids." May 17. <cbc.ca/news/health/seniors-opioids-1.4666951>.
Canadian Cancer Society. n.d. "Cannabis and Cannabinoids for Medical Purposes."
____ 2023. *Analyzing Hospice Palliative Care Across Canada*. Available through <cancer.ca/en/about-us/media-releases/2023/palliative-care-report>.
Canadian Centre for Architecture. 2016. "The Architecture of Death." June 6. <cca.qc.ca/en/issues/9/let-us-assure-you/1167/the-architecture-of-death>.
Canadian Coalition for Seniors Mental Health. 2019. "Canadian Guidelines on Opioid Use Among Older Adults." <ccsmh.ca/wp-content/uploads/2019/11/Canadian_Guidelines_Opioid_Use_Disorder_ENG.pdf>.
Canadian Drug Policy Commission. 2012. "What Is Naloxone?" August 29. <drugpolicy.ca/what-is-naloxone/>.
Canadian Funerals Online. 2021. "Why Is Cremation on the Increase in Canada." <canadianfunerals.com/cremations.html>.
____ 2025. "Cremation Costs by Province and City." <canadianfunerals.com/cremation-costs-in-canada>.
Canadian Hospice Palliative Care Association. 2005. *What Is Hospice Palliative Care?* <chpca.ca/education/what-is-hospice-palliative-care/>
____ 2018. "Palliative Care and MAID: Co-Existing in the New Environment" November 18. <https://www.virtualhospice.ca/Assets/MAiD_Report_Final_October_15_2018_20181218165246.pdf>.
____ 2024. "Fact Sheet: Hospice Palliative Care in Canada." June. <chpca.ca/wp-content/uploads/2024/06/2023-Fact-Sheet-CHPCA-EN.pdf>.
Canadian Institute for Health Information. 2018. "Framework on Palliative Care in Canada." <canada.ca/en/health-canada/services/health-care-system/reports-publications/palliative-care/framework-palliative-care-canada.html>.
____ 2023. "Access to Palliative Care in Canada 2023." <cihi.ca/sites/default/files/document/access-to-palliative-care-in-canada-2023-report-en.pdf>.
Canadian Integrative Network for Death Education and Alternatives. n.d. "The Emerging Modern Pan-Death Movement." <cindea.ca/pan-death.html>.
____ n.d. "Music Thanatology." <cindea.ca/resources-elsewhere.html#MUS>.
Canadian Mental Health Association. 2018. "Care Not Corrections: Relieving the Opioid Crisis in Canada." <cmha.ca/wp-content/uploads/2021/07/Summary-Report.pdf>.
Canadian Mental Health Coalition. 2018. "Opioids-CNDN Mental Health." <ccsmh.ca/areas-of-focus/opioids>.

Canadian Network of Palliative Care for Children. <cnpcc.ca>.
Canadian Plasma Resources, Compensation. 2017. <giveplasma.ca/become-a-donor/compensation>.
Canadian Psychiatric Association. 2016. "Psychiatrists Welcome Cautious Approach to Mental Illness and Medical Assistance in Dying." <cpa-apc.org/psychiatrists-welcome-cautious-approach-to-mental-illness-and-medical-assistance-in-dying/>.
Canadian Public Health Association. 2025. *First Nations, Inuit, and Métis Peoples Health | Canadian Public Health Association*. <www.cpha.ca/indigenous-health>.
Canada Royal Commission on Aboriginal Peoples. 1995. "Choosing Life-Special Report Suicide among Aboriginal Peoples." Ottawa, Ontario: Minister of Supply and Services.
Canadian Virtual Hospice. 2017. "Advance Care Planning in Canada." <virtualhospice.ca/en_US/Main+Site+Navigation/Home/Topics/Topics/Decisions/Advance+Care+Planning+Across+Canada.aspx>.
_____ 2025. "About Us." <virtualhospice.ca/en_US/Main+Site+Navigation/Home+Navigation/About+Us.aspx>.
Canen, J.M., and Brausch, A.M. 2024. "Minority Stressors and Suicidal Ideation in Sexual Minority Individuals Across Adulthood." *Suicide and Life-Threatening Behavior* 54, 4: 702–712. <doi.org/10.1111/sltb.13080>.
Cardany, A.B. 2018. "Mitigating Death Anxiety: Identifying Music's Role in Terror Management." *Psychology of Music* 46, 1: 3–17. <doi.10.1177/0305735617690600>.
Carroll, N. 2001. *Beyond Aesthetics: Philosophical Essays*. Cambridge University Press.
Carteret, M. 2010. "Cultural Aspects of Death and Dying." November 3. <www.scribd.com/document/444192901/Cultural-Aspects-of-Death-and-Dying>.
Castillo, M. 2017. "In 'Coco' Death Is the Point." *New York Times*. <nytimes.com/2017/12/08/movies/coco-pixar.html>.
Castleden, H., Crooks, V.A., Sloan Morgan, V., et al. 2009. "Dialogues on Aboriginal-Focused Hospice-Palliative Care in Rural and Remote British Columbia, Canada." <unbc.ca/sites/default/files/sections/neil-hanlon/2009_hanlon_dialoguesfinalreport.pdf>.
Cate, S. 2024. "How Much Are Your Organs Worth on the Black Market." *The Hearty Soul*, August 9. <theheartysoul.com/organ-trafficking-black-market-worth>.
Celestial Memorial Spaceflights. n.d. <celestis.com/experiences-pricing/#service-Earth-Rise>.
Cerel, J., McIntosh, J., Neimeyer, R., et al. 2014. "The Continuum of 'Survivorship': Definitional Issues in the Aftermath of Suicide." April 7. <doi.10.1111/sltb.12093>.
Chambers, S. 2016. "Assisted Dying: A History of Ethical Principles." *Impact Ethics*, June 13. <impactethics.ca/2016/06/13/assisted-dying-a-history-of-ethical-principles>.
Chang, I.-C. 2005. "Theatre as Therapy, Therapy as Theatre Transforming the Memories and Trauma of the 21September 1999 Earthquake in Taiwan." *Research in Drama Education: The Journal of Applied Theatre and Performance* 10, 3: 285–301.
Cheechov, S. 2016. "Theatre Group Spotlights Mental Health Sexuality in New Musical." *Daily Bruin*, May 30. <dailybruin.com/2016/05/30/theater-group-spotlights-mental-health-sexuality-in-new-musical>.
China Organ Harvest Research Center. n.d. "Plastinated Bodies." <chinaorganharvest.org/report/findings/appendix-admissions/plastinated-bodies>.
Chochinov, H., and Wilson, K. 1995. "The Euthanasia Debate: Attitudes, Practices and Psychiatric Considerations." *Canadian Journal of Psychiatry*, 40. <doi.org/10.1177/070674379504001005>.
Chodorow, J., Govine, B., Gould, S., and Verebes, A. 1999. "Honoring and Remembering Trudi Schoop." *American Journal of Dance Therapy* 21, 2: 113–116. <doi.10.1023/A:1022108704098>.

Cianconi, P., Betrò, S., and Janiri, L. 2020. "The Impact of Climate Change on Mental Health: A Systematic Descriptive Review." *Frontiers in Psychiatry* Mar. 6, 11: 74, <doi:10.3389/fpsyt.2020.00074>.

Claxton-Oldfield, S. 2018. "The Changing Face of Volunteering in Palliative Care in Canada." In Scott and Howlett (eds.) *Palliative Care: An International Perspective*. Oxford, UK: Oxford University Press.

Claxton-Oldfield, S., and Beaudette, S. 2021. "Hospice Palliative Care Volunteers' Attitudes, Opinions, Experiences, and Perceived Needs for Training Around Medical Assistance in Dying (MAID)." *American Journal of Hospice Palliative Care*, 38, 11: 1282–1290. <doi.10.1177/1049909114523826>.

Claxton-Oldfield, S., and Miller, K. 2015. "A Study of Canadian Hospice Palliative Care Volunteers' Attitudes Toward Physician-Assisted Suicide." *American Journal of Hospice and Palliative Medicine* 32, 2: 305–312. <doi.10.1177/1049909114523826>.

Cockburn, D. 1989. "People and the Paranormal." In Berger, Badham, Kutscher, et al., *Perspectives on Death and Dying*. Philadelphia: Charles Press.

Coleman, T.A., Chee, K., Chin-see, R., et al. 2024. "Minority Stressors, Social Provisions, and Past-Year Suicidal Ideation and Suicide Attempts in a Sample of Sexual Orientation and Gender Identity/Expression Minority People in Canada." *LGBT Health* 11, 7: 539–551. <doi.org/10.1089/lgbt.2022.0344>.

College of Physicians and Surgeons of Nova Scotia. 2017. "College Endorses New Canadian Guidelines for Opioid Prescribing." May 31. <cpsns.ns.ca/college-endorses-new-canadian-guideline-for-opioid-prescribing>.

____ 2018. "Professional Standards Regarding Medical Assistance in Dying." <cpsns.ns.ca/wp-content/uploads/2018/12/ProfessionalStandard_MedicalAssistanceInDying_Dec2018.pdf>.

Conejero, I., Olié, E., Courtet, P., and Calati, R. 2018. "Suicide in Older Adults: Current Perspectives." *Clinical Interventions in Aging* 13: 691–699. <doi:10.2147/CIA.S130670>.

Contro, N., and Sourkes, B. 2012. "Opportunities for Quality Improvement in Bereavement Care at a Children's Hospital Assessment of Interdisciplinary Staff Perspectives." *Journal of Palliative Care* 28, 1: 28–35.

Corr, C.A. 2014. "The Death System According to Robert Kastenbaum." *Omega-Journal of Death and Dying* 70, 1: 13–25. <doi:10.2190/OM.70.1.c. >.

Corr, C., Nabe C. and Corr D. 1997. *Death and Dying, Life and Living*. Brooks/Cole Publishing.

Costa, A.C., and Viegas Abreu, M. 2018. "Expressive and Creative Writing in the Therapeutic Context: From the Different Concepts to the Development of Writing Therapy Programs." *Journal: Psychologica* 61, 1: 69–86. <doi.10.14195/1647-8606_61-1_4>.

Costa, M.C. 2019. "Unspeakable: The Truth about HIV-Tainted Blood in Canada." *The Lancet* 19, 9. <doi.10.1016/S1473-3099(19)30434-7>.

Cousins, N. 1989. *The Healing Heart*. New York: Avon Press.

Cox, M., Garrett, E., and Graham, J.A. 2005. "Death in Disney Films: Implications for Children's Understanding of Death." *OMEGA-Journal of Death and Dying* 50, 4: 267–280. <doi.10.2190/Q5VL-KLF7-060F-W69V>.

Cramer, R.J., and Kapusta, N.D. 2017. "A Social-Ecological Framework of Theory, Assessment, and Prevention of Suicide." *Frontiers in Psychology* 8: 1756. <doi.org/10.3389/fpsyg.2017.01756>.

Cremation Association of North America (CANA). 2024. *Annual Statistics Report*.

____ n.d. "Alkaline Hydrolysis." <www.cremationassociation.org/alkalinehydrolysis.html>.

Crosthwait, G. 2020. "The Afterlife as Emotional Utopia in Coco." *Animation: An Interdisciplinary Journal* 15, 2: 179–192. <doi.10.1177/1746847720937443>.

Cryonics Institute. n.d. "Why Choose Cryonics?" <cryonics.org>.

Cummins, L. 2004. "The Funeral of Froggy the Frog: The Child as Dramatist, Designer and Realist." *YC Young Children* 59, 4: 87–91. <https://www.jstor.org/stable/42730144>.

Curl, J.S. 1993. *A Celebration of Death: An Introduction to Some of the Buildings, Monuments, and Settings of Funerary Architecture in Western European Tradition*. London: T.B. Batsford.

Dalhousie University. n.d. "Human Body Donation Program." <medicine.dal.ca/departments/department-sites/medical-neuroscience/about/donation-program.html>.

Daoust, R., Paquet, J., Moore, L., et al. 2018. "Recent Opioid Use and Fall-Related Injuries Among Older Patients with Trauma." *Journal of the Canadian Medical Association* 190, 16: e500-e506. < doi.10.1503/cmaj.171286>.

David, J., and Jaffray, B. 2022. "Homicide in Canada, 2021." Juristat: Canadian Centre for Justice Statistics, November 21, 1, 3-30. <proquest.com/scholarly-journals/homicide-canada-2021/docview/2769626624/se-2>.

Davis, C., and Breede, D. 2018. *Talking Through Death: Communicating About Death in Interpersonal, Mediated, and Cultural Contexts*. Routledge.

Davis, C.S., and Crane, J.L. 2015. "A Dialogue with (Un) Death: Horror Films as a Discursive Attempt to Construct a Relationship with the Dead." *Journal of Loss and Trauma* 20, 5: 417–429. <doi.10.1080/15325024.2014.935215>.

Davis, C., and Warren-Findlow, J. 2011. "Coping With Trauma Through Fictional Narrative Ethnography: A Primer." *Journal of Loss and Trauma* 16, 6: 563–572. <doi.10.1080/15325024.2011.578022>.

de Guzman, A.B. Satuito, J.C.B., Satumba, M.A.E., et al. 2011. "Filipino Arts Among Elders in Institutionalized Care Settings." *Educational Gerontology* 37, 3: 248–261.

de Mendonça Lima, C.A., De Leo, D., Ivbijaro, G., and Svab, I. 2021. "Suicide Prevention in Older Adults." *Asia-Pacific Psychiatry* 13, 3: 1–12. <doi.org/10.1111/appy.12473>.

Death Café. <deathcafe.com/>.

Death Doula Association of Canada. n.d. "What Is a Death Doula: Let's Start the Conversation." <endoflifedoulaassociation.org>.

Deuter, K., Procter, N., and Evans, D. 2020. "Protective Factors for Older Suicide Attempters: Finding Reasons and Experiences to Live." *Death Studies* 44, 7: 430–439. <doi.org/10.1080/07481187.2019.1578303>.

Devandas Aguilar, C. 2019. "Report of the Special Rapporteur on the Rights of Persons with Disabilities on Her Visit to Canada: Comments by the State." <digitallibrary.un.org/record/3848188?ln=enandv=pdf >.

DeVita, Michael. A. 2001. "The Death Watch: Certifying Death Using Cardiac Criteria." *North American Transplant Coordinators Organization*.

Devlin, J., Richardson, D.C., Hogan, J., and Nuttall, H. 2017. "Audience Members' Hearts Beat Together at the Theatre." *UCL Psychology and Language Sciences*, Lancaster University. <ucl.ac.uk/brain-sciences/news/2017/nov/audience-members-hearts-beat-together-theatre#:~:text=New%20research%20led%20by%20the,Joe%20Devlin%2C%20Dr%20Daniel%20C>.

Dickerman, L. 2024. "The Last Sculptures (For Richard Serra). *MIT Press*, 189, Summer: 203–219. <doi.10.1162/octo_a_00532>.

Diefenbach, D.L., and West, M. 2007. "Television and Attitudes toward Mental Health Issues: Cultivation Analysis and the Third-Person Effect." *Journal of Community Psychology* 35, 2: 181–195. <doi.10.1002/jcop.20142>.

Díez-Gómez, A., Sebastián-Enesco, C., Pérez-Albéniz, A., et al. 2024. "The PositivaMente Program: Universal Prevention of Suicidal Behaviour in Educational Settings." *School Mental Health: A Multidisciplinary Research and Practice Journal* 16, 2: 455–466. <doi.org/10.1007/s12310-024-09650-0>.

Dignitas. n.d. "Countries with End-of-life Help Laws and/or Regulations." <dignitas.ch/index.php?option=com_contentandview=articleandid=54andlang=en>.

Dignity Memorial. n.d. "Living Funerals: Celebrating Life Before You Die." <dignitymemorial.com/en-ca/memorial-services/planning-a-funeral/what-is-a-living-funeral>.

Djelantik, A.M.J., Aryani, P., Boelen, P.A., et al. 2021. "Prolonged Grief Disorder, Post-traumatic Stress Disorder, and Depression Following Traffic Accidents Among Bereaved Balinese Family Members: Prevalence, Latent Classes, and Cultural Correlates." *Journal of Affective Disorders* 292: 773–781. <doi.10.1016/j.jad.2021.05.085>.

Doka, K.J. 1989. *Disenfranchised Grief*. Lexington, MA: Lexington Press.

———2002. *Disenfranchised Grief: New Directions. Challenges and Strategies for Practice*. Champaign, IL: Research Press.

Donor Alliance. 2025. "What Is the Time Frame for Transplanting Organs?" February 21. <donoralliance.org/newsroom/donation-essentials/what-is-the-time-frame-for-transplanting-organs/>.

Downie, J. 2004. *Dying Justice: A Case for Decriminalizing Euthanasia and Assisted Suicide in Canada*. Toronto: University of Toronto Press.

Downie, J., and Chandler, J. 2018. *Interpreting Canada's Medical Assistance in Dying Legislation*. Institute for Research and Public Policy, Ottawa. <irpp.org/wp-content/uploads/2018/03/Interpreting-Canadas-Medical-Assistance-in-Dying-Legislation-MAiD.pdf>.

Dransart, D.A.C. 2016. "Reclaiming and Reshaping Life: Patterns of Reconstruction after the Suicide of a Loved One." *Qualitative Health Research* 27, 7: 994–1005. <doi.org/10.1177/1049732316637590>.

Dubinsky, K. 2022. Some Canadian Med Schools Are Running Low on a Precious Resource — Cadavers. *CBC News*. June 28. <www.cbc.ca/news/canada/london/human-cadaver-shortage-1.6503714>.

Duke, D.F. (ed.). 2006. *Canadian Environmental History: Essential Readings*. Canadian Scholars' Press.

DuLong, J. 2024. "Why Do We Die? The Latest on Aging and Immortality from a Nobel Prize-Winning Author." *CNN*, April 9. <cnn.com/2024/04/09/health/aging-death-why-we-die-wellness>.

Dunbar-Ortiz, R. 2014. *An Indigenous Peoples History of the United States*. Beacon Press. <sackett.net/An-Indigenous-Peoples-History-of-the-United-States-Ortiz.pdf>.

Dunfield, A, 2024. "Women Are Changing the Face of the Death Care Industry." *Globe and Mail*, February 13.

Dunn, N.S., McVittie, J., Ansloos, J., and Peltier, S. 2024. "Suicide Risk Assessment With Indigenous Peoples: Exploring Providers' Knowledge and Experiences." *Practice Innovations* 9, 3: 223–239. <doi.org/10.1037/pri0000236>.

Dunphy, K., Baker, F.A., Dumaresq, E., et al. 2019. "Creative Arts Interventions to Address Depression in Older Adults: A Systematic Review of Outcomes, Processes, and Mechanisms." *Frontiers in Psychology* January 8, 9: 02655. <doi.org/10.3389/fpsyg.2018.02655>.

Durkheim, É. 1951 [1897]. *Suicide: A Study in Sociology* (translated by J.A. Spaulding and G. Simpson). Glencoe, IL: Free Press.

Düzgün, G., and Karadakovan, A. 2024. "Effects of Music on Pain in Cancer Patients in Palliative Care Service: A Randomized Controlled Study." OMEGA—*Journal of Death and Dying* 88, 3: 1085–1100. <doi.10.1177/00302228211059891>.

Dying with Dignity. 2016. "What Types of MAID Are Available in Canada?" <dyingwithdignity.ca/get_the_facts_assisted_dying_law_in_canada>.

____ n.d. "Your Rights and the Law." <dyingwithdignity.ca/know_your_rights>.

Ebert, R. 2012. "Films That Are Not for Dying so Much." <rogerebert.com/roger-ebert/films-that-are-not-for-the-dying-so-much>.

Elias, N. 2001. *Loneliness of the Dying*. London, UK: Bloomsbury Publishing.

Emanual, E.J. 1994. "The History of Euthanasia in the United States and Britain." *Annals of Internal Medicine* 121, 10: 793–802.

Emanual, L., and Emanuel, E.J. 1989. "The Medical Directive." *Journal of the American Medical Association* 261, 22: 3288–93.

End of Life Doula Association of Canada. n.d. "Become a Doula." <eoldac.org/become-a-doula/>.

End of Life Planning Canada. 2016. "Patient Rights Booklet: Your Rights and Options at the End-of-Life." April. <d3n8a8pro7vhmx.cloudfront.net/dwdcanada/pages/709/attachments/original/1474555815/patient-rights-booklet_2016_elpc1.pdf?1474555815>.

Engel, S. 2016. "Death Doulas Are Transforming How We Die in Canada." *Global News*, June 10. <globalnews.ca/news/2754795/death-doulas-transforming-how-we-die-in-canada>.

Erizanu, P. 2018. "The Biodegradable Burial Pod That Turns Your Body Into a Tree." *CNN*, January 11. <cnn.com/2017/05/03/world/eco-solutions-capsula-mundi>.

Erlangsen, A., Banks, E., Joshy, G., et al. 2021. "Physical, Mental, and Social Wellbeing and Their Association with Death by Suicide and Self-Harm in Older Adults: A Community-Based Cohort Study." *International Journal of Geriatric Psychiatry* 36, 5: 647–656. <doi.org/10.1002/gps.5463>.

Eternal Reefs. n.d. "What Is an Eternal Reef?" <eternalreefs.com/the-eternal-reef-story/what-is-an-eternal-reef>.

Faigin, D., and Stein, C.H. 2010. "The Power of Theatre to Promote Individual Recovery and Change." *Psychiatric Services* 61, 3: 306–08. <doi.10.1176/ps.2010.61.3.306>.

Fair Funerals Program. n.d. "What Is Funeral Poverty?" <fairfuneralscampaign.org.uk/content/what-funeral-poverty>.

Family Caregivers Alliance. n.d. "Caregiver Stories." <caregiver.org/caregiver-stories>.

Fässberg, M.M., Cheung, G., Canetto, S.S. et al. 2016. A Systematic Review of Physical Illness, Functional Disability, and Suicidal Behaviour Among Older Adults. *Aging & Mental Health*, 20, 2. <doi.org/10.1080/13607863.2015.1083945>.

Favel, M. 2024. "This Sask. First Nation Will Be One of Few in Canada to Have Its Own Funeral Home." *CTV News*, August 7. <ctvnews.ca/regina/article/this-sask-first-nation-will-be-one-of-few-in-canada-to-have-its-own-funeral-home>.

Favril, L., Shaw, J., and Fazel, S. 2022. "Prevalence and Risk Factors for Suicide Attempts in Prison." *Clinical Psychology Review* 97: 1–10. <doi.org/10.1016/j.cpr.2022.102190>.

Ferlatte, O., Dromer, E., Salway, T., et al. 2024. "Self-Perceived Reasons for Suicide Attempts in Sexual and Gender Minorities in Canada." *Journal of Homosexuality*. <doi.org/10.1080/00918369.2024.2384939>.

First Nations Health Authority. 2025. "Our History, Our Health." <fnha.ca/wellness/wellness-for-first-nations/our-history-our-health>.

Flett, G.L., and Heisel, M.J. 2021."Aging and Feeling Valued Versus Expendable During the COVID-19 Pandemic and Beyond: A Review and Commentary of Why Mattering Is Fundamental to the Health and Well-Being of Older Adults." *International Journal of Mental Health and Addiction* 19, 6: 2443–2469. <doi.org/10.1007/s11469-020-00339-4>.

Flint, A., Merali, Z., and Vaccarino, F. (eds.). 2018. *Substance Use in Canada: Improving Quality of Life: Substance Use and Aging.* Ottawa: Canadian Centre on Substance Use and Addiction. <www.ccsa.ca/sites/default/files/2022-04/CCSA-Substance-Use-and-Aging-Report-2018-en%20%28ID%2023186%29.pdf>.

Freese, R.A., Canada, K.E., Nichols, P.M., and McNamara, B. 2023. "Suicide in Prisons: Describing Trends and Staff Knowledge and Preparedness to Address Suicide." *International Journal of Prisoner Health* 19, 3: 427–439. <emerald.com/insight/content/doi/10.1108/ijph-02-2022-0011/full/html>.

Freud, S. 1957. "Mourning and Melancholia." In Strachey (ed. and trans.), *The Standard Edition of the Complete Psychological Works of Sigmund Freud* (Vol.14: 152–v170). London: Hogarth Press.

Froese, J., McDermott, L., and Iwasaki, Y. 2020. "The Other Side of Suicide Loss: The Potential Role of Leisure and Meaning-Making for Suicide Survivors." *Annals of Leisure Research* 23,3. <doi:10.1080/11745398.2019.1616572>.

Fulton, G., and Metress, E. 1995. *Perspectives on Death and Dying.* Boston: Jones and Bartlett.

Funeral Resources.org. 2023. "Body Disposition: What Does It Mean in the Context of a Funeral?" <funeralresources.org/funeral-planning/body-disposition>.

Funerals360. n.d. "Alternatives to Embalming." <funerals360.com/blog/cremations/alternatives-to-embalming>.

———. 2022. "7+ Alternatives to Traditional Burial and Cremation." <everloved.com/articles/funeral-planning/7-alternatives-to-burial-cremation/>.

Gaind, K.S. 2020. "What Does 'Irremediability' in Mental Illness Mean?" *Canadian Journal of Psychiatry* 65, 9: 604–606. <doi:10.1177/0706743720928656>.

Garbay, M., Gay, M.C., and Claxton-Oldfield, S. 2015. "Motivations, Death Anxiety, and Empathy in Hospice Volunteers in France." *American Journal of Hospice and Palliative Medicine* 32, 5: 521–527. <doi.10.1177/1049909114536978>.

Gawande, A. 2017. *Medicine and What Matters in the End.* Northampton, ME: Metropolitan Books.

Gerbner, G. 1970. "Cultural Indicators: The Case of Violence in Television Drama." *The Annals of the American Academy of Political and Social Science* 388, 1: 69–81.

Germaine, A., and Moore, M. 2024. "These Unclaimed Bodies Are Stuck in Limbo in Freezers Outside the Health Sciences Centre." *CBC News,* March 6. <cbc.ca/news/canada/newfoundland-labrador/health-sciences-centre-cold-storage-bodies-1.7132964>.

Ginicola, M.M., Smith, C., and Trzaska, J. 2012. "Counselling Through Images: Using Photography to Guide the Counselling Process and Achieve Treatment Goals." *Journal of Creativity in Mental Health* 7, 4: 310–329.

Givler, A., Bhatt, H., and Maani-Fogelman, P.A. 2018. "The Importance of Cultural Competence in Pain and Palliative Care." In *Care at the Close of Life* by the National Library of Medicine. National Institutes of Health. <ncbi.nlm.nih.gov/books/NBK493154/>.

Gizmodo. n.d. "What Is Your Body Worth?" <gizmodo.com/5904129.heres-how-much-body-parts-cost-on-the-black-market>.

Glaser, B., and Strauss, A. 1965. *Awareness of Dying.* Chicago: Aldine.

Goffman, E. 1959. *The Presentation of Self in Everyday Life.* New York: Anchor Press.

_____ 1961. *Asylums: Essays on the Social Situations of Mental Patients and Other Inmates.* New York: Anchor.

_____ 1963. *Stigma: Notes on the Management of Spoiled Identity.* Englewood Cliff, NJ: Prentice-Hall.

_____ 1967. *Interaction Ritual: Essays on Face-to-Face Behavior.* New York: Pantheon Books. <https://eclass.uoa.gr/modules/document/file.php/PPP860/Erving%20Goffman%20-%20Interaction%20Ritual_%20Essays%20on%20Face-to-Face%20Behavior%20-Pantheon%20%281982%29.pdf>.

Gorer, G. 1965. "The Pornography of Death." In G. Gorer (ed.) *Death, Grief and Mourning.* London: Cresset Press.

Government of Canada. n.d. "Explore the Full Spectrum of Palliative Care." <canada.ca/content/dam/hc-sc/documents/services/publications/health-system-services/infographic-explore-full-spectrum-palliative-care/explore-full-spectrum-palliative-care.pdf>.

_____ n.d. "Organ and Tissue Donation." <canada.ca/en/health-canada/services/healthy-living/blood-organ-tissue-donation/organ-tissue.html>.

_____ n.d. "Palliative Care: Overview." <canada.ca/en/health-canada/services/health-services-benefits/palliative-care.html>.

_____ n.d. "Supervised Consumption Explained: Types of Sites and Services." <canada.ca/en/health-canada/services/substance-use/supervised-consumption-sites/explained.html>.

_____ 2014. "A Three-Year Review of Federal Inmates Suicides (2011–2014)." September 10. <oci-bec.gc.ca/en/content/backgrounder-three-year-review-federal-inmate-suicides-2011-2014>.

_____ 2016a. "Understanding the New Access to Cannabis for Medical Purposes Regulations." August. <canada.ca/en/health-canada/services/publications/drugs-health-products/understanding-new-access-to-cannabis-for-medical-purposes-regulations.html>.

_____ 2016b. "Blood, Organ and Tissue Donation." <canada.ca/en/public-health/services/diseases/blood-organ-tissue-donations.html>.

_____ 2016c. "Immigration and Ethnocultural Diversity: Key Results from the 2016 Census." October 25. <www150.statcan.gc.ca/n1/daily-quotidien/171025/dq171025b-eng.htm>.

_____ 2016d. "An Act to Amend the Criminal Code and to Make Related Amendments to Other Acts (Medical Assistance in Dying)." <laws-lois.justice.gc.ca/PDF/2016_3.pdf>.

_____ 2017. *2nd Interim Report on Medical Assistance in Dying in Canada.* <canada.ca/en/health-canada/services/publications/health-system-services/medical-assistance-dying-interim-report-sep-2017.html>.

_____ 2019. "Apparent Opioid Related Deaths in Canada. Public Health Agency." <health-infobase.canada.ca/datalab/national-surveillance-opioid-mortality.html>.

_____ 2021. "New Medical Assistance in Dying Legislation Becomes Law." Department of Justice. March 17. <canada.ca/en/department-justice/news/2021/03/new-medical-assistance-in-dying-legislation-becomes-law.html>.

_____ 2022. *The Canadian Census: A Rich Portrait of the Country's Religious and Ethnocultural Diversity.* <www150.statcan.gc.ca/n1/daily-quotidien/221026/dq221026b-eng.htm>.

_____ 2023a. *Fourth Annual Report on Medical Assistance in Dying in Canada, 2022.* October. <canada.ca/en/health-canada/services/publications/health-system-services/annual-report-medical-assistance-dying-2022.html>.

_____ 2023b. *The Framework on Palliative Care in Canada: Five Years Later: A Report on the State of Palliative Care in Canada*. December 15. <canada.ca/en/health-canada/services/publications/health-system-services/framework-palliative-care-five-years-later.html>.

_____ 2024a. *Fifth Annual Report on Medical Assistance in Dying in Canada, 2023*. December 11. <canada.ca/en/health-canada/services/publications/health-system-services/annual-report-medical-assistance-dying-2023.html>.

_____ 2024b. *Opioid Use Disorder and Treatment*. <canada.ca/en/health-canada/services/opioids/opioids-use-disorder-treatment.html>.

_____ 2024c. "Medical Assistance in Dying: Overview." Updated October 28. <canada.ca/en/health-canada/services/health-services-benefits/medical-assistance-dying.html>.

_____ 2024d. *Suicide Prevention in Indigenous Communities*. <sac-isc.gc.ca/eng/1576089685593/1576089741803>.

_____ 2025a. "Opioid- and Stimulant-Related Harms in Canada." March 7. <health-infobase.canada.ca/substance-related-harms/opioids-stimulants/>.

_____ 2025b. "Supervised Consumption Sites: Dashboard." <health-infobase.canada.ca/supervised-consumption-sites/>.

_____ 2025c. "Blood, Organ and Tissue Donation." <canada.ca/en/health-canada/services/healthy-living/blood-organ-tissue-donation.html>.

Green Burial Society of Canada. n.d. "Certified Sites." <greenburialcanada.ca/directory>.

Grow, B., and Shiffman, J. 2017. "In the U.S. Market for Human Bodies, Almost Anyone Can Dissect and Sell the Dead." Reuters, October 24. <reuters.com/investigates/special-report/usa-bodies-brokers>.

Guy, T. 1993. "Exploratory Study of Elementary-Aged Children's Conception of Death through the Use of Story." *Death Studies* 17, 1: 27–54.

Habenstein, R.W., and Lamers, W.M. 1960. *The History of American Funeral Directing*. Milwaukee: Bullfinch.

Halifax Hospice Society. <hospicehalifax.ca>.

Hamdan, S., Berkman, N., Lavi, N., et al. 2020. "The Effect of Sudden Death Bereavement on the Risk for Suicide: The Role of Suicide Bereavement." *Crisis: The Journal of Crisis Intervention and Suicide Prevention* 41, 3: 214–224. <doi.org/10.1027/0227-5910/a000635>.

Hansen, N., Janz, H., and Sobsey, D. 2008. "21 Century Eugenics?" *The Lancet*, Special Issue 372: S104–107.

Harker, A. 2012. "Landscape of the Dead: An Argument for Conservation Burial." *Berkeley Planning Journal* 25, 1: 150–159

Harrawood, L.K., Doughty, E., and Wilde, B. 2011. "Death Education and Attitudes of Counsellors-in-Training Toward Death: An Exploratory Study." *Counselling and Values* 56, 1–2: 83–95.

Harrington-LaMorie, J., Jordan, J.R., Ruocco, K., and Cerel, J. 2018. "Surviving Families of Military Suicide Loss: Exploring Postvention Peer Support." *Death Studies* 42, 3: 143–154. <doi.org/10.1080/07481187.2017.1370789>.

Hartley, G., and Hartley, N. (eds.). 2008. *Dying, Bereavement and the Healing Arts: Creative Responses to Death*. London: Jessica Kingsley Publishers.

He, Y., Wong, A., Zhang, Y., et al. 2024. "Effects of Mozart-Orff Parent-Child Music Therapy Among Mothers and Their Preschool Children with Autism Spectrum Disorder: A Mixed Methods Randomized Controlled Trial." *BMC Pediatrics* 24, 1: 665–714.

Health Canada. 2005. "Opioid- and Stimulant-Related Harms in Canada: Key Findings." March 7. <health-infobase.canada.ca/substance-related-harms/opioids-stimulants/>.

_____ n.d. "Explore the Full Spectrum of Palliative Care." Infographic. <https://www.canada.ca/content/dam/hc-sc/documents/services/publications/health-system-services/infographic-explore-full-spectrum-palliative-care/explore-full-spectrum-palliative-care.pdf>.

_____ 2023. "Government of Canada Highlights Key Progress in Support of Organ Donation and Transplantation." Sept. 15. <www.canada.ca/en/health-canada/news/2023/09/government-of-canada-highlights-key-progress-in-support-of-organ-donation-and-transplantation.html>.

Health Law Institute. n.d. "End-of-Life Law and Policy in Canada." <eoldev.law.dal.ca/?page_id=231>.

Heartlight Magazine. 1997. "What Can I Say?" <heartlight.org/feature/feature_070396_whatcan.html>.

Hebb, M. 2018. *Let's Talk About Death (Over Dinner)*. Grand Central Printing.

Heller, J., and Peterson, C. 2017. "Human Enhancement and Nanotechnology." *Foresight Institute*. <linkedin.com/pulse/can-we-enhance-human-body-eric-mc-farlane>.

Hemer, S.R. 2010. "Grief as Social Experience: Death and Bereavement in Lihir, Papua New Guinea." *The Australian Journal of Anthropology* 21, 3: 281–297.

Henderson, C. 2024. "Assisted Dying 'Abused' in Canada, Admits Group that Helped Legalise It." *The Telegraph*, October 26. <telegraph.co.uk/us/news/2024/10/26/assisted-dying-abused-canada-admits-group-legalised/>.

Henderson, G. 1973. *Hunters in the Barrens: The Naskapi on the Edge of the White Man's World*. Toronto: University of Toronto Press.

Hermann, E., Morgan, M., and Shanahan, J. 2021. "Television, Continuity, and Change: A Meta-Analysis of Five Decades of Cultivation Research." *Journal of Communication* 71, 4: 515–544. <doi.org/10.1093/joc/jqab014>.

Heuser, C., and Howe, J. 2019. "The Relation Between Social Isolation and Increasing Suicide Rates in the Elderly." *Quality in Ageing and Older Adults* 20, 1: 2–9. <doi.org/10.1108/QAOA-06-2018-0026>.

Hilberdink, C.E., Ghainder, K., Dubanchet, A., et al. 2023. "Bereavement Issues and Prolonged Grief Disorder: A Global Perspective." *Cambridge Prisms: Global Mental Health*, 10, e32. <doi: 10.1017/gmh.2023.28>.

Hobson, E. 2014. "Introducing the 'Drive-Thru' Funeral Home." *Global News*, September 15. <globalnews.ca/news/15646101/introducing-the-drive-thru-funeral-home>.

Hofer, M. 2013. "Appreciation and Enjoyment of Meaningful Entertainment: The Role of Mortality Salience and Search for Meaning in Life." *Journal of Media Psychology: Theories, Methods, and Applications* 25, 3: 109–117.

Holford, A. 2021. "Eight Ways That Music Can Support Young People's Wellbeing and Learning." Center for World Music. <centerforworldmusic.org/2021/08/music-wellbeing-and-learning/>.

Hollander, S.A., Dykes, J.C., Chen, S., et al. 2017. "The End-of-Life Experience of Pediatric Heart Transplant Recipients." *Journal of Pain and Symptom Management* 53, 5: 927–931. <doi:10.1016/j.jpainsymman.2016.12.334>.

Honeycutt, A., and Praetorius, R.T. 2016. "Survivors of Suicide: Who They Are and How Do They Heal?" *Illness, Crisis and Loss* 24, 2: 103–118. <doi.org/10.1177/1054137315587646>.

Hop Wo, N.K., Anderson, K.K., Wylie, L., and MacDougall, A. 2020. "The Prevalence of Distress, Depression, Anxiety, and Substance Use Issues Among Indigenous Post-Secondary Students in Canada." *Transcultural Psychiatry* 57, 2: 263–274. <doi.org/10.1177/1363461519861824>.

Hospice in the Weald. "The Vital Role of Volunteers in Hospice Care." <www.hospiceintheweald.org.uk/news-and-stories/the-vital-role-of-volunteers-in-hospice-care/.

Houle, S.A., Pollard, C., Jetly, R., and Ashbaugh, A.R. 2022. "Barriers and Facilitators of Help Seeking Among Morally Injured Canadian Armed Forces Veterans and Service Members: A Qualitative Analysis." *Journal of Military, Veteran and Family Health* 8, 3: 58–71. <doi.org/10.3138/jmvfh-2021-0093>.

Houlihan, P.J. 1998. *Life Without End: The Transplant Story*. Toronto: N.C. Press.

Howarth, G. 1996. *Last Rites: The Work of the Modern Funeral Director*. New York: Baywood.

Howlett, K. 2017. "Perdue Pharma Agrees to Settle Oxycontin Class-Action Suit." *Globe and Mail*, May 1. <theglobeandmail.com/news/national/purdue-pharma-agrees-to-settle-oxycontin-class-action-suit/article34861736>.

Hsu, M.T., Kahn, D.L., Yee, D.H., and Lee, W.L. 2004. "Recovery Through Reconnection: A Cultural Design for Family Bereavement in Taiwan." *Death Studies* 28, 8: 761–786.

Huertes-Del Arco, A., Izquierdo-Sotorrío, E., Carrasco, M.A., et al. 2024. "Suicidal Ideation in Adolescents and Young Adults: The Role of Defeat, Entrapment, and Depressive Symptoms—From a Systematic Review to a Tentative Theoretical Model." *Behavioral Sciences* 14, 12: 1145. <doi.org/10.3390/bs14121145>.

Igboin, B.O., 2022. "Beliefs and Venerations on Ancestors." In I.S. Aderibigbe and T. Falola (eds.), *The Palgrave Handbook of African Traditional Religion*. Palgrave Macmillan. <doi.org/10.1007/978-3-030-89500-6_7>.

In the Light Urns. n.d. "The Mushroom Coffin: An Eco-Friendly Option for Burial." <inthelighturns.com/funeral-information/the-mushroom-coffin-an-eco-friendly-option-for-burial>.

Indigenous Services Canada. 2023. "An Update on the Socio-Economic Gaps Between Indigenous Peoples and the Non-Indigenous Population in Canada: Highlights from the 2021 Census." <sac-isc.gc.ca/eng/1690909773300/1690909797208>.

International Association for Hospice and Palliative Care. <hospicecare.com/home>.

International Association for the Philosophy of Death and Dying. <philosophyofdeath.org>.

Isenberg, A.C. 2020. *The Destruction of the Bison: An Environmental History, 1750–1920*. Cambridge University Press.

Jackson, A., and Eve, A. 1997. "'97 Directory of Hospice and Palliative Care Services." London, England: Hospice Information Services, St, Christopher's Hospice.

Johnston, B. 1995. "*The Manitous: The Spiritual World of the Ojibway*." New York: Harper Collins Publisher.

Johnston, R.B. 1979. "Notes on Ossuary Burial Among the Ontario Iroquois." *Canadian Journal of Archaeology/Journal Canadien d'Archéologie* 3: 91–104.

Jovanovic, M. 2011. "Cultural Competency and Diversity Among Hospice Palliative Care Volunteers." *American Journal of Hospice and Palliative Medicine* 29, 3:165–170. <doi:10.1016/j.jpainsymman.2016.12.334>.

Kahlor, LA., and Eastin, M.S. 2011. "Television's Role in the Culture of Violence Toward Women: A Study of Television Viewing and the Cultivation of Rape Myth Acceptance in the United States." *Journal of Broadcasting and Electronic Media* 55, 2: 215–231. <doi.org/10.1080/08838151.2011.566085>.

Kalish, R.A. 1989. "Death Education." In R. Kastenbaum and B. Kastenbaum, (eds.), *Encyclopedia of Death*. Phoenix, AZ: Oryx.

Kasperkevic, J. 2014. "How Much Can You Get for Selling Your Body (Parts)?" January 31. <theguardian.com/money/us-money-blog/2014/jan/31/flu-government-sell-egg-sperm-body>.

Kastenbaum, R. 2001. *Death, Society, and Human Experience*. 7th edition. Boston: Allyn and Bacon.

Kelly, L., Linkewich, B., Cromarty, H., et al. 2009. "Palliative Care of First Nations People: A Qualitative Study of Bereaved Family Members." *Canadian Family Physician* 55, 4: 394–395.

Kelner, M. 1995. "Activists and Delegators: Elderly Patients' Perceptions about Control and the End of Life." *Social Sciences and Medicine* 41, 4: 537–545.

Kim, E.H., and Lee, E. 2009. "Effects of a Death Education Program on Life-Satisfaction and Attitudes Towards Death in College Students." *Journal of Korean Academy on Nursing* 39, 1: 1–9.

Kim, H. 2015. "Making Relations, Managing Grief: The Expression and Control of Emotions in Japanese Death Rituals." *The Asia Pacific Journal of Anthropology* 16, 1: 17–35. <doi.org/10.1080/14442213.2014.985605>.

Kim, SH., and Lee, S. 2023. "Effects of an Orff Music Activity Intervention Program on the Ego-Resilience, Peer Relationships, Happiness, Interpersonal Care Awareness, Anxiety and Stress of Children from Multicultural Families in the Republic of Korea." *Healthcare* 11, 14: 1–14. <doi:10.5388/aon.2024.24.4.165>.

Kirkey, S. 2023. "Why Some People Are Freezing Their Bodies and Hoping for Resurrection." *National Post*, August 30. <nationalpost.com/feature/cryopreservation-cryonics>.

Kjølseth, I., Ekeberg, Ø., and Steihaug, S. 2010. "Elderly People Who Committed Suicide—Their Contact with the Health Service. What Did They Expect, and What Did They Get?" *Aging Mental Health* 14, 8: 938–946. <doi.org/10.1080/13607863.2010.501056>.

Klonsky, E.D., and May, A.M. 2015. "The Three-Step Theory (3ST): A New Theory of Suicide Rooted in the 'Ideation-to-Action' Framework." *International Journal of Cognitive Therapy* 8, 2: 114–129. <doi.org/10.1521/ijct.2015.8.2.114>.

Knapp, S. 2023. "The Essentials of Creating Effective Safety Planning-Type Interventions for Suicidal Patients." *Practice Innovations* 8, 2: 131–140. <doi.org/10.1037/pri0000205>.

Kneer, J., and Rieger, D. 2016. "The Memory Remains: How Heavy Metal Fans Buffer Against the Fear of Death." *Psychology of Popular Media Culture* 5, 3: 258–272. <https://doi.org/10.1037/ppm0000072>.

Knoll, G. and Mahoney, J. 2004. "How to Improve Organ Donation Rates." *Canadian Medical Journal* 170, 3: 319. <cmaj.ca/content/170/3/319.1.full>.

Kovac, Sathya D. 2022. Obituary Sathya Dhara Kovac. *Winnipeg Free Press Passages*. <passages.winnipegfreepress.com/passage-details/id-311052/KOVAC_SATHYA>.

Králová, J., and Walter, T. (eds.). 2018. *Social Death: Questioning the Life-Death Boundary*. Oxon, UK: Routledge Press.

Kübler-Ross, E. 1969. *On Death and Dying*. London: Tavistock.

Kumar, M.B., and Tjepkema, M. 2019. "Suicide Among First Nations People, Métis and Inuit (2011–2016): Findings from the 2011 Canadian Census Health and Environment Cohort (CanCHEC)." June 28. <www150.statcan.gc.ca/n1/pub/99-011-x/99-011-x2019001-eng.htm>.

Landecker, H. 2007. "Tissue Economies: Blood, Organs and Cell Lines in Late Capitalism." *Journal of the History of Medicine and Allied Science* 62, 2: 270–272.

Landry, F. 2023. "How Do We Define Death? Canada Now Has Clear Clinical Guidelines." May 31. <muhc.ca/news-and-patient-stories/news/how-do-we-define-death-canada-now-has-clear-clinical-guidelines>

Latimer, E.J. 1995. "Caring for the Dying in Canada." *Canadian Family Physician* 41 (March): 362–65. <pmc.ncbi.nlm.nih.gov/articles/PMC2148018/>.

Lavalley, J., Kastor, S., Valleriani, J., and McNeil, R. 2018. "Reconciliation and Canada's Overdose Crisis: Responding to the Needs of Indigenous Peoples." *Canadian Medical Association Journal* 190, 50: e1466-1467. <doi.org/10.1503/cmaj.181093>.

Leerhson. C., and Peyser, M. 1992. "The Saddest Song." *Newsweek* 119, 12: 52.

Leming, M.R., and Dickinson, G.E. 1988. *Understanding Dying, Death and Bereavement*, first edition. Orlando, FL: Harcourt Brace.

Levi-Belz, Y., Ben-Yehuda, A., and Zerach, G. 2023. "Suicide Risk Among Combatants: The Longitudinal Contributions of Pre-Enlistment Characteristics, Pre-Deployment Personality Factors and Moral Injury." *Journal of Affective Disorders* 324, 1: 624–631. <doi.org/10.1016/j.jad.2022.12.160>.

Ley, D., and van Bommel, H. 1994. *The Heart of Hospice*. Toronto: NC Press.

Li, C., Wang, P., Martin-Moratinos, M., et al. 2024. "Traditional Bullying and Cyberbullying in the Digital Age and Its Associated Mental Health Problems in Children and Adolescents: A Meta-Analysis." *European Child and Adolescent Psychiatry* 33, 9: 2895–2909. <doi.org/10.1007/s00787-022-02128-x>.

Liebmann, M. 2021. "Colonialism and Indigenous Population Decline in the Americas." In L. Panich and S. Gonzalez (eds.), *Routledge Handbook of the Archaeology of Indigenous-Colonial Interaction in the Americas*. Routledge.

Littlewood, J. 1993. "The Denial of Death and Rites of Passage in Contemporary Societies." In David Clark (ed.), *The Sociology of Death*. London: Blackwell.

Living Urn. "Urns for Ashes: Tree Burial and Cremation Urns." <thelivingurn.com>.

Llewllyn, N. 1991. "The Art of Death." London: Reaction Books.

Longboat, D.M. 2002. "Ian Anderson Continuing Education Program: Indigenous Perspectives on Death and Dying." University of Toronto. <cpd.utoronto.ca/endoflife/Modules/Indigenous%20Perspectives%20on%20Death%20and%20Dying.pdf>.

MacNeil, A., Findlay, B., and Bimman, R. 2021. "Exploring the Use of Virtual Funerals During the COVID-19 Pandemic: A Scoping Review." *Omega-Journal of Death and Dying* 88, 2: 425–448. <doi:10.1177/00302228211045288>.

MacQueen, K. 2015. "Saskatchewan's HIV Epidemic." *Maclean's*, July 22. <macleans.ca/news/canada/saskatchewans-hiv-epidemic>.

Manitoba Law Reform Commission. 1974. *Report on the Statuary Definition of Death*. Issue 16, Province of Manitoba. <manitobalawreform.ca/pubs/pdf/fullreports/16-full_report.pdf>.

Marks, R.B., Moreira, N., O'Connell, K.L., et al. 2024. "Suicide While Locked Up in Texas: Risk Factors for Death by Suicide in Custody." *Journal of Interpersonal Violence* 39, 23/24: 4896–4923. <doi.org/10.1177/08862605241243366>.

Marsh, I. 2016. "Critiquing Contemporary Suicidology." In J. White, I. Marsh, M.J. Kral, and J. Morris (eds.), *Critical Suicidology: Transforming Suicide Research and Prevention for the 21st Century*. UBC Press.

Maté, G. 2015. "Gabor Maté: How to Build a Culture of Good Health." *Yes! Journalism for People Building a Better World*. <yesmagazine.org/issue/good-health/2015/11/16/gabor-mate-how-to-build-a-culture-of-good-health>.

Maxwell, R.J., and Silverman, P. 1989. "Geronticide." In R. Bolton (ed.), *The Context of Culture: Constants and Constraints*. CT: Bergin and Harvey.

Mayer, R.A. 1996. *Embalming History: Theory and Practice*. 2nd edition. Norfolk: CT: Appleton and Lange.

McClatchey, I.S., and King, S. 2015. "The Impact of Death Education on Fear of Death Anxiety Among Human Services Students." *OMEGA-Journal of Death and Dying* 71, 4: 343–361. <doi.10.1177/0030222815572606>.

McGill, K., Bhullar, N., Batterham, P.J., et al. 2023. "Key Issues, Challenges, and Preferred Supports for Those Bereaved by Suicide: Insights from Postvention Experts." *Death Studies* 47, 5: 624–629. <doi.org/10.1080/07481187.2022.2112318>.

McGill University. n.d. "Palliative Social Work." <mcgill.ca/palliativecare/education-and-traiing/interdisciplinary-education-team/palliative-social-work>.

McGill University Health Centre Research Institute. 2023. *How Do We Define Death? Canada Now Has Clear Clinical Guidelines.* <https://rimuhc.ca/-/how-do-we-define-death-canada-now-has-clear-clinical-guidelines>.

Meili, R., and Dutt, M. 2014. "Why We Shouldn't Pay Canadians to Donate Blood." *Globe and Mail,* May 12. <theglobeandmail.com/opinion/why-we-shouldnt-pay-canadians-to-donate-blood/article18123479>.

Memorial Society of BC. n.d. <memorialsocietybc.org>.

Menzies, R.E and Menzies, R.G. 2020. "Death Anxiety, in the Time of COVID-19: Theoretical Explanations and Clinical Implications." June 11. <doi:10.1017/S1754470X20000215>.

Mian, R., and Rejnö, A. 2024. "The Meaning of Culture in Nursing at the End of Life." *BMC Palliative Care* 23, 166. <doi.org/10.1186/s12904-024-01493-5>.

Michalak, E.E., Livingstone, J.D., Maxwell, V., et al. 2014. "Using Theatre to Address Mental Illness Stigma: A Knowledge Translation Study in Bipolar Disorder." *International Journal of Bipolar Disorders* 21, 2: 1. <doi.10.1186/2194-7511-2-1>.

Modern Loss. n.d. "Social Media and Technology." <modernloss.com/tag/social-media-and-technology>.

Monette, E.M. 2021. "Cultural Considerations in Palliative Care Provision: A Scoping Review of Canadian Literature." *Palliative Medicine Reports* 2, 1: 146–156. <doi.org/10.1089/pmr.2020.0124>.

Moody, R. 1975. *Life After Life.* Harper One.

Morgan, J.D. 1986. *Death Education in Canada.* Toronto, ON: Kings College.

Morrisseau, M. 2024. *Opioid Crisis Devastates Indigenous Communities in Canada.* October 3. <yellowheadinstitute.org/wp-content/uploads/2024/10/YI-Brief-Opiod-Crisis-10.24-1-1.pdf>.

Mount, B. 1992. "Volunteer Support Services: A Key Component in Palliative Care." *Journal of Palliative Care* 8, 1: 59–64. <doi.10.1177/082585979200800113>.

Mournet, A.M., Bower, E., and Van Orden, K.A. 2020. "Domains of Functional Impairment and Their Associations with Thwarted Belonging and Perceived Burden in Older Adults." *Clinical Gerontologist* 43, 1: 95–103. <doi.10.1080/07317115.2019.1650406>.

Mroz, E., Bluck, S. and Smith. K. 2020. "Young Adults' Perspectives on Advance Care Planning: Evaluating the Death Over Dinner Initiative." *Death Studies* 46, 2: 381–390. <doi.org/10.1080/07481187.2020.1731015>.

Music Thanatology Association International. n.d. "Music—Thanatology?" <mtai.org>.

Muslim Hope. 2009. "Sects of Islam." <muslimhope.com/SectsofIslam.htm>.

Nan, J.K.M., Pang, K.S.Y., Lam, K.K.F., et al. 2020. "An Expressive-Arts-Based Life-Death Education Program for the Elderly: A Qualitative Study." *Death Studies* 44, 3: 131–40. <doi.10.1080/07481187.2018.1527413>.

Native Women's Association of Canada. 2022. *Misconduct, Missing and Murdered: The Experiences of Anti-Indigenous Racism in Reproductive Healthcare among Indigenous*

Women, Girls, Two-Spirit, Transgender, and Gender Diverse People, and the MMIWG2S+ Genocide. <nwac.ca/assets-knowledge-centre/9-Dec-Racism-in-Healthcare.pdf>.

Nayfeh, A. 2023. "Exploring the Quality and Experience of Care at the End of Life for Patients from Ethnocultural Minority Backgrounds." Dissertation, University of Toronto. <utoronto.scholaris.ca/server/api/core/bitstreams/c7b22645-4ba6-4c45-9ba1-08105dce67d8/content>.

Near Death Foundation. n.d. "Near Death." <www.nderf.org>.

Neilson, S.J., and Reeves, A. 2019. "The Use of a Theatre Workshop in Developing Effective Communication in Paediatric End of Life Care." *Nurse Education in Practice* 36: 7–12. <doi.org/10.1016/j.nepr.2019.02.014>.

Neimeyer, R.A. 1998. "Death Anxiety Research: The State of the Art." *OMEGA—Journal of Death and Dying* 36, 2: 97–120.

Nelson, F. 2017. "What Is Grief?" <virtualhospice.ca/en_US/Main+Site+Navigation/Home/Topics/Topics/Emotional+Health/Moving+through+Grief.aspx>.

Netzley, S.B. 2010. "Visibility That Demystifies: Gays, Gender, and Sex on Television." *Journal of Homosexuality* 57, 8: 968–86.

Nguyen, A., Taylor, R., Chatters, L., et al. 2017. "Extended Family and Friendship Support and Suicidality Among African Americans." *Social Psychiatry and Psychiatric Epidemiology* 52, 3: 299–309. <doi.org/10.1007/s00127-016-1309-1>.

Niu, L., Jia, C., Ma, Z., et al. 2020. "Loneliness, Hopelessness and Suicide in Later Life: A Case-Control Psychological Autopsy Study in Rural China." *Epidemiology and Psychiatric Sciences*, 29, e119. <doi.org/10.1017/S2045796020000335>.

Norris, D., Fancey, P., Power, E., and Ross, P. 2013. "The Critical-Ecological Framework: Advancing Knowledge, Practice, and Policy on Older Adult Abuse." *Journal of Elder Abuse and Neglect* 25, 1: 40–55. <doi.10.1080/08946566.2012.712852>.

Nuland, S., 1995. *How We Die: Reflections on Life's Sufferings*. New York: Knopf.

Obuobi-Donkor, G., Nkire, N., and Agyapong, V.I.O. 2021. "Prevalence of Major Depressive Disorder and Correlates of Thoughts of Death, Suicidal Behaviour, and Death by Suicide in the Geriatric Population—A General Review of Literature." *Behavioral Sciences* 11, 11: 142. <doi.org/10.3390/bs11110142>.

Oliffe, J.L., Kelly, M.T., Montaner, G.G., et al. 2021. "Segmenting or Summing the Parts? A Scoping Review of Male Suicide Research in Canada." *The Canadian Journal of Psychiatry / La Revue canadienne de psychiatrie* 66, 5: 433–445. <doi.org/10.1177/07067437211000631>.

Oo, K., and Paperny, A.M. 2024. "In Canada, Bodies Go Unclaimed as Costs Put Funerals Out of Reach." *Reuters*, May 18. <reuters.com/world/americas/canada-bodies-go-unclaimed-costs-put-funerals-out-reach-2024-05-18>.

Ordal, C.C. 1980. "Death as Seen in Books for Young Children." *Death Education* 4, 3: 223–236.

Orkibi, H. 2011. "Using Intermodal Psychodrama to Personalize Drama Students' Experience: Two Case Illustrations." *The Journal of Aesthetic Education* 45, 2:

Otaegui, A. 2021. "'In Those Times She Was Strong': Singing the Grief Among the Ayoreo from the Paraguayan Chaco." *Death Studies* 45, 1: 9–18. <doi.10.1080/07481187.2020.1851886>.

Oxford English Dictionary. n.d. "Bibliotherapy." <oed.com/search/dictionary/?scope=Entriesandq=bibliotherapy>.

____ 2001. "Memento Mori." <oed.com/dictionary/memento-mori_n?tab=factsheet#13403426>.

Paolino, A., and Lummis, G.W. 2015. "Orff-Schulwerk as a Pedagogical Tool for the Effective Teaching of Italian to Upper Primary Students in Western Australia." *Babel (Parkville, Australia)* 50, 1: 12–23.

Paperny, A.M. 2015. "Canada's Organ Donor Rate Lags Other Countries. How Do You Fix It?" *Global News*, April 24. <globalnews.ca/news/1956708/canadas-rogan-donor-rate-lages-behind-other-countries-how-do-you-fix-it>.

Pappas, S. 2011. "After Death: 8 Burial Alternatives That Are Going Mainstream." *Live Science*, September 9. <livescience.com/15980-death-8-burial-alternatives.html>.

Parachute. 2016. "The Canadian Association for Suicide Prevention (CASP)." October 24. <https://phecanada.ca/teaching-tools/teach-resiliency/resources/canadian-association-for-suicide-prevention-casp>.

Park, J. 2021. "Mortality Among First Nations People, 2006 to 2016." *Health Reports* 32, 10. <doi.org/10.25318/82-003-x202101000001-eng>.

Parkes, C.M. 1975. "Determinants of Outcomes Following Bereavement." *Omega* 6, 4: 303–323.

———. 1987. *Recovery from Bereavement*. New York: Basic Books.

———. 1993. "Bereavement as a Psychosocial Transition: Processes of Adaptation to Change." In M. Stroebe, W. Stroebe and Hanson (eds.), *Handbook of Bereavement Theory, Research and Intervention*. New York: Cambridge University Press.

Parkes, C.M., and Young, B. 2015. *Death and Bereavement Across Cultures*. Second edition. London, England: Routledge.

Parry, K.J., Hicken, B.L., Chen, W., et al. 2023. "Impact of Moral Injury and Posttraumatic Stress Disorder on Health Care Utilization and Suicidality in Rural and Urban Veterans." *Journal of Traumatic Stress* 36, 1: 117–128. <doi.org/10.1002/jts.22889>.

Pastrana, T., De Lima, L., Pettus, K. et al. 2021. "The Impact of COVID-19 on Palliative Care Workers Across the World: A Qualitative Analysis of Responses to Open-Ended Questions." *Palliative and Supportive Care*, 19, 2 (April). Published online by Cambridge University Press, March 2: 187–192. <doi:10.1017/S1478951521000298>.

Pentaris, P., and Yerosimou, M. 2020. "The Functional Role of Music in Communicating Death through/in YouTube Videos." *Journal of Education Culture and Society* 5: 206–217. <doi.10.15503/jecs20141.206.217>.

Pernick, M.S. 1988. "Back from the Grave: Reocurring Controversies over Defining and Diagnosing Death in History." In Richard M Zaner (ed.), *Death Beyond Whole Brain Criteria*. New York: Kluner Academic Publishers.

Petracek, H. 2024. "N.S. Woman Opens up About Her Decision to Die and Having a 'Living Funeral.'" Global News, October 9. <globalnews.ca/news/10802641/medically-assisted-death-nova-scotia-MAID/>.

Pfaffenwimmer, B. 2014. "Bibliodrama—Ein Handlungsraum Zur Veränderung von Perfekt-Spirituellen Rollenerwartungen." *Zeitschrift Für Psychodrama Und Soziometrie* 13, 1: 83–93.

Pharr, J.R., and Batra, K. 2024. "Social–Ecological Determinants of Suicidal Ideation Among Sexual and Gender Minority Adults: A Cross-Sectional Study in the United States." *Healthcare* 12, 24: 2540. <doi.org/10.3390/healthcare12242540>.

Phillips, D. 2024. "Legislative Summary of Bill C-62: An Act to Amend an Act to Amend the Criminal Code (Medical Assistance in Dying)." No. 2. Preliminary Version Unedited, Library of Parliament. <lop.parl.ca/sites/PublicWebsite/default/en_CA/ResearchPublications/LegislativeSummaries/441C62E#:~:text=1%20The%20bill%20was%20passed,2024%20to%2017%20March%202027.>.

Phillips, N. 2018. "Skin and Bones: The Decimation of the Plains Buffalo." *Mount Royal Undergraduate Humanities Review (MRUHR)* 5. <mrujs.mtroyal.ca/index.php/mruhr/article/view/463>.

Pine, V.R. 1975. *Caretakers of the Dead: The American Funeral Director.* New York: Lexington.

Power, T.L., and Smith, S.M. 2008. "Predictors of Death and Self Mortality: An Atlantic Canadian Perspective." *Death Studies* 32, 3: 253–271. <doi.10.1080/07481180701880935>.

Principe de Joyce. 2024. "Joyce's Principle." <principedejoyce.com/en/index>.

Pringle, R. 2017. "3D Printed 'Third Thumb' a Handy Extra Digit with Bluetooth Connection." *CBC News,* July 24. <cbc.ca/news/technology/third-thumb-prosthetic-1.4218622>.

Prout, W. 2024. "What Is a Drive Thru Funeral." Titan Caskets, April 16. <titancasket.com/blogs/funeral-guides-and-more/why-and-where-do-drive-thru-funerals-exist?srsltid=AfmBOorYBgnTYFu0OEv9JyDM70JHGapAMWuN85MWPeOFhYrgvyXRdL2b>.

Public Health Agency of Canada. 2018. *Key Health Inequalities in Canada: A National Portrait.* Ottawa: Public Health Agency of Canada. <canada.ca/content/dam/phac-aspc/documents/services/publications/science-research/key-health-inequalities-canada-national-portrait-executive-summary/hir-full-report-eng.pdf>.

____ 2024a. "Statement from the Minister of Mental Health and Addictions and Associate Minister of Health on the Overdose Crisis." March 27. <canada.ca/en/public-health/news/2024/03/statement-from-the-minister-of-mental-health-and-addictions-and-associate-minister-of-health-on-the-overdose-crisis.html>.

____ 2024b. "Suicide in Canada." September 16. <canada.ca/en/public-health/services/suicide-prevention/suicide-canada.html>.

____ 2024c. "The National Suicide Prevention Action Plan 2024–2027." <publications.gc.ca/site/eng/9.937473/publication.html?wbdisable=true>.

Public Health Officer of Canada. 2016. *Health Status of Canadians 2016, Report of the Chief Public Health Officer, What Is Influencing Our Health?* <canada.ca/en/public-health/corporate/publications/chief-public-health-officer-reports-state-public-health-canada/2016-health-status-canadians.html>.

Rando, T. 1984. *Grief, Dying and Death.* Champaign, IL: Research Press.

____ 1986a. *Loss and Anticipatory Grief.* MA: Lexington Books.

____ 1986b. *Parental Loss of a Child.* Champaign, IL: Research Press.

____ 1988. *How to Go on Living when Someone You Love Dies.* New York: Bantam.

____ 1993. *Treatment of Complicated Mourning.* Champaign, IL: Research Press.

Rankanen, M. 2016. "Clients' Experiences of the Impacts of an Experiential Art Therapy Group." *The Arts in Psychotherapy* 50: 101–10. <doi.org/10.1016/j.aip.2016.06.002>.

Rawlinson, R. 2012. "A Brief History of the Undertaker," *The Funeral Guide,* August 3. <goodfuneralguide.co.uk/2012/08/a-brief-history-of-undertakers>.

Razack, S., 2015. *Dying from Improvement: Inquests and Inquiries into Indigenous Deaths in Custody.* University of Toronto Press.

Reidpath, D.D., and Allotey, P. 2003. "Infant Mortality Rate as an Indicator of Population Health." *Journal of Epidemiology and Community Health* 57, 5: 344–346.

Riemer, Rabbi J. n.d. "Writing and Reading Ethical Wills: On the Jewish Custom of Leaving a Written Spiritual Legacy for One's Children." *My Jewish Learning.* <myjewishlearning.com/article/writing-and-reading-ethical-wills>.

Rettner, R. 2014. "How Long Will a Brain-Dead-Person's Body Keep Working?" January 3. <huffingtonpost.com/2014/01/03/brain-dead-body-alive_n_4537750.html>.

Reynolds, A. 2021. "One of Stephen Sondheim's Last Interviews: Reporter's Notebook" <https://abcnews.go.com/Entertainment/stephen-sondheims-interviews-reporters-notebook/story?id=81501990&utm_source=chatgpt.com>.

Richardson, N.M., and Lamson, A.L. 2022. "Understanding Moral Injury: Military-Related Injuries of the Mind, Body, and Soul." *Spirituality in Clinical Practice* 9, 3: 145–158. <doi.org/10.1037/scp0000270>.

Richardson, R., Connell, T., Foster, M., et al. 2024. "Risk and Protective Factors of Self-Harm and Suicidality in Adolescents: An Umbrella Review with Meta-Analysis." *Journal of Youth and Adolescence* 53, 6: 1301–1322. <doi.10.1007/s10964-024-01969-w>.

Richardson, S.C., and Gunn, L.H. 2024. "Factors Associated with Suicide Risk Behavior Outcomes Among Black Middle School Adolescents." *Journal of the American Academy of Child and Adolescent Psychiatry* 63, 12: 1215–1224. <doi.org/10.1016/j.jaac.2024.03.019>.

Riddle, K., and Martins, N. 2022. "A Content Analysis of American Primetime Television: A 20-Year Update of the National Television." *Journal of Communication* 72, 1: 33–58. <doi.org/10.1093/joc/jqab043>.

Rieger, D., and Hofer, M. 2017. "How Movies Can Ease the Fear of Death: The Survival or Death of the Protagonists in Meaningful Movies." *Mass Communication and Society* 20, 5: 710–733. <doi.org/10.1080/15205436.2017.1300666>.

Rinpoche, S. 1993. *The Tibetan Book of The Dead*. San Francisco: Harper.

Roberts, M. 2025. How Much Does a Funeral Cost in Canada in 2025? | MyChoice January 15. <www.mychoice.ca/blog/how-much-does-funeral-cost-canada/>.

Robson, P., and Walter, T. 2013. "Hierarchies of Loss: A Critique of Disenfranchised Grief." *OMEGA—Journal of Death and Dying* 66, 2: 97–119.

Ronconi, L., Biancalani, G., Medesi, G.A., et al. 2023. "Death Education for Palliative Psychology: The Impact of a Death Education Course for Italian University Students." *Behavioral Sciences* 13, 2: 182. <doi.org/10.3390/bs13020182>.

Rosenblatt, P.C. 2008. "Grief Across Cultures: A Review and Research Agenda." In M.S. Stroebe, R.O. Hansson, H. Schut, and W. Stroebe (eds.), *Handbook of Bereavement Research and Practice: Advances in Theory and Intervention*. American Psychological Association. <doi.org/10.1037/14498-000>.

Rossiter, K., Kontos, P., Colantonio, A., et al. 2008. "Staging Data: Theatre as a Tool for Analysis and Knowledge Transfer in Health Research." *Social Science and Medicine* 66, 1: 130–146.

Rousu, M.C. 2018. "Using Show Tunes to Teach about Free (and Not-so-Free) Markets." *Journal of Private Enterprise* 33, 4: 111–128.

Rowan, M., Poole, N., Shea, B., et al. 2014. "Cultural Interventions to Treat Addictions in Indigenous Populations: Findings from a Scoping Study." *Substance Abuse Treatment, Prevention, and Policy* 9: 34. <doi.186/1747-597X-9-34>.

Rowlinson, R. 2012. "A Brief History of the Undertaker." *The Good Funeral Guide*, August 3. <goodfuneralguide.co.uk/2012/08/a-brief-history-of-undertakers>.

Roy, J., and Marcellus, S. 2019. "Homicide in Canada 2018." Statistics Canada. <www150.statcan.gc.ca/n1/pub/85-002-x/2019001/article/00016-eng.htm>.

Royal Canadian Mounted Police. n.d. "What Is Fentanyl?" <rcmp-grc.gc.ca/en/what-is-fentanyl>.

Ruby, J. 1988 "Portraying the Dead." *Omega*, 19, 1: 1–20.

Rudd, M.D. 2006. "Fluid Vulnerability Theory: A Cognitive Approach to Understanding the Process of Acute and Chronic Suicide Risk." In T.E. Ellis (ed.), *Cognition and Suicide: Theory, Research, and Therapy*. American Psychological Association. <doi.org/10.1037/11377-016>.

Rugo-Cook, K.F., Kerig, P.K., Crowell, S.E., and Bryan, C.J. 2021. "Fluid Vulnerability Theory as a Framework for Understanding the Association Between Posttraumatic

Stress Disorder and Suicide: A Narrative Review." *Journal of Traumatic Stress* 34, 6: 1080–1098. <doi.org/10.1002/jts.22782>.

Rusch, R., Greenman, J., Scanlon, C., et al. 2020. "Bibliotherapy and Bereavement: Harnessing the Power of Reading to Enhance Family Coping in Pediatric Palliative Care." *Journal of Social Work in End-of-Life and Palliative Care* 16, 2: 85–98. <doi.10.1080/15524256.2020.1745728>.

Russell, C.A., and Buhrau, D. 2015. "The Role of Television Viewing and Direct Experience in Predicting Adolescents' Beliefs about the Health Risks of Fast-Food Consumption." *Appetite* 92: 200–206. <doi.org/10.1016/j.appet.2015.05.023>.

Sadler, N., Pedlar, D., and Ursano, R. 2024. "Suicide in Military and Veteran Populations: A View Across the Five Eyes Nations." *Psychiatry: Interpersonal and Biological Processes* 87, 2: 161–164. <doi.org/10.1080/00332747.2024.2306794>.

Sakashita, T., and Oyama, H. 2019. "Developing a Hypothetical Model for Suicide Progression in Older Adults with Universal, Selective, and Indicated Prevention Strategies." *Frontiers in Psychiatry* 10. <doi.org/10.3389/fpsyt.2019.00161>.

Sathya, C. 2014. "Organ Donation After Cardiac Death: More Organ Donations Possible if Brain Death Not the Only Option." *CBC News*, March 18. <cbc.ca/news/health/organ-donation-after-death-1.2577269>.

Saunders, C. 1978. "Hospice Care." *American Journal of Medicine* 65, 5: 726–728. <doi.org/10.1016/0002-9343(78)90789-1>.

Saunders, M.G. 1974. "Determining the Presence of Death: A Medical, Legal and Ethical Problem." *Manitoba Law Journal* 2: 327–329.

Scheper-Hughes, N. 2002. "The Ends of the Body: Commodity Fetishism and the Global Traffic in Organs." *SAIS Review* 22, 1: 61–80.

―――― 2014. "Human Traffic: Exposing the Brutal Organ Trade." *New Internationalist*, May 1. <newint.org/features/2014/05/01/organ-trafficking-keynote>.

Schiappa, E., Gregg, P.B., and Hewes, D.E. 2004. "Can a Television Series Change Attitudes About Death? A Study of College Students and *Six Feet Under*." *Death Studies* 28, 5: 459–474. <https://pubmed.ncbi.nlm.nih.gov/15152651>.

Schmutte, T., Olfson, M., Maust, D.T., et al. 2022. "Suicide Risk in First Year After Dementia Diagnosis in Older Adults." *Alzheimer's and Dementia: The Journal of the Alzheimer's Association* 18, 2: 262–271. <doi.10.1002/alz.12390>.

Schoop, T. 1974. *Won't You Join the Dance? — A Dancer's Essay into the Treatment of Psychosis*. National Press.

Schultz, N.W., and Huet, L.M. 2001. "Sensational! Violent! Popular! Death in American Movies." *OMEGA—Journal of Death and Dying* 42, 2: 137–149. <www.sci-hub.in/10.2190/6GDX-4W40-5B94-MX0G>.

Scott, R., and Howlett, S. 2018. *The Changing Face of Volunteering in Palliative Care: An International Perspective*. Oxford, UK, Oxford University Press.

Selby, D., Chan, B., and Nolan, A. 2021. "Characteristics of Older Adults Accessing Medical Assistance in Dying (MAID): A Descriptive Study." *Canadian Geriatrics Journal* 24, 4. <doi:10.5770/cgj.24.520>.

Sellick, S., Charles, K., Dagsvik, J., and Kelley, M. 1996. "Palliative Care Provider's Perspectives on Service and Education Needs." *Journal of Palliative Care* 12, 2: 34–38.

Seneca, L.A. C.4B.C.-65 A.D. Hercules (Etaeus, 930). Cited in James Stevens Curl, 1993, *A Celebration of Death*. London: B.T. Basford.

Shakespeare, W. 1958. "The Complete Works, Macbeth." Act IV, Scene III, p. 939. London: Hamlyn Group.

Shamrock, M. 1997. "Orff-Schulwerk: An Integrated Foundation: This Article on the Methodologies and Practices of Orff-Schulwerk." *Music Educators Journal* 83, 6: 41–44. <doi.org/10.2307/3399024>.

Shaver, A. 1990. *Teen Suicide*. Ottawa: Library of Parliament Research Branch. <publications.gc.ca/Pilot/LoPBdP/BP/bp236-e.htm>.

Shea, J.B. 2003. "Non-Heart-Beating Organ Donation." <https://www.lifeissues.net/writers/she/she_21nonheartbeating.html>.

Shemie, S.D., Wilson, L.C., Hornby, L., et al. 2023. "A Brain-Based Definition of Death and Criteria for Its Determination After Arrest of Circulation or Neurologic Function in Canada: A 2023 Clinical Practice Guideline." *Canadian Journal of Anesthesia* 70, 4: 483–557. <doi.org/10.1007/s12630-023-02431-4>.

Sherman, M.D., Larsen, J.L., and Levy, R. 2021. "Shining a Spotlight on Issues of Mental Health" in Musical Theater and Ways Psychologists Can Help: Perspectives of Theater Professionals." *Professional Psychology: Research and Practice* 52, 6: 579–587. <doi.org/10.1037/pro0000393>.

Sherry, W., and Tremblay, B. 2025. "Organ and Tissue Donation FAQs." Canadian Blood Services. <professionaleducation.blood.ca/en/organs-and-tissues/resources/organ-tissue-donation-faqs-multiple-language-brochures>.

Shimazono, Y. 2007. "The State of the International Organ Trade: A Provisional Picture Based on Integration of Available Information." *Bulletin of the World Health Organization* 85, 12: 955–962. <iris.who.int/handle/10665/269908>.

Shneidman, E.S. 1993. *Suicide as Psychache: A Clinical Approach to Self-Destructive Behavior*. NJ, Aronson Publishers.

Silverman, G.S. 2021. "Saying Kaddish: Meaning-Making and Continuing Bonds in American Jewish Mourning Ritual." *Death Studies* 45, 1: 19–28. <doi.org/10.1080/07481187.2020.1851887>.

Silverman, G.S., Baroiller, A., and Hemer, S.R. 2021. "Culture and Grief: Ethnographic Perspectives on Ritual, Relationships, and Remembering." *Death Studies* 45, 1: 1–8. <doi.org/10.1080/07481187.2020.1851885>.

Simon, G. 2021. "Should We Hide the Eyes of the Dead? Continuing Bonds in Kanaké, Paicî-Camuki Country." *Death Studies* 45, 1: 29–39. <doi.org/10.1080/07481187.2020.1851888>.

Skelly, S. 2024. "AI Immortality: How Deathbots Are Changing the Way We Grieve." *The Lighthouse*. McQuarrie University. <lighthouse.mq.edu.au/article/june-2024/can-deathbots-affect-the-way-we-experience-grief>.

Skye, E.P., Wagenschutz, H., Steiger, J.A., and Kumagai, A.K. 2014. "Use of Interactive Theater and Role Play to Develop Medical Students' Skills in Breaking Bad News." *Journal of Cancer Education* 29, 4: 704–708. <doi.10.1007/s13187-014-0641-y>.

Smith, M., Cui, R., Odom, J.V., et al. 2020. "Giving Support and Suicidal Ideation in Older Adults with Vision-Related Diagnoses." *Clinical Gerontologist* 43, 1: 17–23. <doi.org/10.1080/07317115.2019.1659465>.

Smith, S. 2025. "Christopher Sakezles's Synthetic Humans Are the Future of Medical Testing and Training." *Startup Savant*, August 8. <startupsavant.com/news/christopher-sakezles>.

Sokolovsky, J. (ed.). 1997. *Cultural Context of Aging: World Wide Perspectives*. CT: Bergin and Garvey.

Solomon R. Guggenheim Museum. <guggenheim.org/artwork/17143>.

Sourkes, B. 1995. *Armfuls of Time: The Psychological Experiences of the Child with a Life-Threatening Illness*. Pittsburgh: University of Pittsburgh Press.

_____ 1996. "The Broken Heart: Anticipatory Grief in the Child Facing Death." *Journal of Palliative Care* 12, 3: 56–59.

_____ 2018. "Children's Experience of Symptoms: Narratives through Words and Images." *Children* 5, 4: 53.

Sourkes, B., Frankel, L., Brown, M., et al. 2005. "Food, Toys and Love: Paediatric Palliative Care." *Current Problems in Pediatrics and Adolescent Health Care* 35, 9: 350–385.

South, A.L., and Elton, J. 2017. "Contradictions and Promise for End-of-Life Communication among Family and Friends: Death over Dinner Conversations." *Behavioral Sciences* 7, 20: 24. <doi:10.3390/bs7020024>.

South, A.L., Elton, J., and Lietzenmayer, A.M. 2020. "Communicating Death with Humor: Humor Types and Functions in Death Over Dinner Conversations." *Death Studies* 46, 4: 851–860. <doi.10.1080/07481187.2020.1716883.

Spade, K. 2016. "When I Die, Recompose Me." March. <ted.com/talks/katrina_spade_when_i_die_recompose_me>.

Spafford, S.G., Silverman, M.M., and Gutierrez, P.M. 2024. "What Is Known About Suicide Prevention Gatekeeper Training and Directions for Future Research." *Suicide and Life-Threatening Behavior* 55, 1. <doi.org/10.1111/sltb.13130>.

Spafford, S.G., McWhirter Boisen, M.R., Tanner-Smith, E.E., et al. 2024. "The Effects of Suicide Prevention Gatekeeper Training on Behavioral Intention and Intervention Behavior: A Systematic Review and Meta-Analysis." *Prevention Science* 25, 6: 978–988. <doi.org/10.1007/s11121-024-01710-w>.

Stack, S. 2002. "Opera Subculture and Suicide for Honor." *Death Studies* 26, 5: 431–437.

Staples, L.O. and Gonzalez, C.O. 2023. *Aanjikiing/Changing Worlds: Anishinaabe Traditional Funeral*. Minnesota Historical Society Press.

Statista. 2024. "Number of Deaths in Canada Between 2023 and 2024, by Age Group." December. <statista.com/statistics/444903/number-of-deaths-in-canada-by-age-group>.

_____ 2025a. "Number of Opioid Overdose Deaths in Canada in 2023, by Province." March 27. <statista.com/statistics/812260/number-of-deaths-from-opioid-overdose-canada-province>.

_____ 2025b. "Distribution of the Leading Causes of Death in Canada in 2023." June 25. <statista.com/statistics/437880/proportion-of-deaths-in-canada-by-disease>.

Statistics Canada. 2016. "Aboriginal Peoples: Fact Sheet for Canada." <www150.statcan.gc.ca/n1/pub/89-656-x/89-656-x2015001-eng.htm>.

_____ 2018. "Estimates of the Components of Demographic Growth, Annual." <www150.statcan.gc.ca/t1/tbl1/en/tv.action?pid=1710000801>.

_____ 2022. "The Canadian Census: A Rich Portrait of the Country's Religious and Ethnocultural Diversity." October 26. <www150.statcan.gc.ca/n1/daily-quotidien/221026/dq221026b-eng.htm>.

_____ 2023. *Top 10 Leading Causes of Death*. <www150.statcan.gc.ca/n1/daily-quotidien/250305/t001a-eng.htm>.

_____ 2024. "Health Care Access and Experiences Among Indigenous people." *The Daily*. <www150.statcan.gc.ca/n1/daily-quotidien/241104/dq241104a-eng.pdf>.

_____ 2025. "Number of Deaths in Canada from 2001 to 2024." <statista.com/statistics/443061/number-of-deaths-in-canada/>.

_____ 2025. Provisional Deaths in Canada Dashboard. <www150.statcan.gc.ca/n1/en/catalogue/71-607-X2024004>.

Steele, R., Davies, B., Collins, J., and Cook, K. 2005. "End of Life Care in a Children's Hospice Program." *Journal of Palliative Care* 12, 1.

Steeves, S. 2023. "N.B. Death Doula Helps Families Open Up About End-of-Life Discussions." *Global News*, March 8. <globalnews.ca/news/9536864/n-b-death-doula-helps-families-open-up-about-end-of-life-discussions>.

Steffens, B. 2019. *Thinking Critically: Teen Suicide*. San Diego, CA: Reference Point Press.

Steinhauer D., and Lamouche J. 2015 "Miyo Pimâtisiwin 'A Good Path': Indigenous Knowledges, Languages, and Traditions in Education and Health." In M. Greenwood, S. de Leeuw, N. Lindsay, and C. Reading (eds.), *Determinants of Indigenous Peoples' Health in Canada: Beyond the Social*. Toronto: Canadian Scholars' Press.

Stephen Lewis Foundation. 2018. "Grandmothers to Grandmothers Campaign." <grandmotherscampaign.org>.

Stewart, C. 1999. "Syncretism and Its Synonyms: Reflections on Cultural Mixture." *Diacritics* 29, 3: 40–62.

Stroebe, M. 2018. "The Poetry of Grief: Beyond Scientific Portrayal." *OMEGA—Journal of Death and Dying* 78, 1: 67–96.

Suzuki, D. 1989. "Euthanasia." *The Nature of Things*. CBC, October 17.

Swidler, A. 1986. "Culture in Action: Symbols and Strategies." *American Sociological Review* 51, 2: 273–286.

Szostak, M. 2022. "Revival of Tufts Musical Theatre Continues with 'Spring Awakening.'" *Tufts Daily*. <tuftsdaily.com/article/2022/03/weekender-revival-of-tufts-musical-theater-continues-with-spring-awakening>.

Tamor, G. 2005. *Growing Up Without You: Young People Growing Up with Loss and Its Effects*. London: Jessica Kingsley Publishers.

Tareen, A. 2024. "Disclosure Practices in Muslim Patients and the Impact on End-of-Life Care: A Narrative Review." *American Journal of Hospice and Palliative Medicine* 30, 1: 10–20. <doi.org/10.1177/10499091241303684>.

Tateo, L. 2023. "Cultural Mediation of Grief: The Role of Aesthetic Experience." *Culture & Psychology* 29, 3. <doi.org/10.1177/1354067X221145901>.

Testoni, I., Biancalani, G., Ronconi, L., and Varani, S. 2021. "Let's Start with the End: Bibliodrama in an Italian Death Education Course on Managing Fear of Death, Fantasy-Proneness, and Alexithymia with a Mixed-Method Analysis." *OMEGA—Journal of Death and Dying* 83, 4: 729–579. <doi.10.1177/0030222819863613>.

Testoni, I., Cichellero, S., Kirk, K., et al. 2019. "When Death Enters the Theater of Psychodrama: Perspectives and Strategies of Psychodramatists." *Journal of Loss and Trauma* 24, 5–6: 516–532. <doi.org/10.1080/15325024.2018.1548996>.

Testoni, I., Iacona, E., Fusina, S., et al. 2018. "'Before I Die I Want to … ': An Experience of Death Education among University Students of Social Service and Psychology." *Health Psychology Open* 5, 2: 1–9. <doi.10.1177/2055102918809759>.

Testoni, I., Ronconi, L. Biancalani, G., et al. 2021. "My Future: Psychodrama and Meditation to Improve Well-Being Through the Elaboration of Traumatic Loss Among Italian High School Students." *Frontiers in Psychology* 11: 544661. <doi.org/10.3389/fpsyg.2020.544661>.

Testoni, I., Ronconi, L., Palazzo, L., et al. 2018. "Psychodrama and Moviemaking in a Death Education Course to Work Through a Case of Suicide Among High School Students in Italy." *Frontiers in Psychology* 10, 9: 441. <doi.10.3389/fpsyg.2018.00441>.

Testoni, I., Tronca, E., Biancalani, G., et al. 2020. "Beyond the Wall: Death Education at Middle School as Suicide Prevention." *International Journal of Environmental Research and Public Health* 17, 7: 1–12. <doi.10.3390/ijerph17072398>.

Thatcher, C. 2022. "In Dialogue: How Writing to the Dead and the Living Can Increase Self-Awareness in Those Bereaved by Addiction." *OMEGA—Journal of Death and Dying* 86, 2: 434–456. <doi.0.1177/0030222820976277>.

Thomas, D. 2023. "'A Show About Death Brought Back to Life': Beetlejuice Arrives at Denver Center for the Performing Arts." September 5. <cbsnews.com/colorado/news/colorado-beetlejuice-arrives-denver-center-performing-arts>.

Tipper, S. 1989. "Cremation Is an Opportunity for Funeral Directors." *Canadian Funeral News*, August 10–11.

Topel, F. 2021. "Ben Platt: No Way to Anticipate Emotional Reaction to 'Evan Hansen.'" *United Press International*, September 24. <upi.com/Entertainment_News/Movies/2021/09/24/Ben-Platt-Dear-Evan-Hansen/2261632416294>.

Townes, C. 2023. "The Body After Death: A Brief Guide to Disposition Options." *Memento Therapy*, December 4. <mementotherapy.com/post/the-body-after-death-a-brief-guide-to-disposition-options#:~:text=Choosing%20a%20body%20disposition%20option,respect%20you%20and%20your%20values.>.

Trabor, M. 1992. "Death and the Media: An Introduction." *Media Development* 4. 3-5.

Trillium Gift of Life Network. n.d. <giftoflife.on.ca/en>.

Tsiris, G., Tasker, M., Lawson, V., et al. 2012. "Music, Arts and Death Education—The St Christopher's Health Promotion Project." *BMJ Supportive and Palliative Care* 2: A113. </doi.org/10.1136/bmjspcare-2012-000196.332.

Twist, L. 2022. *Human Organ Trafficking Around the World*. <https://storymaps.arcgis.com/stories/b24a8c9acb564467a97fc705d4448ec6>.

United Nations. 2024. *World Drug Report 2024*. <unodc.org/unodc/data-and-analysis/world-drug-report-2024.html>.

US Department of Health and Human Services. n.d. "What Can Be Donated?" <organdonor.gov/about/what.html>.

Valley Hospice Foundation. <valleyhospice.ca>.

Van Orden, K.A., and Conwell, Y. 2016. "Issues in Research on Aging and Suicide." *Aging and Mental Health* 20, 2: 240–251. <doi.org/10.1080/13607863.2015.1065791>.

Van Orden, K.A., Witte, T.K., Cukrowicz, K.C., et al. 2010. "The Interpersonal Theory of Suicide." *Psychological Review* 117, 2: 575–600. <doi.org/10.1037/a0018697>.

Vancouver Hospice Palliative Care Program. n.d. "Bereavement Walking Group." <vancouverhospice.org/services/grief-support/bereavement-walking-group/>.

Vibes, J. 2016. "Alan Rickman Was Also an Activist Who Once Said That Actors Are Agents of Change." *True Activist*, January 14. <trueactivist.com/alan-rickman-was-also-an-activist-who-once-said-that-actors-are-agents-of-change/?s=rickman>.

Vincent, D., Moore, H., Miller, J., and Grassau, P. 2024. "Quality of Care During the COVID-19 Pandemic: A Qualitative Exploration of Bereavement Caregivers Experiences at a Hospice Residence." *Journal of Palliative Medicine* 27, 9: 1156–1162. <doi.10.1089/jpm.2023.0469>.

Wachowski, W., and Sullivan, K. 2021. *Metonymies and Metaphors for Death Around the World*, 1st ed. New York: Routledge.

Walker, R.S. 2017. "After Suicide: Coming Together in Kindness and Support." *Death Studies* 41, 10: 635–638. <doi.10.1080/07481187.2017.1335549>.

Walker, S. 2019. "The Persistence of Place: Hunter-Gatherer Mortuary Practices and Land-Use in the Trent Valley, Ontario." *Journal of Anthropological Archaeology* 54: 133–148. <doi.org/10.1016/j.jaa.2019.03.002>.

Wallace, E.R., O'Neill, S., and Lagdon, S. 2024. "Risk and Protective Factors for Suicidality Among Lesbian, Gay, Bisexual, Transgender, and Queer (LGBTQ2+) Young People, from Ecological Model: A Scoping Review." *Journal of Adolescence* 96, 5: 897–924. <doi.org/10.1002/jad.12308>.

Walter, T. 1991. "Modern Death: Taboo or Not Taboo?" *Sociology (Oxford)* 25, 2: 293–310.

―――― 1996. "A New Model of Grief: Bereavement and Biography." *Mortality* 1, 1: 7–25.

―――― 1994-95. "Natural Death and the Noble Savage." *Omega—Journal of Death and Dying* 30, 4: 237–248.

―――― 2003. "Historical and Cultural Variations on the Good Death." *BMJ* 26, 327: 218–20. <doi.org/10.1136/bmj.327.7408.218>.

―――― 2012a. "How People Who Are Dying or Mourning Engage with the Arts." *Music and Arts in Action* 4, 1: 73–98.

―――― 2012b. "Why Different Countries Manage Death Differently: A Comparative Analysis of Modern Urban Societies1: Why Different Countries Manage Death Differently." *The British Journal of Sociology* 63, 1: 123–145.

Ware, B. 2019. *The Top Five Regrets of the Dying: A Life Transformed by the Dearly Departing*. Carlsbad, CA: Hay House, Inc.

Watersong, A. 2008. "The Magic of Surplus Reality." Thesis for Australian and New Zealand Psychodrama Association. <aanzpa.org/wp-content/uploads/theses/118.pdf>.

Watters, H. 2015. "Nova Scotia Funeral Homes Increasingly Run by Women 80% of NSCC Funeral Directors Are Women." *CBC News* April 17. <cbc.ca/news/canada/nova-scotia/nova-scotia-funeral0homes-increasingly-run-by-women-1.3036818>.

Westefeld, J.S., Casper, D., Galligan, P., et al. 2015. "Suicide and Older Adults: Risk Factors and Recommendations." *Journal of Loss and Trauma* 20, 6: 491–508. <doi:10.1080/15 325024.2014.949154>.

Whalley Hammell, K.R. 2020. *Engagement in Living: Critical Perspectives on Occupation, Rights, and Wellbeing*. Ottawa, ON: CAOT.

Whipple, V. 2006. *Lesbian Widows: Invisible Grief*. New York: Harrington Press.

White, J. 2017. "What Can Critical Suicidology Do?" *Death Studies* 41, 8: 472–480. <doi.org/10.1080/07481187.2017.1332901>.

Woodgate, R.L. 2006. "Living in a World Without Closure: Reality in Parents Who Have Experienced the Death of a Child." *Journal of Palliative Care* 22, 2: 75–82.

Worden, J.W. 2008. *Grief Counselling and Grief Therapy: A Handbook for the Mental Health Practitioner*, 4th edition. New York: Springer.

World Health Organization. n.d. "WHO Definition of Palliative Care." <who.int/cancer/palliative/definition/en>.

―――― n.d. "COVID-19 Cases, World." <data.who.int/dashboards/covid19/cases?n=c>.

―――― 2020a. "Palliative Care Key Facts." August 5. <who.int/news-room/fact-sheets/detail/palliative-care>.

―――― 2020b. International Standards for the Treatment of Drug Use Disorders, Revised Edition Incorporating Results of Field-Testing." March 31. <who.int/publications/i/item/international-standards-for-the-treatment-of-drug-use-disorders>.

―――― 2023. *Addressing Human Trafficking Through Health Systems: A Scoping Review* <www.who.int/europe/publications/i/item/9789289058827>.

―――― 2024a. "HIV/AIDS data." <who.int/data/gho/data/themes/hiv-aids>.

―――― 2024b. "Harms of World Drug Problems Continue to Mount amid Expansions in Drug Use and Markets." June 26. <unodc.org/unodc/en/press/releases/2024/June/unodc-world-drug-report-2024_-harms-of-world-drug-problem-continue-to-mount-amid-expansions-in-drug-use-and-markets.html>.

―――― 2025. *World Health Statistics 2025: Monitoring Health for the SDGs, Sustainable Development Goals*. <https://www.who.int/publications/i/item/9789240110496>.

World Population Review. 2025. "Countries Where Euthanasia Is Legal 2025?" <worldpopulationreview.com/country-rankings/where-is-euthanasia-legal>.

Worldwide Hospice Palliative Care Alliance. <thewhpca.org>.

Youth Music. 2024. "Sound of the Next Generation 2024." <youthmusic.org.uk/sound-of-the-next-generation-2024>.

Zhang, J. 2019. "The Strain Theory of Suicide." *Journal of Pacific Rim Psychology* January. <https://doi.org/10.1017/prp.2019.19>.

INDEX

abandonment, 2, 19
Aboriginal; *see* Indigenous Peoples
abuse and addiction, 9, 21, 30, 37, 96, 100–105, 128, 138, 139, 143, 173, 182, 188, 193, 211
   of alcohol, 9, 30
   of drugs, 9, 21, 30, 37, 95, 96, 100, 104, 105, 115, 138
   Opioid Use Disorder (OUD), 103
activities, 3, 35, 50, 77, 93, 96, 173, 174, 177, 184, 185, 192, 194
adaptation, 66, 120, 131, 135, 178
adults, 2, 38, 103, 163, 169, 173, 176–78, 185, 195, 202, 204
advisors, 9, 78, 130
advocacy, 44, 69, 86, 157, 162, 197, 198
Afghanistan, 55
Africa, 29, 42, 117, 217
after-death arrangements, 21, 37, 41, 46
   alternative forms of body disposal, 149
   Aquamation, 150
   Capsula Mundi, 149
   Eternal Reefs, 149, 150
   mummification, 39, 41, 42, 132
   mushroom-based coffin, 101, 144, 150
   plastination, 26
   recomposition, 146
   Resomation, 150
   space burials, 144, 150
   Celestis Memorial Spaceflights, 150
   suspended animation, 43
   embalming, 13, 39–41, 89, 144, 146, 152, 154–56
   post-deathcare, 3
afterlife, 45, 109, 133, 158–60, 216
   circle of life, 42, 133
   eternity, 45, 110, 159
   life everlasting, 91, 212
   heaven, 15, 37, 42, 45, 52, 86, 109, 159, 196

   hell, 15, 19, 37, 45, 52, 94, 128
   reincarnation, 42, 52, 108, 196, 217
   spirits, 94, 101, 109, 114, 132–34, 217
aging, 4, 27, 76, 80, 103, 204, 209
   anti-aging, 213
AIDS; *see* HIV/AIDS
Alberta, 101, 105, 117, 148, 163
Alzheimer's, 4, 21, 195
ancestors, 90, 109, 114, 117, 133, 134, 212, 216, 217
ancient, 14, 39, 42, 93, 110
angels, 158, 159
anger, 51, 147, 182, 183, 188, 193, 198, 201
animals, 13, 90, 159, 167, 169, 203
anthropology, 8, 10, 132, 135
anxiety, 2, 11, 45, 46, 83–85, 87, 92, 95, 98, 179, 182–84, 199
   death, 11, 17, 86, 88, 93, 98
   ecoanxiety, 173
   social, 45
archaeology, 10, 14
Arctic, 153
Argentina, 29
artificial intelligence (AI), 215, 216, 218
arts, 10, 14, 37, 98, 107, 109, 158, 159, 167, 200
   animation, 90
   artwork, 83
   bibliodrama, 92
   dance, 93, 96, 97, 124, 138, 139, 157
   drama, 86, 92, 96
   film and movies, 10, 14, 35, 36, 84, 87, 88, 90, 94, 95, 98, 208, 209
   music, 82, 85–87, 95, 98, 108, 110, 113, 134, 135, 139, 141, 154, 156, 168, 198, 207, 208
   Metallica, 86
   Music-Thanatology, 198
   showtunes, 93
   songs, 85, 86, 93–96, 107, 113, 124, 135, 138, 156, 157, 169

novels, 110
opera, 95, 110, 209
photography, 41, 46, 83–85, 110, 202, 216
PhotoVoice, 84
poetry, 37, 83, 98, 110, 139, 156, 160, 169
sculpture, 83–85, 110, 158
television, 2, 15, 35, 87, 89, 95, 208
soap operas, 209
theatre, 3, 10, 82, 90–93, 98, 157, 167
musical, 88, 90, 93–96
visual, 14, 82, 83, 85, 98
Asia, 100, 117, 121, 217
Atlantic Canada, 68, 210
Australia, 91

babies; see children
Bali, 34, 109, 113
barriers, 58, 63, 126, 181, 205
beliefs, 13, 15, 23, 30, 31, 39, 47, 48, 50, 52, 54, 60, 68, 89, 107–9, 118–22, 135, 158, 162, 164, 165, 177, 193, 196, 217
bereavement, 1, 11, 15, 31, 40, 42, 55, 62–64, 66, 67, 90, 96, 97, 108, 111, 113, 115, 116, 136, 147, 148, 151, 153, 160, 167, 187, 188, 191, 192, 195–97, 200, 201, 203, 204
bodies, 13–15, 22, 23, 26, 27, 29, 31, 32, 39–43, 45, 49, 109, 111, 140, 144, 149, 150, 153, 155, 162, 165, 166, 168, 211, 214
  digital remains, 216
  disposal of, 9, 13, 15, 21, 23, 31, 40, 46, 132, 133, 140, 144, 149–52, 156, 159, 161, 168, 193, 211
  dissection of, 27, 41, 43
  donation of, 26, 162, 211
Bowers-Bryanton, Jenna, 172
brain injury, 24, 49, 182
Brazil, 29
Britain, 5, 6, 34, 37, 38, 41, 42, 44, 46, 50, 51, 53, 59, 65, 115, 117, 121, 145, 155, 156, 158, 202, 208, 209, 218
  Victorian England, 34, 37, 41
British Columbia, 63, 64, 71, 72, 101, 102, 105, 118, 119, 148, 151, 163
bullying, 172, 173, 176, 177, 181, 183
  anti-bullying, 178

burial, 3, 12, 21, 31, 34, 39, 40, 42, 46, 52, 88, 109, 111, 145, 149, 150, 155, 156, 159, 169, 209
  arrangements, 163
  cemeteries, 37, 40, 98, 110, 144, 146, 149, 158–60
  coffins, 6, 40, 42, 45, 85, 110, 144, 149, 150, 155
  columbariums, 150
  crypts, 110
  environmentally friendly, 22, 146, 149, 150
  graves and graveyards, 2, 20, 40, 43, 110, 114, 119, 132, 154, 158–60
  headstones, 119, 154, 159
  mausoleums, 42, 110
  mounds, 132
  ossuaries, 132
  pits, 6
  plots, 22, 37, 110, 154, 156
  pods, 144
  practices and rituals regarding, 38, 40, 52, 144
  premature (live), 19, 43
  sarcophagi, 40
  sites, 14, 22, 39, 119, 153, 158
  tombs, 14, 39, 40, 42, 110
  vaults, 40, 153, 156
Burkina Faso, 113

cadavers; see bodies
Cambodia, 116
Canada, 1–4, 6, 7, 17, 20–23, 25, 27, 30, 34, 36–39, 41, 42, 45–47, 49–51, 53–55, 57–65, 67, 68, 71–78, 80, 85–87, 97, 100–105, 107–11, 117–21, 124–31, 134, 136–38, 144–46, 148, 151–53, 157, 158, 163–68, 171–73, 176, 178, 179, 182, 183, 186, 196–98, 200, 204, 208–11, 214
cancer, 4, 7, 21, 25, 37, 62, 63, 65, 87, 88, 91, 120, 132, 165, 167, 202, 208
cannabis, 101, 104
caregiving, 9, 22, 34, 37, 38, 40, 53, 58, 64, 66–68, 76, 97, 122, 130
  at-home/in-home, 7, 12, 34, 58, 61, 122
  chronic care, 59
  end-of-life care, 1, 38, 66, 67, 80, 92, 120–22, 130, 198

long-term, 2, 53, 58, 59
pastoral care, 8, 55
CBC, 36, 145, 146, 151
children, 2, 5–7, 15, 20, 25, 28, 30, 38, 41, 53, 58, 90, 96, 113–16, 126, 128, 130, 136, 139, 163, 164, 167, 172, 178, 187, 189, 195, 202, 203, 213, 216, 217
China, 26, 34, 41, 110, 111, 113, 116, 117, 121, 217
Colombia, 118
colonialism, 50, 63, 124–26, 131, 132, 134, 136, 137, 139, 140, 179
colonization, 7, 39, 117, 124, 126, 127, 129, 131, 132, 134–36, 138, 140, 179
connections, 30, 31, 33, 35, 40, 41, 46, 51, 82, 112, 114, 173, 178, 181
consciousness, 30, 31, 41, 44, 49, 54, 181, 214
coroners, 10, 128, 145
corpses; *see* bodies
counselling, 8, 9, 11, 13, 31, 62, 66, 69, 86, 90, 97, 98, 116, 184, 194, 196
crises, 1, 2, 20, 53, 100, 102, 104, 109, 126, 185–87
critical-ecological framework, 175
culture, 2–4, 8–13, 15, 20, 21, 30, 34–36, 39, 42, 46, 47, 52–54, 60, 62–64, 69, 82, 87, 95, 101, 107–9, 111–14, 116–18, 120–25, 128–36, 138–42, 153, 154, 172, 175–79, 183, 184, 191, 192, 196, 198, 204, 207, 212, 216–18
  cultural practices, 108, 118, 129, 134, 136, 138, 139
  multiculturalism, 3, 117, 120
cyber
  cyberbullying, 172, 173, 177, 185
  cyber-grieving, 196, 197
  cyborg, 215

Dagara people, 113
death and dying, 1, 3–17, 19–26, 29–62, 64, 66–80, 82–101, 103, 107–11, 113–15, 117, 119–24, 126–34, 136–43, 145–47, 149, 151–63, 166–74, 176, 177, 182, 183, 187, 188, 191–205, 207–14, 216–19
  abortion, 15, 195, 203, 210, 211
  acceptance of, 34, 51, 54, 70, 192
  accidental, 4, 9, 14, 17, 19, 30, 38, 101, 126, 127, 132, 154, 162, 168, 171, 172, 196, 203, 213

ars moriendi, 15
art galleries, 200
assisted dying, 9, 73
  see also Medical Assistance in Dying (MAID)
  see also suicide, assisted
Avoidance of, 11, 88, 90, 92, 93, 110
Awareness of, 2, 10, 19, 22, 31, 41, 87, 91, 95, 107, 120, 122, 138, 200, 208, 210, 211
bad deaths, 12, 52–54, 147
biological death, 12, 30, 51
brain death, 23–25, 30, 49
cafés, 1, 200
care of the dead, 21, 32, 39–41, 46
celebration of, 1, 40, 42, 90, 113, 154
feasts, 129, 133
clinical death, 25, 30, 49, 51, 52
death benefits, 151, 152, 167
death certificates, 52, 108, 154, 211
death-defying, 3, 207
death-denying, 3, 15, 35, 207
death education, 3, 55, 56, 82, 84, 86–93, 199
death songs, 95
denial of, 15, 41, 44, 46, 51, 88, 192
dinners, 1, 198–200
dying alone, 19, 35, 51, 53
dying wishes, 98
euthanasia, 36, 53, 71, 76, 77, 80
execution, 13
financial costs of, 27, 65, 144, 146, 147, 151, 167, 169
financial planning for, 162, 166, 167
goodbyes, 30, 44, 52, 53, 149, 169, 176, 196
good death, 15, 52, 53, 56
guilt regarding, 147, 151, 182, 188, 193, 201, 203
gun-related, 2
infanticide, 30
lethal injections, 77, 212
midwives, 2
miscarriage, 195, 203
murder, 2, 14, 17, 19, 24, 30, 125–27
near-death experiences, 15, 52
overdoses, 19, 100, 101, 105, 115, 127, 138
persistent vegetative state (PVS), 24, 31, 53

pets, 7, 22, 115, 137, 169, 192, 196, 201, 203, 204, 213, 214
plans, 168, 169
prevention of, 2, 9, 36–39, 101, 103, 127, 129, 182
rites and rituals regarding, 3, 13, 15, 16, 18, 21, 33, 37, 38, 41, 45, 46, 48, 50, 54, 101, 107–9, 112–16, 123, 124, 129, 133, 134, 147, 149, 154, 192, 193, 195, 205
celebrations of life, 13, 70, 111, 144, 147, 156, 157, 160, 193
social death, 30, 46, 51, 56
spiritual death, 30, 50
taboos surrounding, 98, 110, 199
dementia, 51, 79, 177
depression, 51, 95, 113, 116, 173, 179, 182–84, 187
diabetes, 4, 126, 127, 132
discrimination, 46, 128, 176, 180, 181, 212
ableism, 76
ageism, 177, 185, 212
gender-based, 48, 96, 100, 177, 181, 212
homophobia, 212
toward Indigenous Peoples, 179
non-discrimination, 125
transphobia, 2
diversity, 116, 117, 120, 122, 172, 216
cultural, 4, 8, 10, 13, 14, 23, 30, 34, 35, 37, 39, 46, 54, 55, 63, 85, 108, 110–17, 120–22, 130, 134, 135, 153, 192, 195, 207, 209, 216
customs, 34, 37, 39, 41, 107, 129, 132, 133, 135, 140, 164, 207
Día de los Muertos, 90, 113
ethnicity, 10, 13, 19, 37, 52, 91, 117, 118, 120, 132, 134, 178, 191
faith-based, 68
infanticide, 30
Tibetan Book of the Dead, 44
doctors, 12, 24, 35, 43, 58, 62, 64, 72, 74, 77, 78, 101, 120, 121, 155, 156, 164, 166, 167, 194, 208
doulas
birth, 130
death, 2, 35, 129–31, 133, 140, 198
end of life, 197
grief, 196, 197
in music thanatology, 198

Ecuador, 114
Egypt, 34, 39, 41, 42, 110, 113
elderly, 6, 36, 51, 59, 60, 103, 121, 125, 209
England; see Britain
ethics, 3, 9, 14, 15, 29, 61, 78, 121, 162, 168, 212, 214, 216
bioethics, 58, 72
Europe, 6, 7, 28, 29, 34, 37–41, 43, 46, 59, 60, 110, 111, 117, 131, 132, 134, 144, 151, 158, 159, 217

family, 1, 5–7, 12–14, 19, 21, 23, 24, 33, 35, 37–42, 44, 47, 53, 55, 58, 59, 61, 64, 66–69, 88–90, 94, 97, 101, 104, 105, 111, 114, 115, 120–22, 129, 130, 132, 133, 135, 136, 139, 145–48, 150–57, 163–65, 167, 168, 171, 173, 175, 176, 178, 180–83, 186–89, 191, 193, 195, 197, 199, 203, 204, 208, 213
Finland, 110
Florida, 26
France, 117
funerals and burial practices, 3, 6, 8, 9, 12, 13, 21, 22, 31, 33, 34, 38, 40–42, 45, 46, 52, 66, 85, 88, 89, 108, 109, 111–13, 115, 129, 133–35, 138, 144–49, 151–59, 163, 167, 168, 192, 193, 198, 201
affordability of, 22, 145, 151, 158, 161, 213
after-burial arrangements, 38
arrangements for, 21, 31, 37, 38, 40, 41, 46, 151, 154, 156, 163, 167
caskets, 145, 154, 156
ceremonies, 45, 107, 114, 132, 136, 138, 139, 153, 179
cooperatives, 151, 167
costs regarding, 9, 61, 102, 137, 144–46, 150–52, 158, 196, 214
cremation, 3, 13, 21, 39, 40, 89, 132, 144, 146, 149, 150, 153, 154, 156, 159, 193, 209
funeral chapels, 129
funeral cooperatives, 151, 167
funeral directors, 9, 12, 37, 40, 41, 45, 120, 146, 147, 152–57, 167
funeral homes, 21, 42, 45, 89, 98, 129–31, 144–46, 148, 149, 151–56, 169, 213

INDEX 253

funeral poverty, 145, 152
funeral pyres, 153, 209
funeral rites, 3, 45, 109, 134
gatherings, 2, 95, 96, 135, 147, 148, 200
libitinarii, 40
livestreaming of, 45, 156
mortuaries, 45, 132, 133, 140, 143
pallbearers, 169
shrouds, 40, 45, 149
undertakers, 37, 39–41, 154–56
urns, 22, 39, 148–50, 154, 156

Gaza, 2
gender, 48, 50, 76, 89, 172–74, 178, 180, 212
genocide, 2, 51, 135, 138, 209
Germany, 86, 114, 117, 139
Greece, 39, 40, 42, 76, 93, 113
grief and bereavement, 1, 2, 7, 8, 11, 14, 15, 30, 31, 33–36, 52, 54, 55, 58, 62, 63, 66, 67, 82–90, 96–98, 107–9, 111–17, 120, 122, 124, 129–32, 134–40, 147–49, 152, 154, 187, 188, 191–98, 200, 202–5, 216
  intergenerational, 138, 139
  Prolonged Grief Disorder (PGD), 116
  sorrow, 34, 84, 86, 108, 113, 115, 116, 191
  wailing, 34, 42, 195
  professional wailers, 34
  weeping, 34, 113, 160

Haiti, 2, 47
healthcare, 7, 12, 31, 38, 46, 47, 58, 61, 64, 65, 68, 72, 76, 80, 91, 102, 103, 105, 120, 126–28, 130, 137, 138, 164, 178–81, 186, 187, 189, 198, 199, 209, 210, 212, 218
HIV/AIDS, 46–48, 60, 94–96, 208
Holocaust, 6, 85, 204, 209
hospices, 1, 5, 6, 12, 17, 21, 24, 31, 34, 36, 44, 46, 53, 54, 57–69, 74, 75, 80, 120–22, 154, 196, 197, 202, 207–10
  Canadian Hospice Palliative Care Association, 53, 58, 60, 62, 64, 208
  Canadian Virtual Hospice, 58, 130, 163, 200
hospitals, 6, 12, 15, 17, 21, 24, 28, 31, 34, 36, 38, 46, 52, 53, 58–61, 65, 66, 68, 98, 102, 103, 121, 128, 154, 156, 166, 171, 198, 210, 213

Hubbard, April, 157
human trafficking, 28, 29
humour, 88, 89, 135, 139, 156, 199

illnesses, 10, 38, 78, 88
  chronic, 4, 7, 38, 76, 103, 127, 176, 188, 195, 210, 212
  terminal, 3, 11, 24, 50, 51, 53, 57–59, 61, 62, 120, 121, 197–99, 213
immortality, 11, 14, 42, 93, 110, 159, 207, 212, 214, 216–18
India, 111, 117
Indigenous Peoples, 2, 4, 7, 39, 42, 50, 63, 64, 102, 117, 124–43, 153, 172, 178–80, 187, 217
  Achuar, 114
  Algonquin, 117
  Anishinaabe, 3, 132–35, 139
  Atikamekw, 128
  Ayoreo, 113
  Chippewas; see Ojibway
  Nawash, 135
  Cree, 64, 117, 129, 135
  Nêhiyawêwin, 135
  Peepeekisis, 129
  end-of-life rituals, 133, 134
  Indian, 20, 125, 131
  Inuit, 102, 124, 126, 128, 130, 140, 179
  Iroquois, 142
  land-based teachings, 124, 125, 136, 138
  lifeways, 126, 131
  Lihir, 113
  Métis, 63, 124, 126, 128, 130, 140, 142, 180
  Mi'kmaq, 117
  off-reserve, 126–28
  Ojibway, 64, 117, 142
  on-reserve, 126, 127, 135
  Potwatomi, 124
  smudging, 134, 135
  Waasigwan, 134
  Wasauksing, 3, 124, 139, 216
Indonesia, 109, 113
internet, 2, 3, 22, 45, 48, 152, 156, 158, 160, 219
  blogs, 200
  virtual care, 66
  virtual funeral, 147, 148
  virtual hospice, 58, 130, 163, 200

websites, 21, 22, 26–28, 35, 42, 52, 58, 59, 110, 129, 130, 148, 150, 151, 156, 160, 163, 165, 166, 196–201, 214, 216
Iran, 107, 108, 110, 111, 113, 114, 120
Iraq, 108
Ireland, 60, 117
Israel, 29, 44
Italy, 43, 93, 108, 113, 115, 117, 149

Japan, 34, 113, 217

Kevorkian, Dr. Jack, 208
Kosovo, 28

Latimer, Robert, 211
legal aspects of death and dying, 9, 21, 31, 79, 80, 162, 168, 182, 188, 208, 211
   advance care planning, 163, 199
   Bills, 71, 73, 104
   death certificates, 23, 24, 29, 43, 52, 108, 154, 162
   directives
      advance, 162, 163, 211
      healthcare, 162–64
      medical, 163, 164, 211
   dying wills, 12
   estate planning, 12, 24, 163, 166–68
   executors, 166, 167
   MAID legalities, 72, 75, 80
   organ and tissue donation legalities, 24, 27, 29, 31, 162
   Supreme Court, 71, 72
   taxes, 162, 166, 167
   trustees, 168
life extension, 27, 212, 213, 216, 217
   Alcor Life Extension Foundation, 213
   biomechatronic, 22, 214, 215
   biomedical, 44
   body modification, 22, 212, 214, 215
   biomechatronics, 215
   bionics, 22, 214, 215
   implants, 22, 214, 215
   nanotechnology, 215
   Neuralink, 215
   plastic surgery, 214
   prosthetics, 22, 212, 214, 215
   cryonic suspension, 22, 212–14
   organ transplantation, 24, 27, 166
   transhumanism, 215, 216

Lithuania, 6
loss, 5, 7, 8, 13, 15, 17, 30, 31, 34–38, 46, 52, 83, 85–87, 89, 90, 96–98, 108, 109, 112, 113, 115, 116, 129, 140, 153–55, 172, 176, 187–89, 191, 192, 194–97, 200–206, 214, 218
   ambiguous, 136, 137
   cultural, 107, 136, 138, 179
   symbolic, 136

Macedonia, 91, 92
Manitoba, 1, 23, 24, 75, 101, 118, 129, 163
Medical Assistance in Dying (MAID), 7, 67, 68, 71–80, 157, 163, 168, 169, 172, 210–12
medication, 8, 10, 26, 33, 57, 58, 72, 77, 78, 101, 104, 105, 121, 131, 132, 168, 178, 184, 198, 211, 215
meditation, 44, 96, 158
Mediterranea, 113
memento vivere, 84
memorialization, 3, 22, 46, 149
   architecture, 40, 42, 110, 160
   archways, 158
   cards, 154, 156, 160
   commemoration, 40–42, 107, 160
   epitaphs, 42
   flowers, 39, 154, 156, 158–60, 168, 207
   jewellery, 22, 132, 144, 150, 156, 168
   marble, 37, 158, 159
   memento mori, 41, 42, 84
   memorial societies, 151
   monuments, 42, 110, 158
   obituaries, 22, 37, 42, 52, 156
   tattoos, 144
   tombstones, 42, 46, 158, 159, 169
   veneration, 119, 217
   video recordings, 41, 46, 156, 164, 216
Mesopotamia, 110
Mexico, 40, 90, 113
Michigan, 45, 213
minorities, 47, 172, 177, 180, 181
Moldova, 29
Morrison, Dr. Nancy, 211
mortality, 37, 82, 83, 85, 87, 88, 90, 91, 95, 98, 107, 122, 158, 182, 198–200, 207
   rates of, 9, 124, 126–29, 131, 132, 138, 140

mourning, 6, 34, 37, 41, 46, 85, 87, 111–15, 133, 137, 147, 148, 152–54, 156, 172, 188, 192, 195, 196, 209, 218
  ceremonies and rituals, 41, 107, 109, 111, 113, 116, 149
  colour black, 37, 41, 110, 111, 113, 114
  mourning clothes, 40
  professional mourners, 40
movements
  death-with-dignity, 77
  hospice care, 54, 60, 67, 68, 121
  midwifery, 54, 208
  palliative care, 53, 61, 207
  pan-death, 3
  right to die, 77, 163, 208
  social, 64, 70, 145, 151
  transhumanism, 215, 216

Netherlands, 139
New Brunswick, 3, 101, 163, 171, 198
Newfoundland and Labrador, 95, 101, 145
New Guinea, 113
North America, 21, 28, 34, 59, 60, 110, 131, 148–50, 155, 156, 202
Northwest Territories, 163
Norway, 83
Nova Scotia, 65, 72, 78, 101, 157, 163
Nunavut, 101
nurses, 10, 24, 31, 35, 55, 58, 61, 62, 65, 74, 78, 92, 122, 208, 209
  nurse practitioners, 58, 72

Ontario, 1, 3, 63, 64, 95, 101, 105, 118, 122, 139, 145, 146, 148, 151, 163, 213, 216
opiates and opioids, 2, 4, 21, 101–4, 121, 211
  drug trafficking, 100, 101
  fentanyl, 100–102
  heroin, 101, 104, 105
  injection sites, 100, 105
  morphine, 57, 101
  naloxone, 101, 104, 105
  opioid crisis, 2, 20, 100, 102, 104
  opium, 101
  over-prescription of, 100–102
  OxyContin, 102
  Purdue Pharma, 102
organs and tissues, 23, 25, 28, 40, 43, 44, 49, 155, 157, 162, 165, 166, 211, 213, 214, 216
  brokers of, 27–29
  buying and selling of, 22, 26–29
  donation of, 15, 24, 25, 27, 29, 3.
  donation of, 15, 24, 25, 27, 29, 32 165
  harvesting of, 24, 26, 28, 29
  preservation of, 155, 213
  retrieval of, 28
  trafficking of, 29
  transplantation of, 24, 27–29, 32, 4. 44, 166

pain, 8, 9, 17, 19, 31, 36, 38, 44, 50, 53, 54, 57, 60, 62, 64, 70, 83, 86, 87, 96, 97, 101–4, 116, 121, 128, 139, 168, 172–74, 176, 188, 191, 192, 194, 198, 209, 211
palaeontology, 14, 131, 132
Palestine, 44
palliative care, 1, 7, 10, 12, 17, 21, 24, 31, 34, 35, 44, 46, 53–55, 57–69, 74, 75, 77, 87, 120, 121, 157, 169, 196, 198, 207–10
  Canadian Hospice Palliative Care Association, 53, 58, 60, 62, 64, 208
  Canadian Palliative Care Nursing Association, 58
  Canadian Society of Palliative Medicine, 58
  home-based palliative care (HPC), 74, 75
  Palliative Care Coalition of Canada, 58
  The Canadian Network of Palliative Care for Children, 58
pandemics, 2, 11, 47, 48, 54, 65–67, 146, 147, 149, 166, 198, 204, 212
Paraguay, 113
Parsons, Rehtaeh, 172
patients, 12, 24, 25, 27, 29, 31, 44, 51, 53, 60–62, 64–68, 74, 77, 79, 87, 91, 92, 96, 97, 101, 103, 120, 121, 163, 164, 166, 195, 202, 209, 213, 214
Persia, 107
pharmaceutical industry, 10, 102
Philippines, 29, 121, 122
philosophy, 3, 13, 14, 43, 53, 60, 153, 160, 191, 209, 214
prisons and jails, 19, 47, 173, 183, 184
psychology, 3, 8–11, 92, 98, 116

United Church, 118, 135
worship, 119, 148, 217
Rodriguez, Sue, 71, 208, 211
Rome, 40, 42, 93
Russia, 44

Saskatchewan, 101, 105, 118, 129, 163
Schiavo, Terri, 211
Scotland, 117
social construct, 4, 11, 13, 36, 54
social media, 12, 21, 42, 87, 98, 197, 208, 216
   Facebook, 21, 197, 214
   Instagram, 88, 197
   Reddit, 110
   Twitter, 21, 78
social supports, 137, 177, 178, 181, 184, 185
social workers, 9, 58, 62, 97, 137
society, 12–14, 21, 33–36, 51–53, 56, 64, 76, 80, 87, 107, 112–16, 129, 132, 135, 137, 139, 153, 157, 159, 167, 176, 177, 180, 181, 189, 201, 203, 214
   colonial, 125
   modern, 54, 88
   traditional, 54
   Western, 15, 44, 46, 122
sociology, 3, 4, 8, 9, 11–13, 16, 22, 49, 51, 64, 65, 107, 111, 122, 168, 174
South Africa, 29
spirituality, 8, 9, 15, 21, 30, 31, 33, 50, 52, 56, 57, 60, 62, 69, 108, 109, 114, 119, 124, 125, 129–33, 138, 156, 164, 165, 169, 177, 179, 193, 196, 198, 207, 217
stigmas, 46, 47, 91–93, 104, 115, 151, 180–82, 185, 188, 204, 210
   anti-stigma, 185
Sudan, 2
suicide, 14, 15, 20, 30, 51, 53, 77, 95, 108, 115, 126, 127, 139, 162, 172–78, 184, 186–89, 196
   2SLGBTQ+, 180
   armed forces and veteran, 181–83
   assisted, 24, 77, 80
   physician-assisted, 77
   attempts, 77, 176, 179, 183–85, 187
   awareness, 140, 184, 186
   Indigenous, 178
   inmates, 183, 184
   interventions, 186

prevention of, 9, 138, 171, 173–76, 178–80, 184–87, 189, 190
rates, 178, 179
risk, 172, 173, 177, 181–84, 189
suicidal ideation, 188
Switzerland, 116, 208

Taiwan, 113
Taylor, Gloria, 72, 188
technology, 24, 37, 41, 43, 44, 66, 153, 197, 213, 215
chatbots, 216
deathbots, 2, 216
medical, 29, 44, 51
reproductive, 211, 212
see also Artificial Intelligence (AI)
teenagers, 20, 79, 88, 93
terrorism, 2, 30, 35, 54
thanatology, 1, 10, 11, 54, 198
therapy, 62, 86, 104, 171, 202
art, 82–85, 202
bibliotherapy, 97
dance/movement therapy (DMT), 96, 97
music, 87, 198, 202
Tibet, 44, 111
Todd, Amanda, 172
traditions, 6, 8, 41, 44, 90, 91, 109, 111–14, 116, 120, 129, 132, 133, 135, 136, 158, 205, 217
trauma, 7, 30, 83, 85, 97, 101, 138, 139, 158, 182, 183, 187, 188
physical, 24, 25, 103, 182
Post-traumatic Stress Disorder (PTSD), 182, 188, 189
sexual, 182, 183

Ukraine, 2, 44, 107, 117
United Kingdom (UK); *see* Britain
United Nations (UN), 47, 76, 100
United States, 2, 15, 20, 26, 27, 29, 38, 41, 46, 51, 52, 54, 88, 102, 116, 121, 148, 150, 151, 155, 208, 209, 215
American, 27, 84, 88, 93, 120, 148, 213, 215

Victorian Order of Nurses (VON), 58, 69, 210
Vietnam, 95

war, 2, 5, 7, 13, 20, 30, 31, 35, 38, 44, 54, 90, 95, 104, 108, 131, 132, 137, 155, 156, 169, 175, 182, 208, 209
anti-war, 110
Crimean War, 156
soldiers in, 54, 137
territorial, 61
US Civil War, 155
Vietnam War, 95
World War II, 5, 7
wills, 12, 52, 108, 162, 163, 167
ethical, 164, 165
World Health Organization (WHO), 2, 28, 47, 49, 105

youth, 95, 172, 173, 177–80, 187, 218
Yukon, 63, 101, 119, 163

257

61,